the protein hit

the protein

Alexander
Hart

100+
protein-packed,
speedy salads to
fuel your day

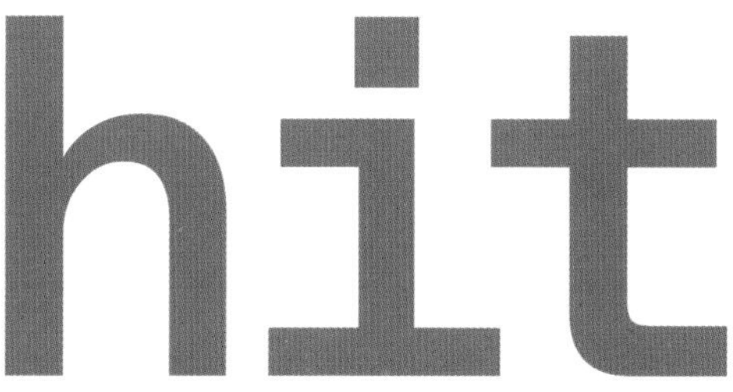

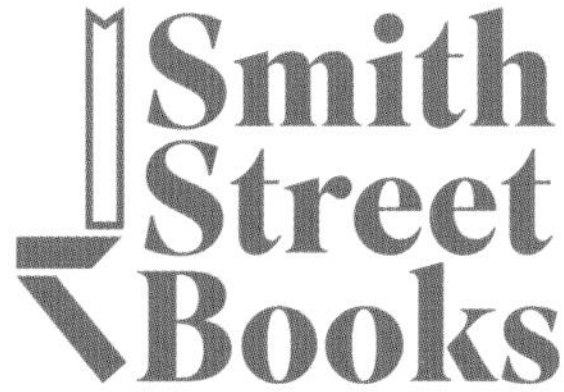

Introduction

Protein is having a real moment. Scroll through social media or wander the aisles of your local supermarket and you'll see it everywhere – in bars, powders, yoghurts, even bread. But you don't need to overhaul your diet or buy a shelf full of supplements to enjoy the benefits of eating more protein.

This book is here to show you how simple it can be to build high-protein meals using everyday ingredients. Each of the 100+ recipes inside delivers at least 25 grams of protein per serve – no maths required. From quick lunches to hearty dinners, you'll find colourful, flavour-packed salads that don't just taste great but also help you feel satisfied.

We start strong with dependable Crowd pleasers (page 13). These salads use all of the reliable protein heroes – think chicken, beef and tuna – in classic flavour combinations. Light & low-carb (page 55) offers a selection of fresher and brighter salads which are perfect for when you're craving something a little gentler. In Leafy & loaded (page 91) you'll find plenty of leaf-forward bowls which are made more substantial with the addition of nuts, grains, cheese or meat. Vegetarians are well looked after in Plant power (page 123), and you'll find plenty of satiating salad bowls full of lentils, quinoa, rice and noodles in Grains & good carbs (page 153). Rounding out the book is Hearty hits (page 191), which features a selection of robust, protein-packed bowls with bold flavour combinations, perfect for dinners.

The goal here isn't to lecture or hand out nutrition rules. Instead, *The Protein Hit* is about celebrating flavour and convenience. Think of protein as the anchor of your salad: it's the element that makes a bowl of leaves and dressing feel like a meal. Add a few simple staples and you've got a dish that's speedy, substantial and delicious.

WHAT IS PROTEIN AND WHY DO WE NEED IT?

Protein is one of the three major macronutrients, alongside carbohydrates and fats. Your body requires these macronutrients in relatively large amounts (compared to micronutrients) to make energy and to maintain a healthy body. Our bodies use the protein we eat through the consumption of meat, fish, eggs, dairy products, legumes, seeds, nuts and wholegrains in many ways, including the growth and repair of muscle and other tissues and supporting immune function.

There are a number of reasons why you may want to increase the amount of protein you consume throughout the day. Protein is essential for building and repairing muscles, especially after exercise, meaning it plays an important role in the diets of people who are looking to maintain and build their muscle mass. Some people find that eating a diet that is higher in protein can increase their sense of satiety (a feeling of fullness that lasts until the next meal) throughout the day, which in turn can help reduce snacking.

The daily recommended amount of protein you will need to eat varies depending on several factors, including your age, gender, whether you are pregnant or breastfeeding, how much you exercise and what your fitness goals are. In general, you will maintain your basic nutritional requirements by consuming at least 0.8 grams of protein per kilogram of body weight (or 0.36 grams per pound) a day. If you have specific goals or if you are concerned about a deficiency, it is always best to consult a doctor, dietician or nutritionist to help.

It is important to note that protein is just one macronutrient that our bodies require to function optimally. As with everything, moderation is key and eating a balanced diet that incorporates a healthy proportion of protein, fat and carbohydrates is essential.

Protein hit essentials

Keep these high-protein staples on hand and you'll never be stuck for a quick, satisfying salad. Each of these ingredients is versatile, affordable, and an easy way to boost your daily protein intake.

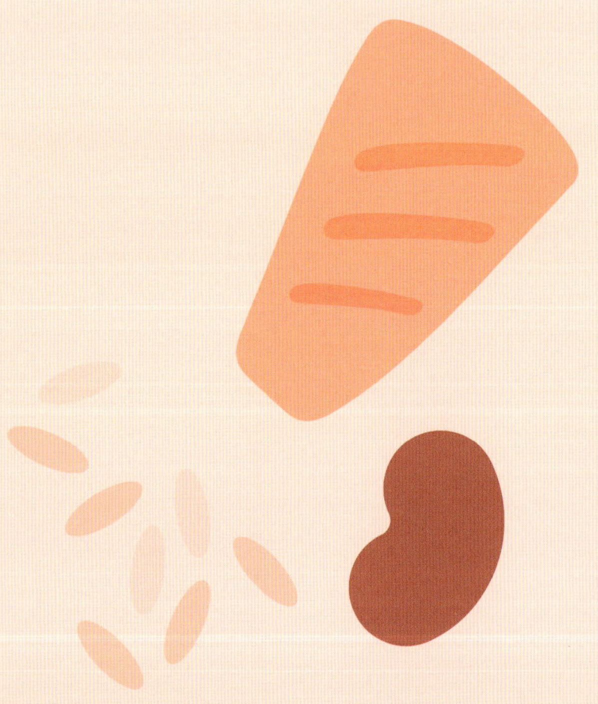

CHEESE	(COTTAGE CHEESE, FETA, PARMESAN, MOZZARELLA) Cheese adds flavour and substance to lighter, leaf-based bowls, or can perfectly accent heartier, grain-based dishes. From crumbly feta to creamy mozzarella, a little can go a long way to bumping up the satiating power of your meals. Cottage cheese is a very popular choice, and for good reason! It's a great source of protein, with a half-cup serving clocking in at just over 13 grams of protein, and it's also relatively low in fat and calories. It can be eaten with sweet and savoury flavours, so it's a versatile way to pump up the protein. Blend it into dressings or dips, or dollop it on top of your dinners like it's yoghurt or sour cream – the possibilities are endless! PROTEIN HIT! ~7-12 G PROTEIN PER 50 G SERVE
CHICKEN	Lean, tasty and endlessly adaptable – chicken is perfect for slicing into strips, shredding, and tossing through noodles and grains. If you're short on time, you can purchase a whole roast chicken, then chop or shred the meat and store it in an airtight container for up to 4 days. Another healthy option (if you have the time) is to poach some chicken breasts to use throughout the week. PROTEIN HIT! ~30 G PROTEIN PER 100 G COOKED CHICKEN
EGGS	Eggs are one of the most nutritious protein sources and are loaded with almost every vitamin and mineral needed by the human body. Boil a batch on Sunday and you've got instant protein that will keep for up to 1 week. Slice into green salads, mash into dressings, or keep a couple on hand for snacks. To boil eggs, place your eggs in a saucepan and cover with cold water. Bring to the boil over medium–high heat, then cover, remove from the heat and set aside for 8–11 minutes (depending on how hard-boiled you like them – 8 minutes will yield a jammier yolk, while 11 minutes will give you a true hard-boiled egg). Drain, cool in iced water and peel just before adding to your salad. PROTEIN HIT! ~13 G PROTEIN PER 2 EGGS

LENTILS & BEANS	Another pantry staple that can quickly pack a powerful protein punch. Tinned lentils, chickpeas (garbanzo beans) or black beans bring bulk, texture and a plant-based boost. They'll quickly soak up the flavour of whatever dressing you're working with, making them an easy flavour bomb, too. PROTEIN HIT! ~8-9 G PROTEIN PER 100 G COOKED LENTILS/BEANS
NUTS & SEEDS	This one might surprise you, but nuts and seeds are a small but mighty source of protein. Sprinkle almonds, pumpkin seeds or sunflower seeds over your salad for crunch and extra substance. PROTEIN HIT! ~5-6 G PROTEIN PER 30 G HANDFUL
QUINOA & BLACK RICE	These grains are nutrient-dense and offer a healthy boost of plant-based protein, along with fibre and other essential minerals. They add chewiness, a nutty flavour, and a useful protein bump that you won't get with white rice. Their mild flavour means they can be used as a hunger-satisfying base in many recipes. PROTEIN HIT! ~4-5 G PROTEIN PER 100 G COOKED QUINOA
SALMON	Whether you're using fresh fillets or hot-smoked salmon, this protein powerhouse adds richness and healthy fats that will support muscle health and overall wellness. PROTEIN HIT! ~25 G PROTEIN PER 100 G COOKED SALMON

TINNED FISH

This is the ultimate convenience protein. Whether you prefer tuna, sardines, mackerel or salmon, tinned fish should be a staple ingredient in your high-protein pantry. Simply open, drain and mix through with pasta, beans or crunchy veg for a filling meal in seconds.

PROTEIN HIT! ~25 G PROTEIN PER 100 G DRAINED TUNA

TOFU & TEMPEH

Tofu and tempeh are excellent sources of plant-based protein, making them great options for vegetarians and vegans. Both are made from soybeans, with tofu being made from soy milk (offering a smoother, milder option), while tempeh is made from whole fermented soybeans (making it a firmer, nuttier option with more fibre).

Simply soak sliced tofu or tempeh in marinades and pan-fry until golden, or cube straight into salads. These are great plant-based all-rounders.

PROTEIN HIT! ~8-19 G PROTEIN PER 100 G (TEMPEH AT THE HIGHER END)

SIMPLE HIGH-PROTEIN SWAPS

Boost your bowls with these easy switches:

- Use Greek-style yoghurt instead of sour cream or creme fraiche
- Use cottage cheese in dressings instead of mayonnaise
- Sub quinoa or black rice for white rice
- Cook legume or pulse pasta instead of regular pasta
- Switch in toasted seeds or roasted chickpeas for croutons

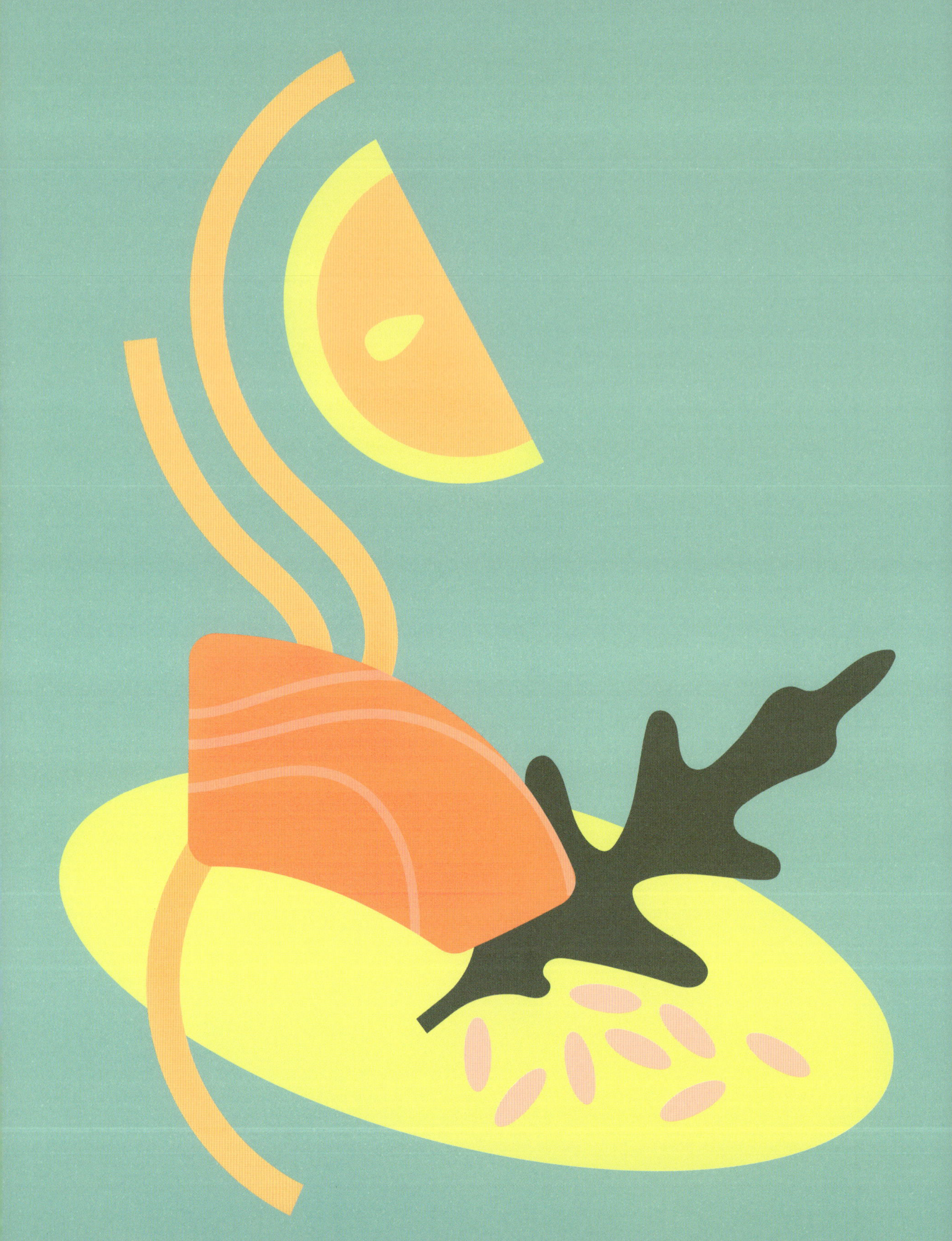

crowd

pleasers

PROTEIN: 38 G NET CARBS: 36 G FAT: 21 G

Teriyaki chicken noodle salad

Chicken delivers a lean protein boost in this Japanese-inspired salad, which is balanced with sweet pineapple and an easy teriyaki–sesame dressing that ties everything together.

- 180 g (6½ oz) cooked ramen noodles, prepared as per packet instructions
- 100 g (⅔ cup) shredded cooked chicken
- 50 g (⅓ cup) chopped pineapple
- 1 small spring onion (scallion), finely sliced
- 1 small carrot, julienned
- 40 g (½ cup) shredded red cabbage
- 2 teaspoons toasted sesame seeds

TERIYAKI-SESAME DRESSING

- 2 teaspoons teriyaki sauce
- 2 teaspoons sesame oil
- 2 teaspoons kecap manis (sweet soy sauce)
- 2 teaspoons rice vinegar
- 1 teaspoon soy sauce

1. Place all the salad ingredients in a bowl and toss lightly.
2. Combine the dressing ingredients in a small bowl.
3. Pour the dressing over the salad just before serving and toss well to coat.

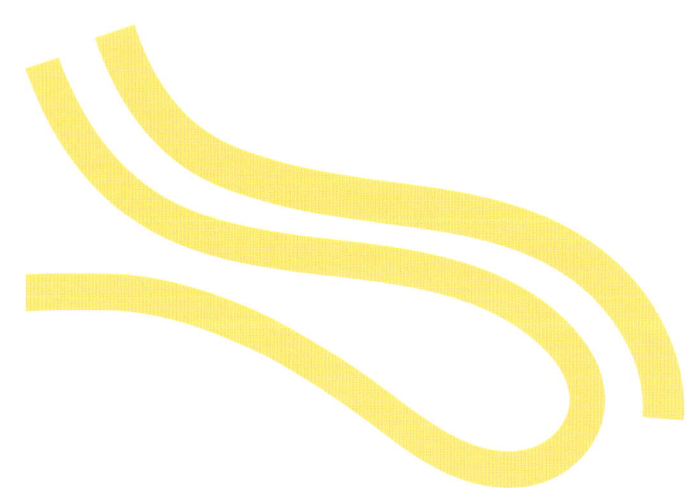

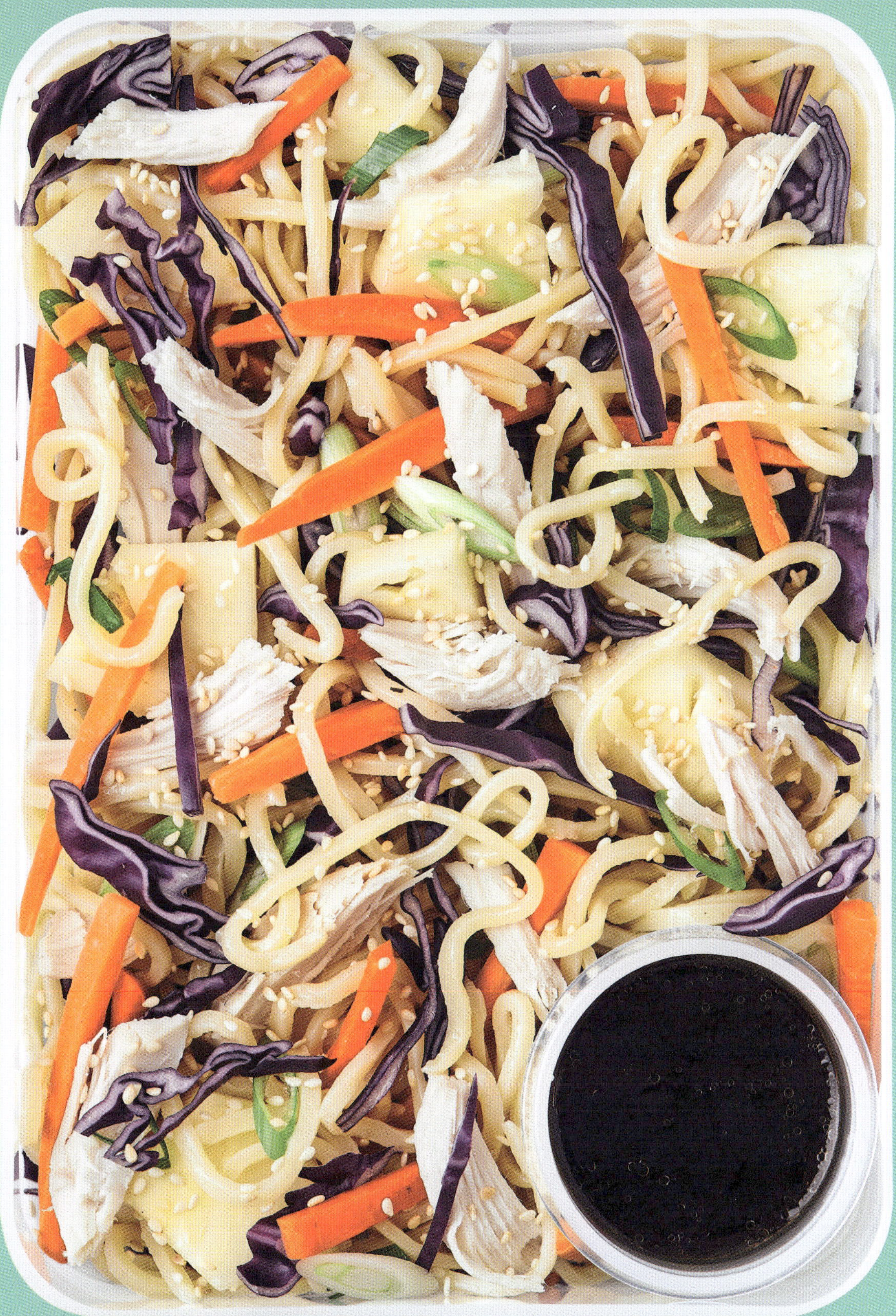

PROTEIN: 43 G NET CARBS: 49 G FAT: 18 G

Deconstructed rice paper rolls

This quick and easy spin on Vietnamese rice paper rolls swaps the rice paper wrapping for a protein-packed chicken and noodle salad, freshened with herbs, sprouts and crunchy peanuts.

80 g (2¾ oz) dried rice vermicelli noodles, prepared as per packet instructions

100 g (⅔ cup) shredded cooked chicken

2-3 iceberg lettuce leaves, shredded

½ carrot, shredded

45 g (½ cup) bean sprouts

small handful of coriander (cilantro) leaves

small handful of Vietnamese mint leaves

2 tablespoons roasted peanuts

lime wedge, to serve

LIME-CHILLI DRESSING

2 tablespoons sweet chilli sauce

1 tablespoon lime juice

1 teaspoon sesame oil

1. Place all the salad ingredients in a bowl, except the lime wedge, and toss lightly.
2. Combine the dressing ingredients in a small bowl.
3. Pour the dressing over the salad just before serving and toss well to coat, then squeeze over the lime.

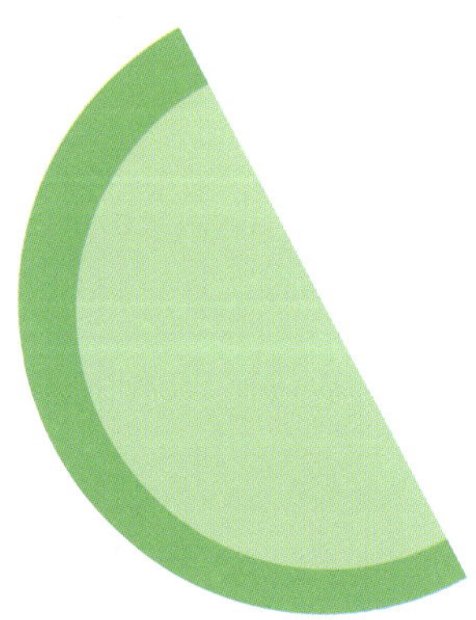

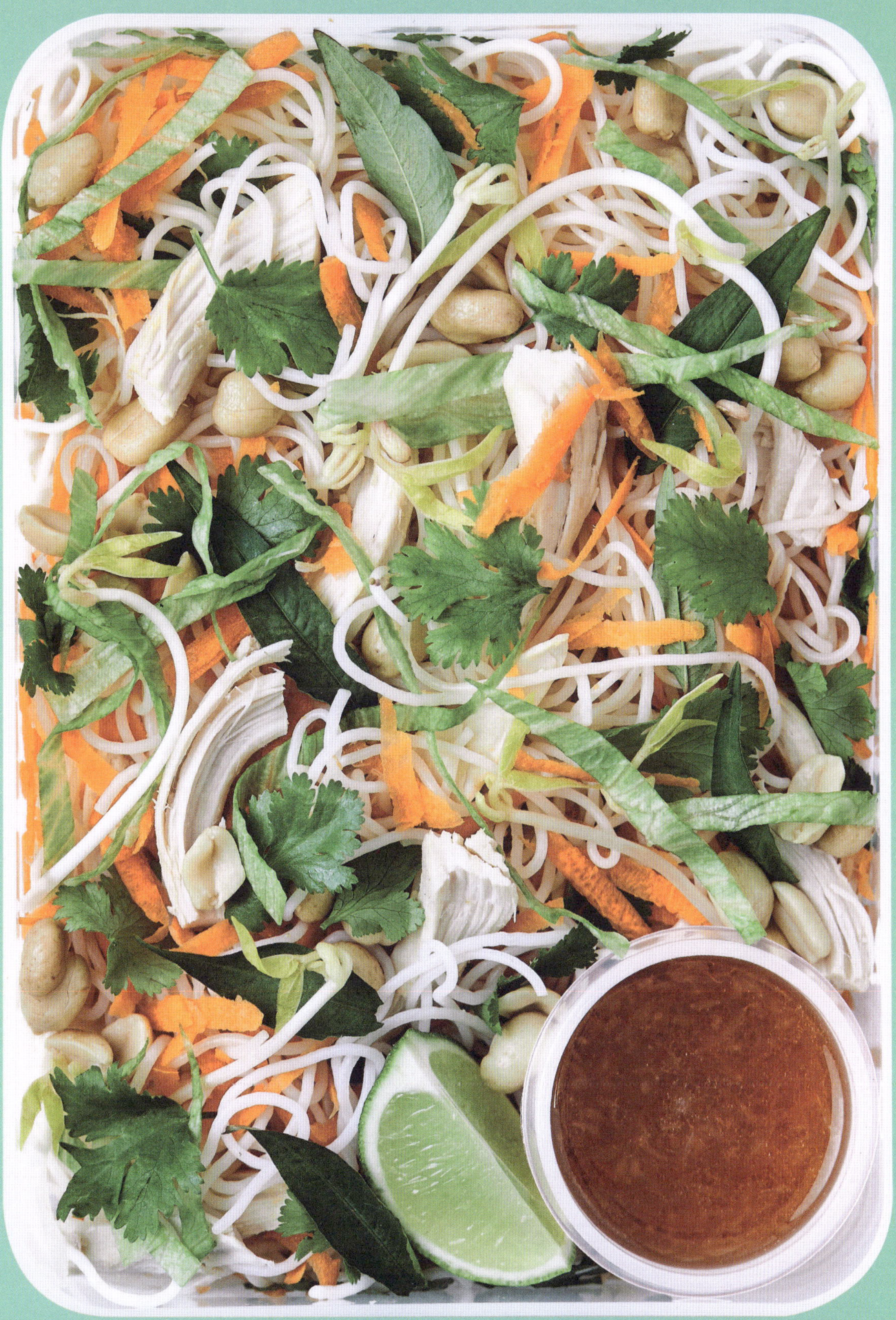

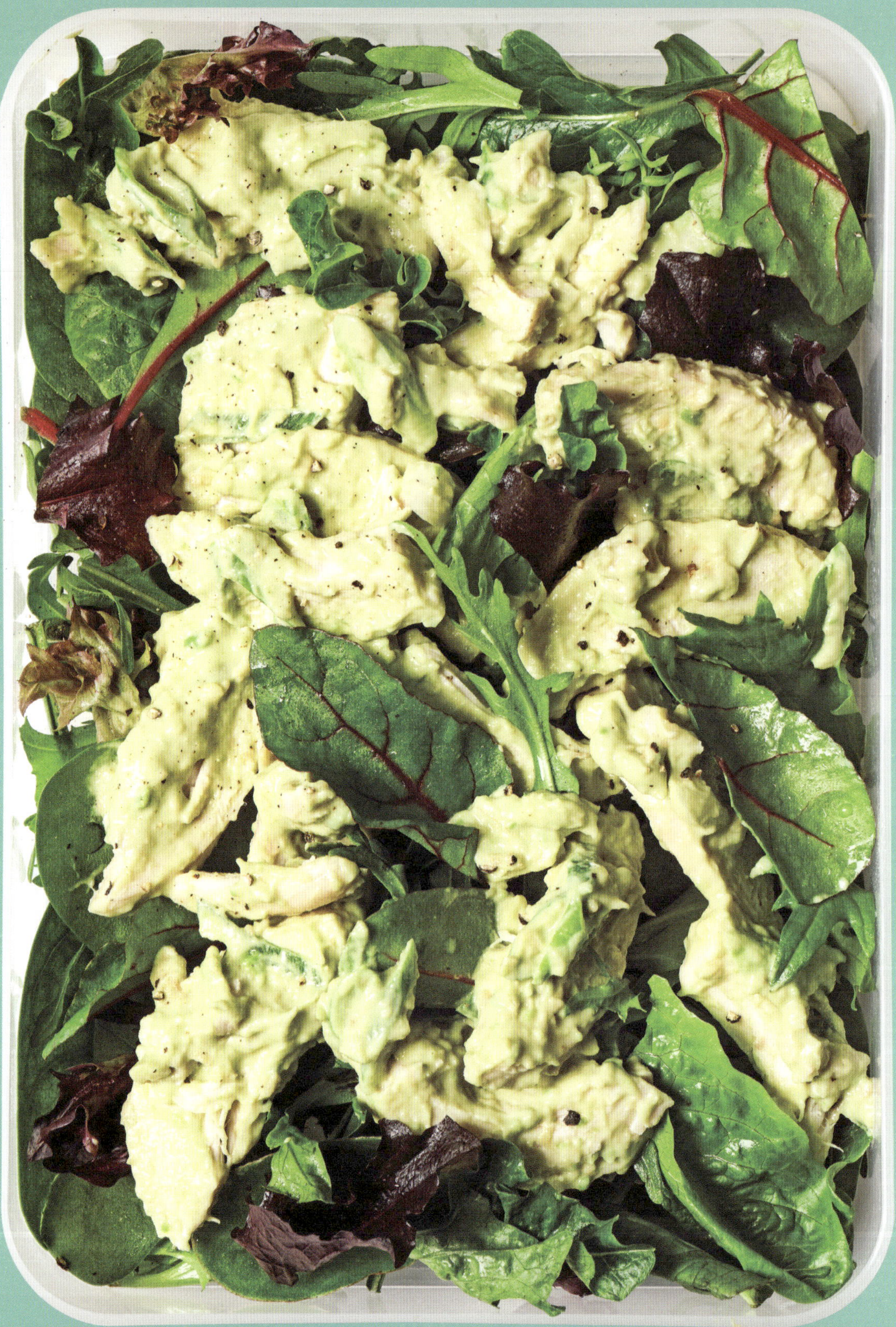

PROTEIN: 36 G NET CARBS: 5 G FAT: 9 G

Green goddess chicken & avo salad

This salad is a combination of two classics: green goddess dressing and chicken salad. Blitzing together avocado and yoghurt makes for the easiest green goddess dressing that's high in healthy fats and protein.

- 100 g (⅔ cup) shredded cooked chicken
- 1 celery stalk, diced
- 1 spring onion (scallion), sliced
- small handful of mixed herbs, such as dill, tarragon, chives and parsley
- 60 g (1½ cups) mixed salad greens

GREEN GODDESS DRESSING

- ¼ avocado, diced
- 2 tablespoons high-protein Greek-style yoghurt
- 2 teaspoons lemon juice

1. Combine the dressing ingredients in a small blender and blitz until smooth and creamy. Season to taste with salt and pepper.
2. Combine the chicken, celery, spring onion and herbs in a bowl. Pour the dressing over and toss together.
3. To serve, place the salad greens in a bowl and top with the chicken mixture.

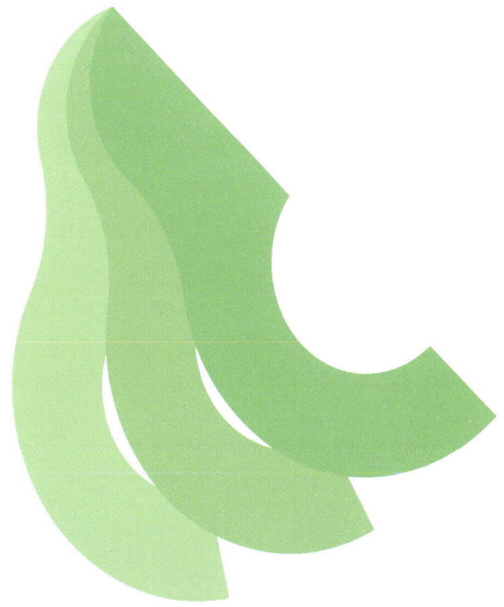

PROTEIN: 54 G NET CARBS: 7 G FAT: 45 G

Cobb salad

A true classic: chicken, bacon, cheese and egg layered over lettuce. Each element adds body in its own way – lean meat, dairy and eggs – making this one of the most reliable 'meal salads' out there.

- 1 tomato, diced
- 100 g (3½ oz) cooked chicken, diced
- ¼ avocado, diced
- 55 g (1½ cups) chopped cos (romaine) lettuce
- 30 g (1 oz) blue cheese, crumbled
- 25 g (1 oz) cooked bacon, chopped
- 1 hard-boiled egg, quartered

ONION & MUSTARD VINAIGRETTE

- 1 tablespoon extra virgin olive oil
- 1 tablespoon chopped red onion
- 2 teaspoons red wine vinegar
- 1 teaspoon dijon mustard

1. Place the salad ingredients in a bowl and toss lightly.
2. Combine the vinaigrette ingredients in a small bowl, then season to taste with salt and pepper.
3. Pour the vinaigrette over the salad just before serving and toss well to coat.

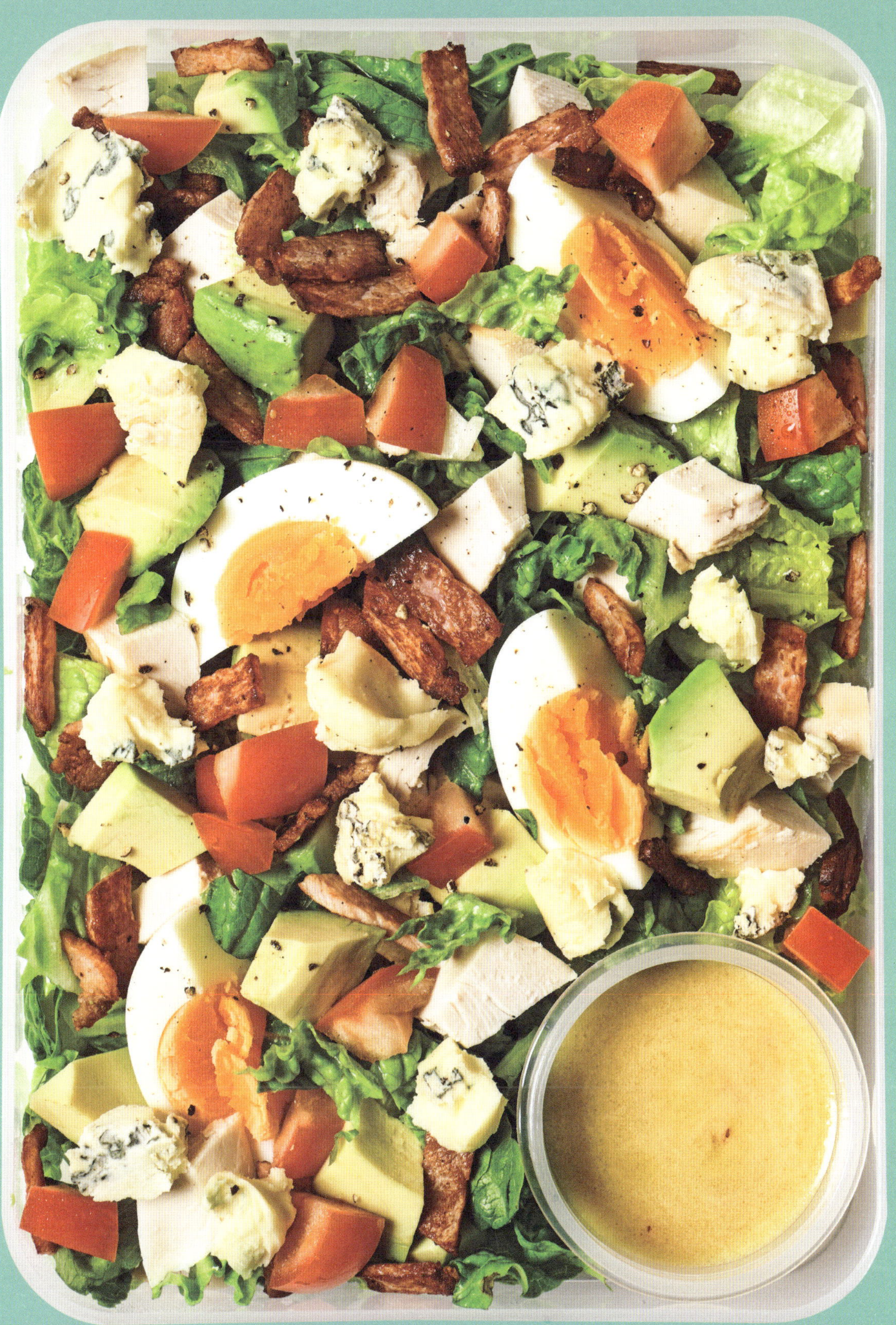

PROTEIN: 46 G NET CARBS: 33 G FAT: 32 G

Chicken, lentil & caper salad

Protein-rich chicken and lentils make a hearty pairing here, with briny capers and a lemony dressing bringing the flavours together. Use left-over roast or poached chicken, or even pre-cooked bought barbecued chicken. To shred it, simply use two forks or clean hands to pull it apart.

- 150 g (5½ oz) tinned lentils, drained and rinsed
- 100 g (⅔ cup) shredded cooked chicken
- 100 g (3½ oz) mixed small heirloom tomatoes, halved
- 2 tablespoons baby capers

PRESERVED LEMON & HONEY DRESSING

- ¼ preserved lemon skin, finely chopped
- juice of ½ lemon
- 1 teaspoon honey
- 1½ teaspoons dijon mustard
- 2 tablespoons extra virgin olive oil

1. Place the salad ingredients in a bowl and toss lightly, then season to taste with salt and pepper.
2. Combine the dressing ingredients in a small bowl.
3. Pour the dressing over the salad just before serving and toss well to coat.

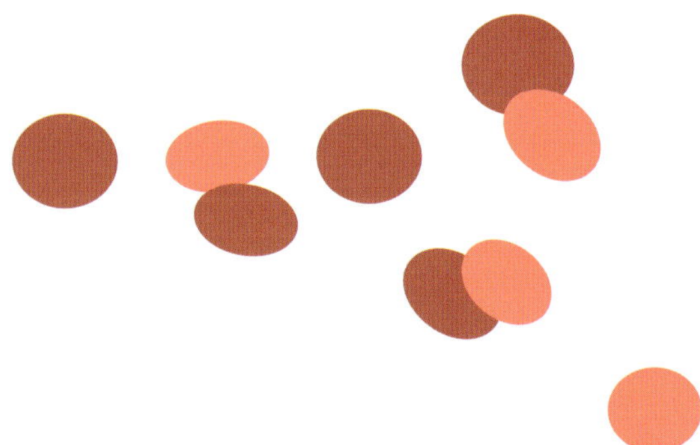

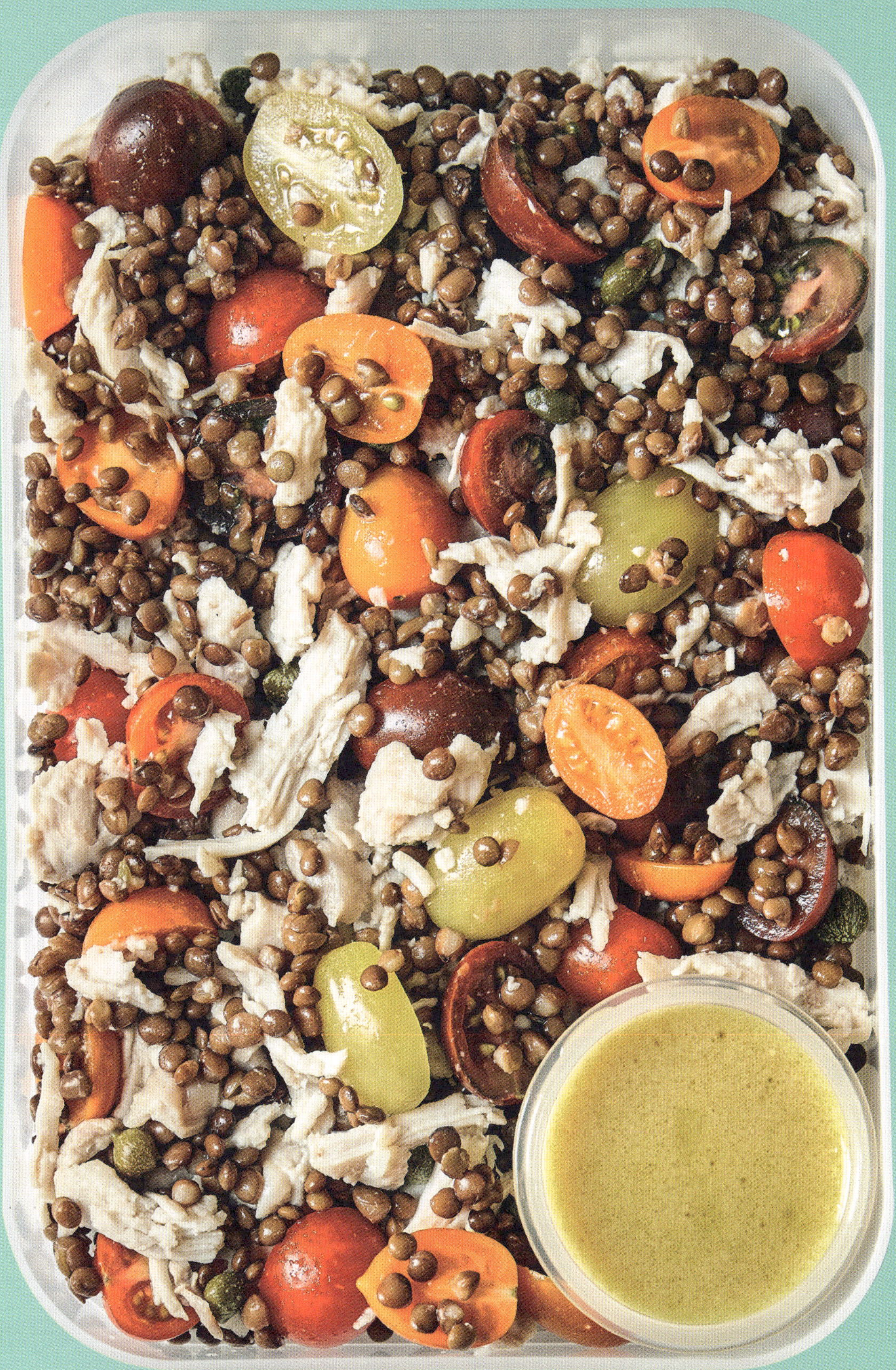

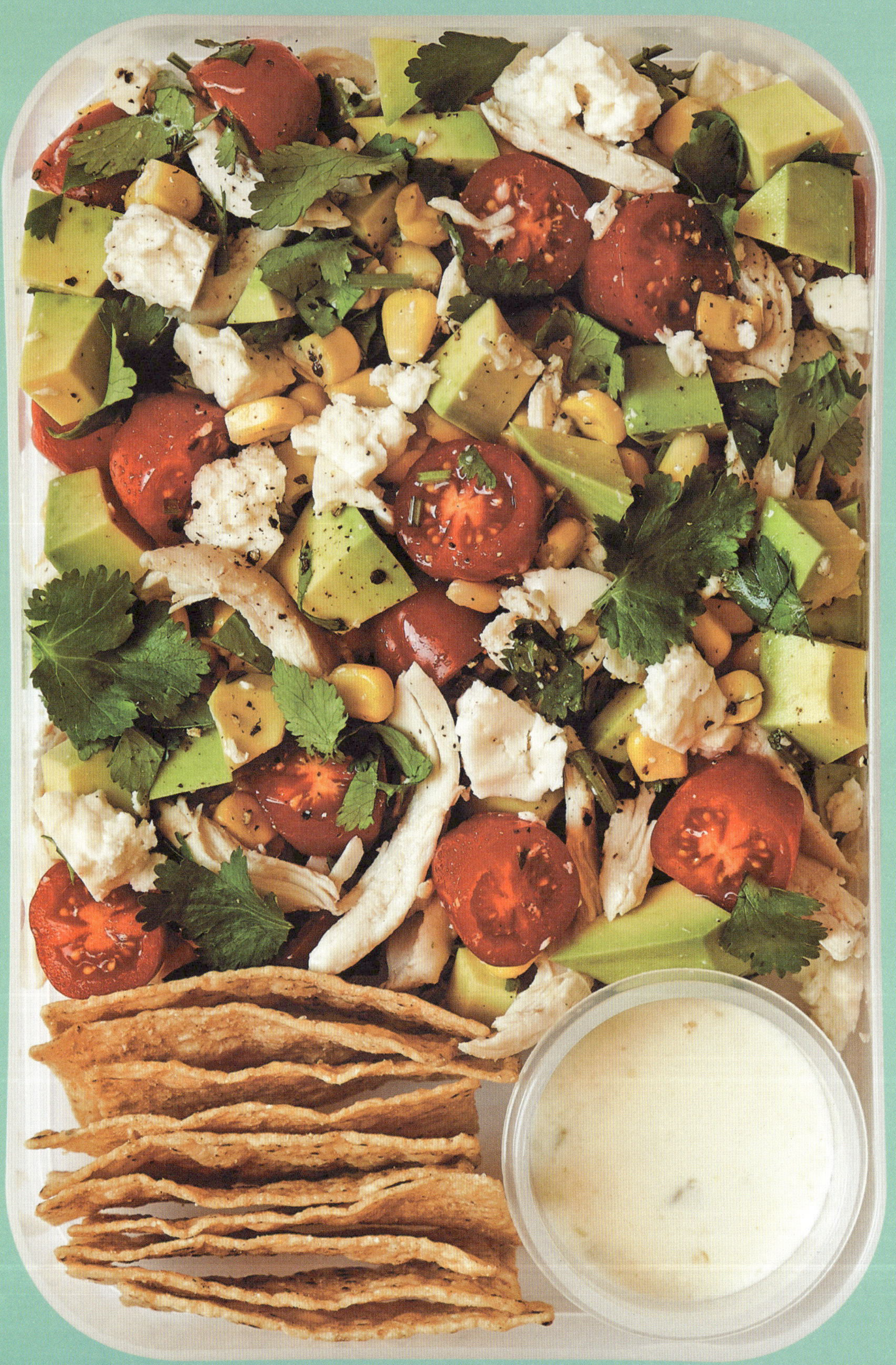

PROTEIN: 42 G NET CARBS: 29 G FAT: 26 G

Chicken taco salad with jalapeño crema

Shredded chicken is the protein hero in this Tex-Mex bowl, complemented by a creamy yoghurt–jalapeño dressing and a crunchy tortilla topping. Queso fresco is a mild-flavoured Mexican cheese, available at Latin grocers and some good supermarkets.

- ½ avocado, diced
- juice of ½ lime
- 100 g (⅔ cup) shredded cooked chicken
- 75 g (2¾ oz) tinned sweet corn kernels, drained and rinsed
- 100 g (3½ oz) grape (baby plum) tomatoes, halved
- 30 g (1 oz) queso fresco, crumbled
- small handful of coriander (cilantro) leaves, roughly chopped
- handful of tortilla chips, roughly broken

JALAPEÑO CREMA DRESSING

- 1 tablespoon lime juice
- 1 tablespoon high-protein Greek-style yoghurt
- 3 slices pickled jalapeños, finely chopped

1. Place the avocado in a bowl and toss in the lime juice. Add the remaining salad ingredients, except the tortilla chips, and toss lightly.
2. Combine the dressing ingredients in a small bowl, then season to taste with salt and pepper.
3. Pour the dressing over the salad just before serving and toss through the tortilla chips.

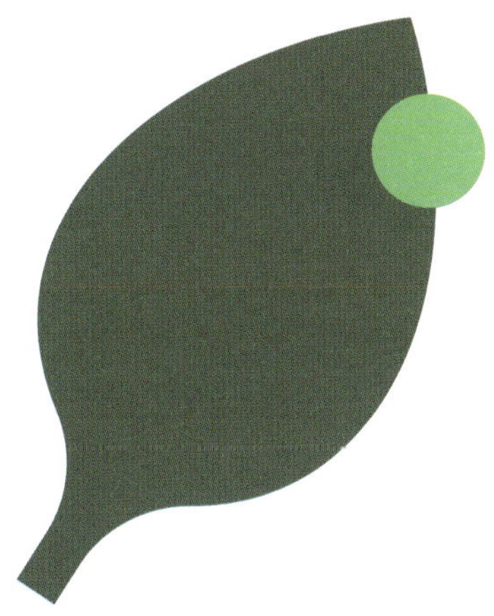

PROTEIN: 39 G NET CARBS: 66 G FAT: 5 G

Chicken & mango noodle salad

Chicken brings satisfying protein to this bright summer salad, with ripe mango and a sweet chilli–lime dressing for a fresh finish.

100 g (3½ oz) cooked, rinsed and drained vermicelli noodles

100 g (⅔ cup) shredded cooked chicken

½ mango, sliced

handful of coriander (cilantro) leaves

SWEET CHILLI & LIME DRESSING

2½ tablespoons sweet chilli sauce

zest and juice of ½ lime

2 teaspoons finely chopped red onion

2 teaspoons finely chopped mint leaves

1 teaspoon minced ginger

1. Place the salad ingredients in a bowl and toss lightly, then season to taste with salt and pepper.
2. Combine the dressing ingredients in a small bowl.
3. Pour the dressing over the salad just before serving and toss well to coat.

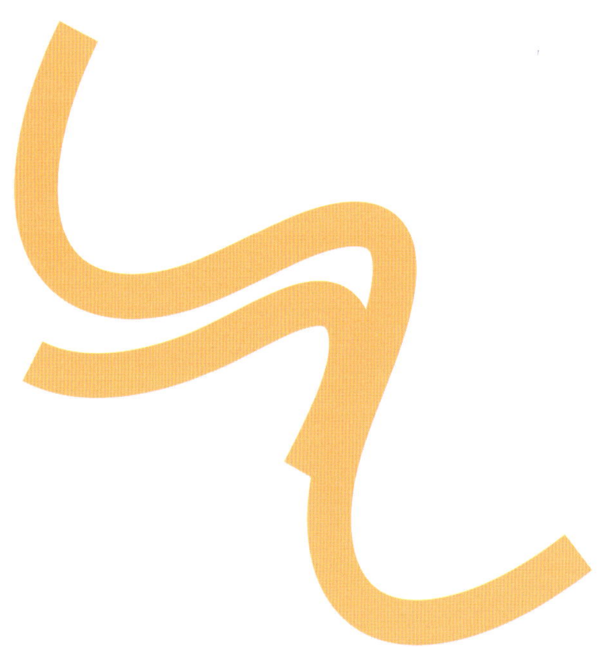

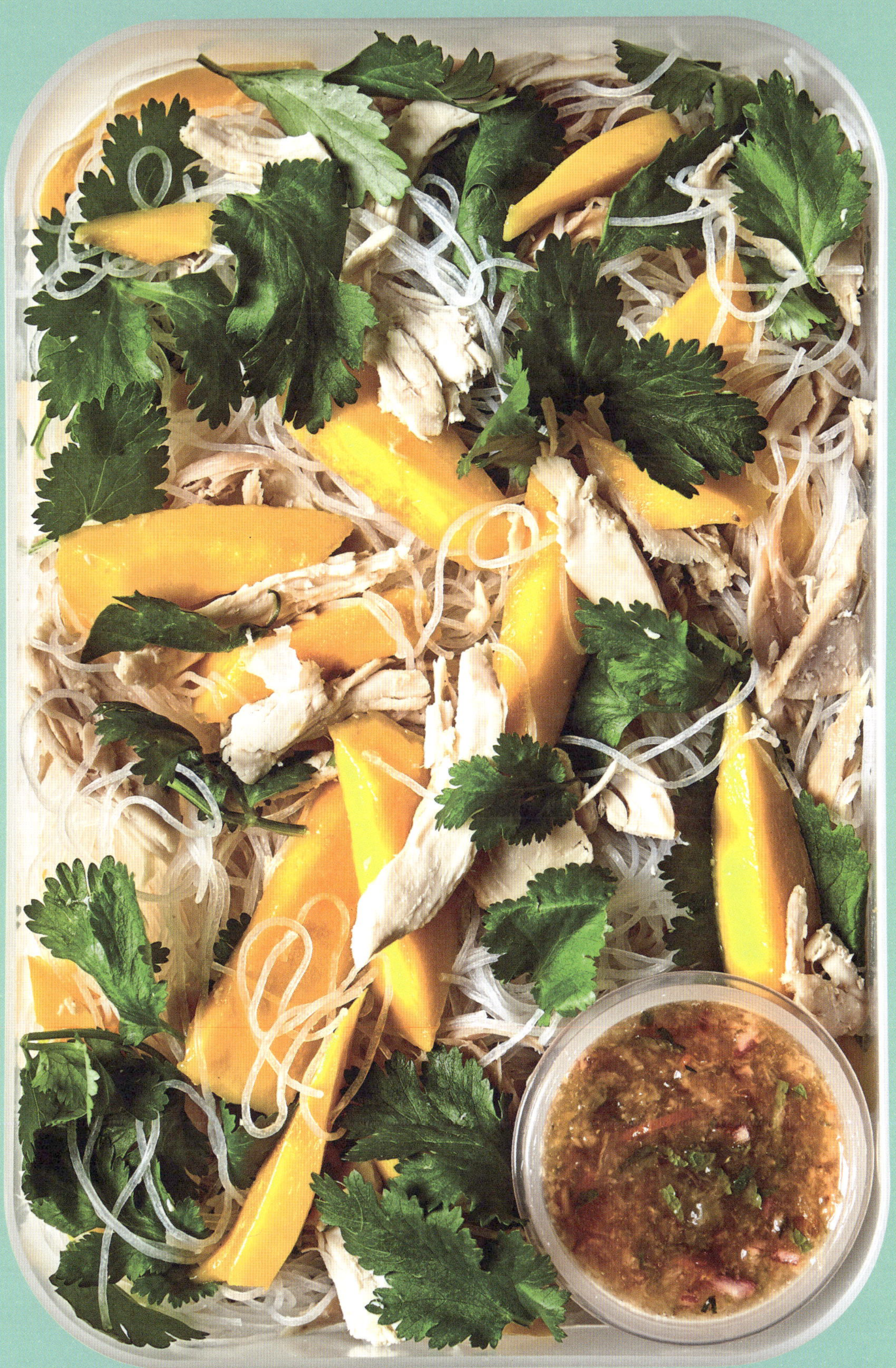

PROTEIN: 35 G NET CARBS: 34 G FAT: 10 G

Thai-style red curry chicken zoodles

Lean chicken paired with spiralised veg and a Thai-inspired curry dressing makes for a lighter, protein-forward take on curry noodles. If you prefer, opt for brown rice noodles instead of the spiralised vegetables.

- 100 g (2/3 cup) shredded cooked chicken
- 1 carrot, spiralised
- 1 zucchini (courgette), spiralised
- handful of mixed Asian herbs, such as Thai basil, Vietnamese mint and coriander (cilantro) leaves

THAI RED CURRY DRESSING

- 2 tablespoons coconut cream
- 1 teaspoon mirin
- 1 teaspoon store-bought Thai red curry paste
- zest and juice of 1/2 lime

1. Place the salad ingredients together in a bowl and toss lightly, then season to taste with salt and pepper.
2. Combine the dressing ingredients in a small bowl.
3. Pour the dressing over the salad just before serving and toss well to coat.

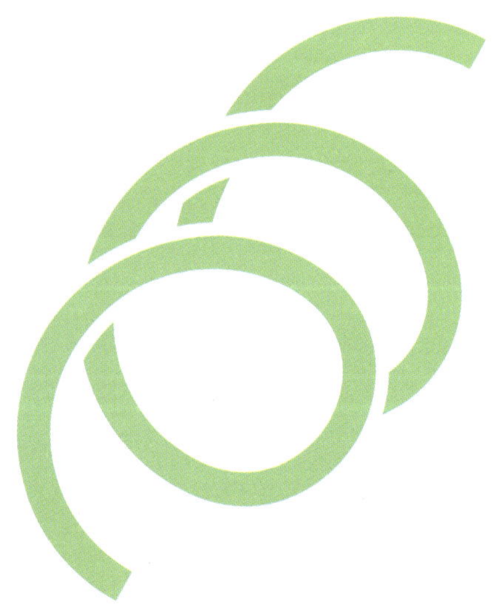

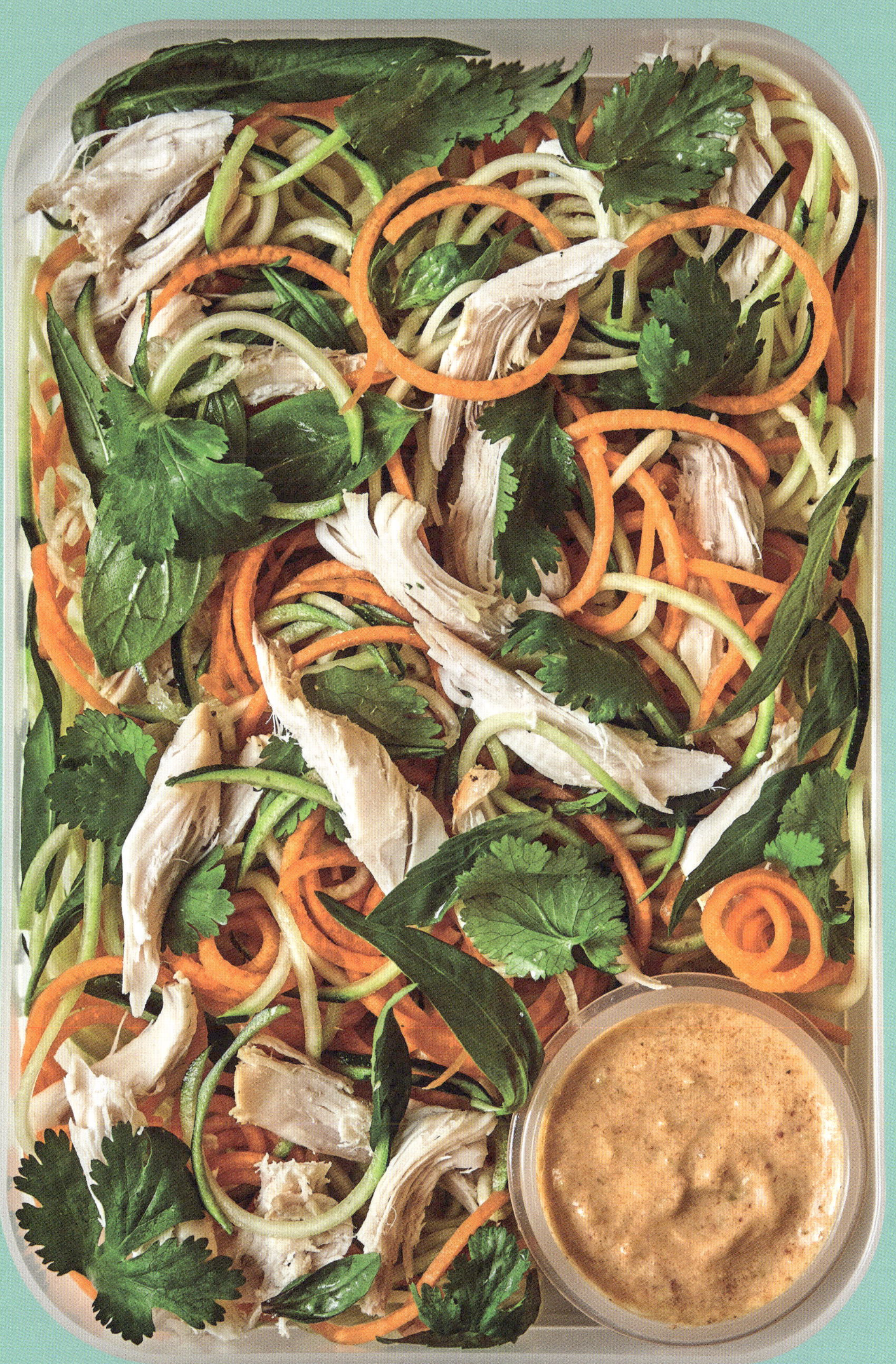

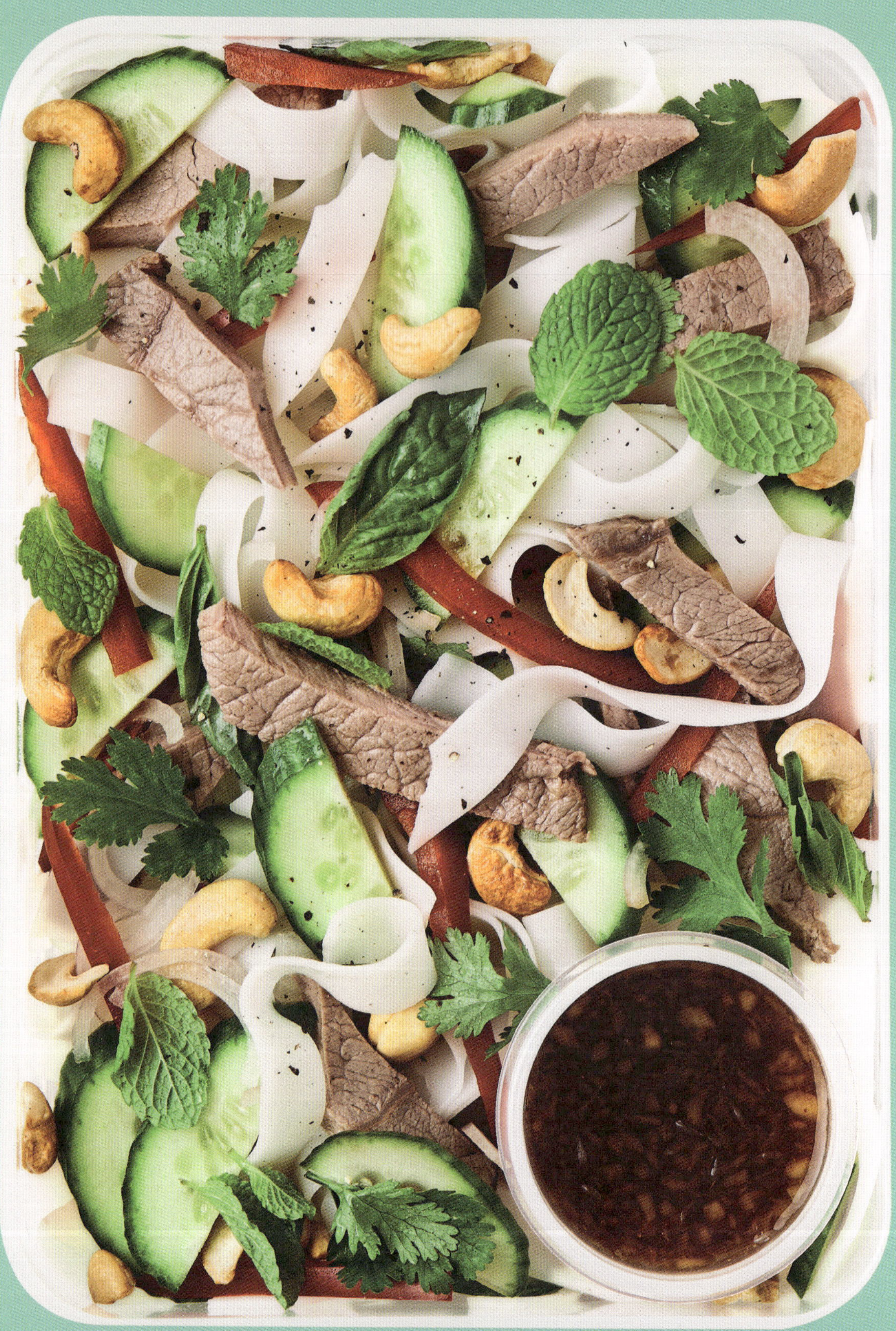

PROTEIN: 41 G NET CARBS: 60 G FAT: 33 G

Thai-style beef noodle salad

Tender beef and rice noodles create a filling, protein-loaded version of Thailand's much-loved beef salad, brightened with herbs and lime.

- 1 teaspoon olive oil
- 100 g (3½ oz) minute steak
- 80 g (2¾ oz) dried wide rice noodles, prepared as per packet instructions
- ½ short cucumber, sliced
- ¼ red bell pepper (capsicum), sliced
- 1 small red Asian shallot, finely sliced
- handful of mixed herbs, such as Thai basil, coriander (cilantro) and mint leaves
- 40 g (¼ cup) roasted cashews

SWEET CHILLI-GINGER DRESSING

- 2½ tablespoons sweet chilli sauce
- 1 teaspoon soy sauce
- zest and juice of ½ lime
- 1 teaspoon minced ginger

1. Drizzle the olive oil over the steak and season with salt and pepper. Place in a non-stick frying pan over high heat and cook for 1–2 minutes on each side, until cooked to your liking. Rest for a few minutes, then slice and allow to cool.
2. Place the steak in a bowl with the remaining salad ingredients and toss lightly.
3. Combine the dressing ingredients in a small bowl.
4. Pour the dressing over the salad just before serving and toss well to coat.

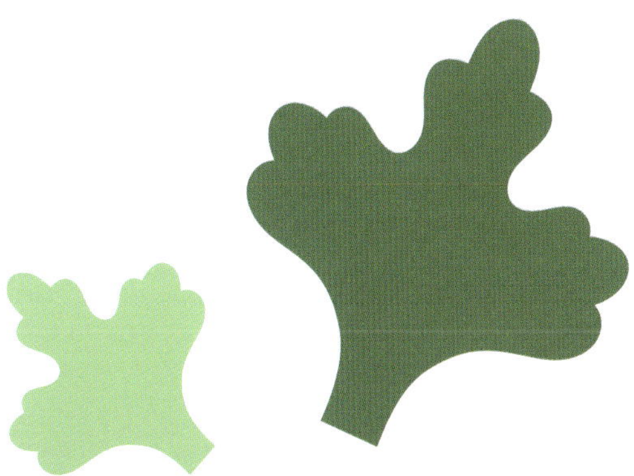

PROTEIN: 25 G NET CARBS: 12 G FAT: 71 G

Antipasto salad

This salad leans on deli staples like salami, bocconcini and olives to provide richness and bite. It's a good reminder that ingredients usually reserved for grazing plates can double as the backbone of a meal. You can dial up the heat by using a spicy salami, if you wish.

- 90 g (3 oz) sliced pork salami
- 60 g (2 cups) rocket (arugula) leaves
- 3 bocconcini, halved
- 70 g (2½ oz) cherry tomatoes, halved
- 30 g (¼ cup) marinated pitted olives
- 3 pepperoncini (marinated hot yellow peppers), sliced, stems discarded

ITALIAN VINAIGRETTE

- 2 tablespoons extra virgin olive oil
- 1 tablespoon red wine vinegar
- 1 tablespoon finely diced red onion
- ½ teaspoon dried Italian herbs

1. Place the salad ingredients in a bowl and toss lightly.
2. Combine the vinaigrette ingredients in a small bowl, then season to taste with salt and pepper.
3. Pour the vinaigrette over the salad just before serving and toss well to coat.

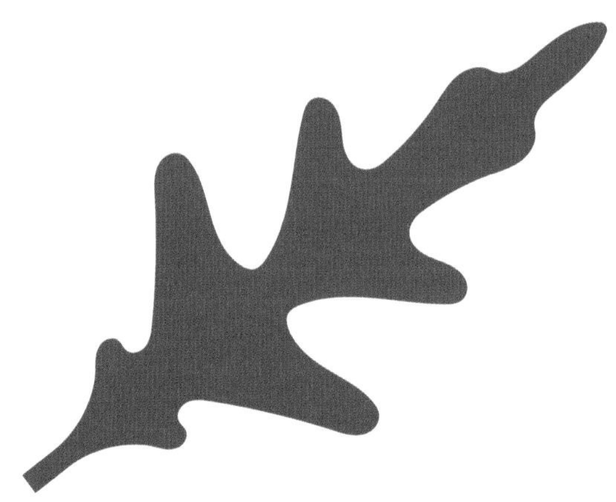

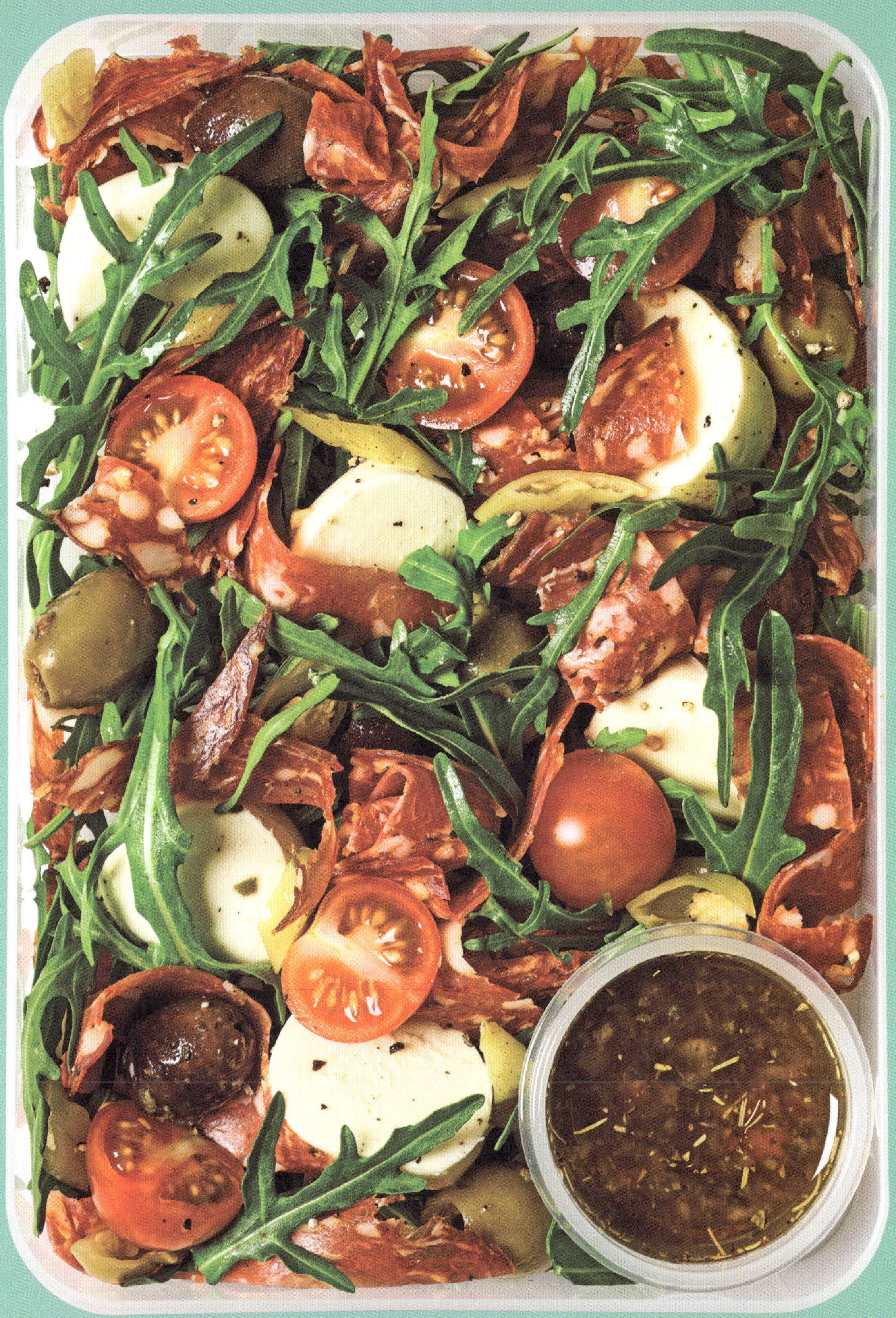

PROTEIN: 36 G NET CARBS: 11 G FAT: 37 G

Classic tuna niçoise

Tuna, egg and anchovy are all excellent sources of protein here. This French favourite is a great reminder that tinned fish and boiled eggs can turn a simple vegetable salad into a filling lunch.

- 100 g (3½ oz) blanched green beans
- 95 g (3¼ oz) tinned tuna in spring water
- ¼ red onion, finely sliced
- 80 g (2¾ oz) grape (baby plum) tomatoes, halved
- 30 g (¼ cup) pitted black olives
- 1 hard-boiled egg, halved
- 3 anchovy fillets, chopped (optional)

FRENCH DRESSING

- 1 tablespoon red wine vinegar
- 2 tablespoons extra virgin olive oil

1. Place the salad ingredients in a bowl and toss lightly, then season to taste with salt and pepper.
2. Combine the dressing ingredients in a small bowl.
3. Pour the dressing over the salad just before serving and toss well to coat.

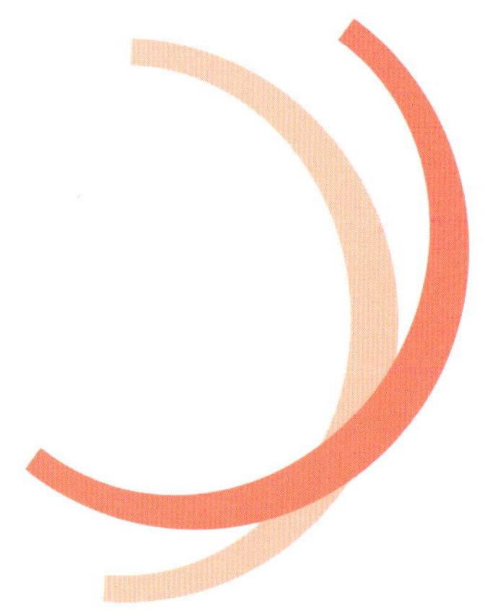

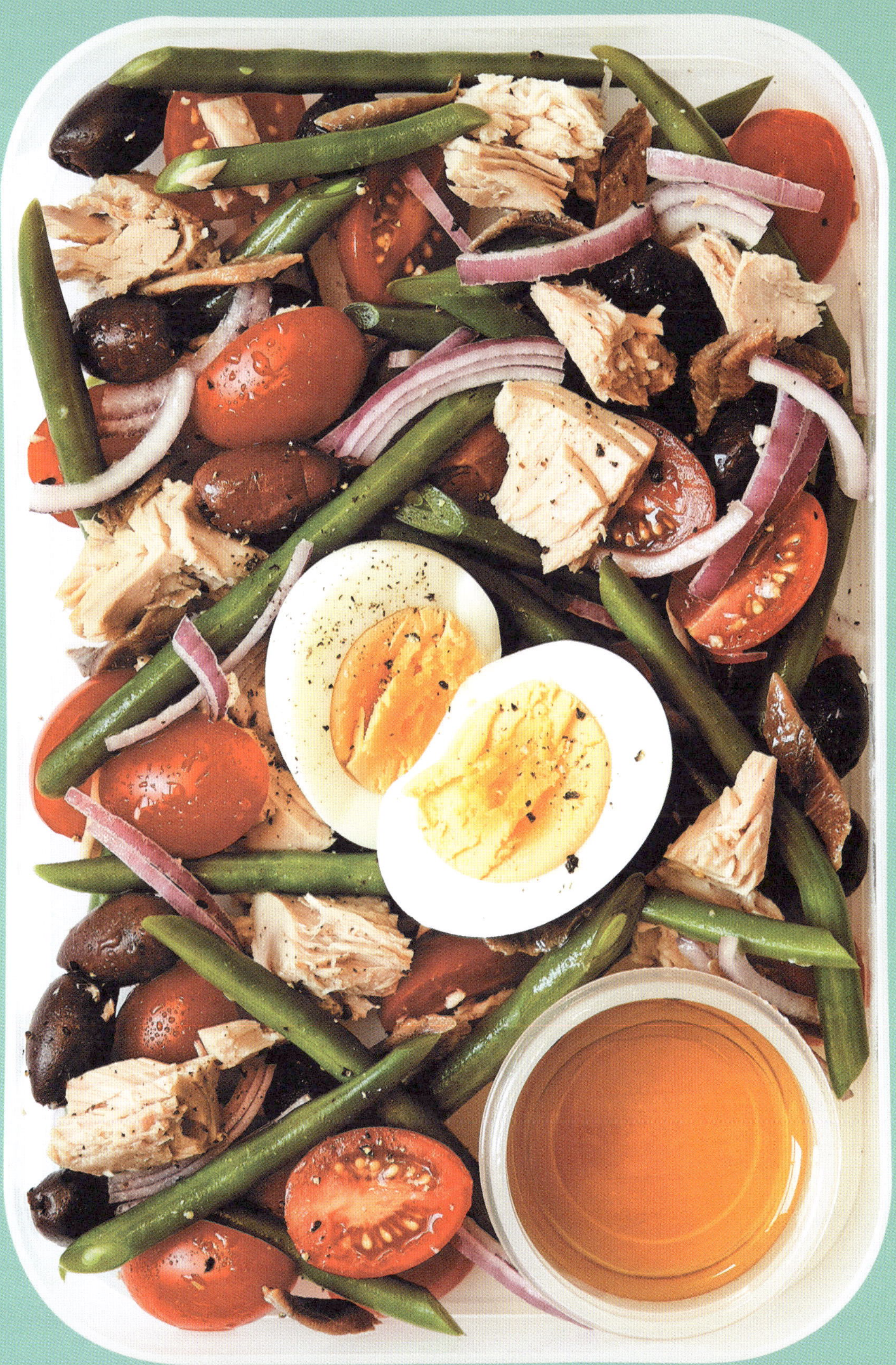

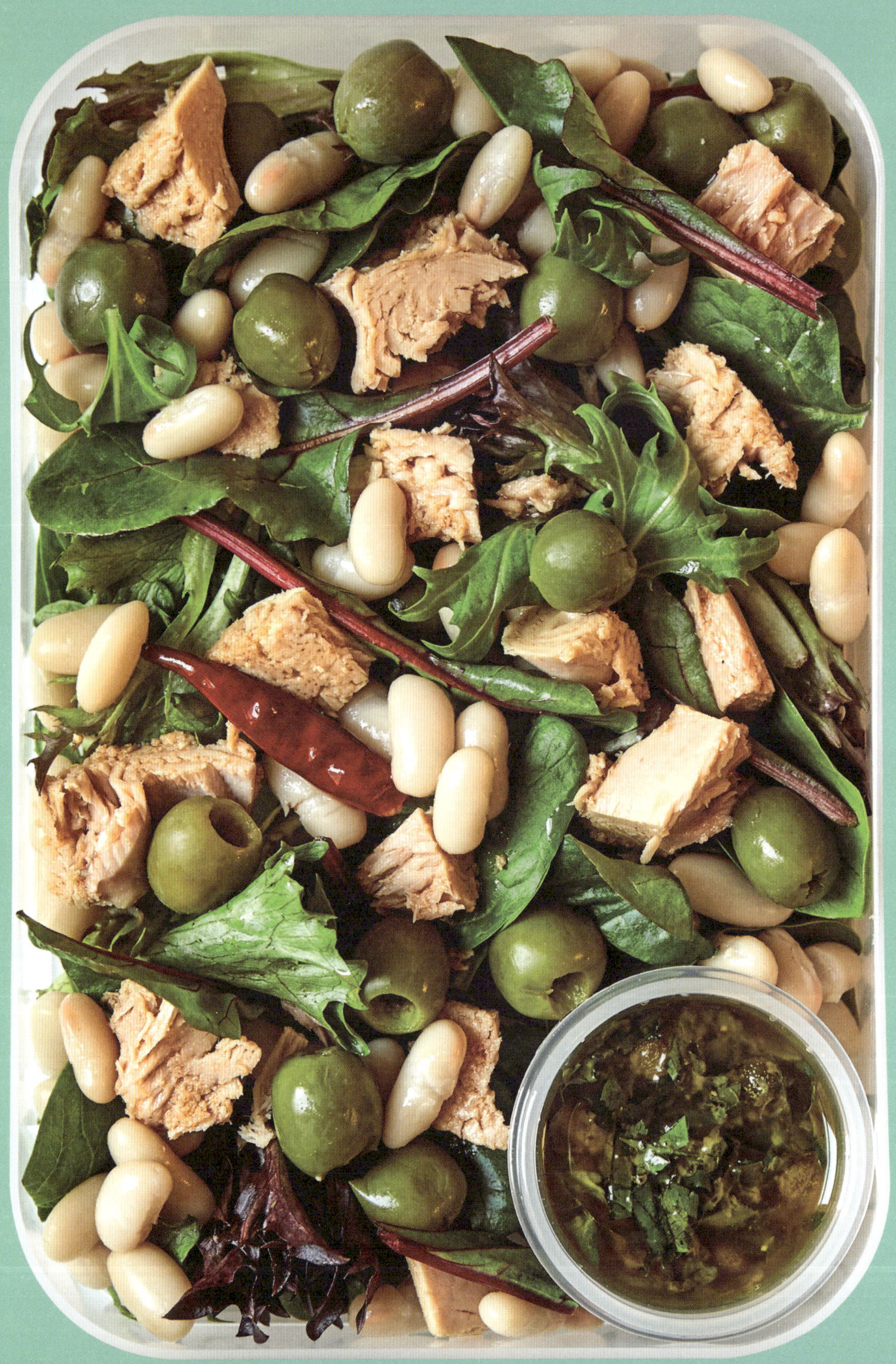

PROTEIN: 35 G NET CARBS: 19 G FAT: 31 G

Italian tuna, olive & cannellini bean salad

Beans are one of the best plant-based ways to add more protein to a salad, and they really sing when paired with tuna. A lemon, caper and parsley dressing ties everything together, with olives adding a buttery finish. If you prefer your tuna without spice, go for tinned tuna in olive oil instead of one infused with chilli.

95 g (3¼ oz) tinned tuna in chilli oil, drained

100 g (3½ oz) tinned cannellini beans, drained and rinsed

20 g (¾ oz) pitted Sicilian green olives

60 g (2 cups) mixed salad greens

PARSLEY & CAPER DRESSING

1½ tablespoons extra virgin olive oil

zest and juice of ½ lemon

3 teaspoons chopped parsley leaves

1 teaspoon baby capers

1. Place the salad ingredients in a bowl and toss lightly, then season to taste with salt and pepper.
2. Combine the dressing ingredients in a small bowl.
3. Pour the dressing over the salad just before serving and toss well to coat.

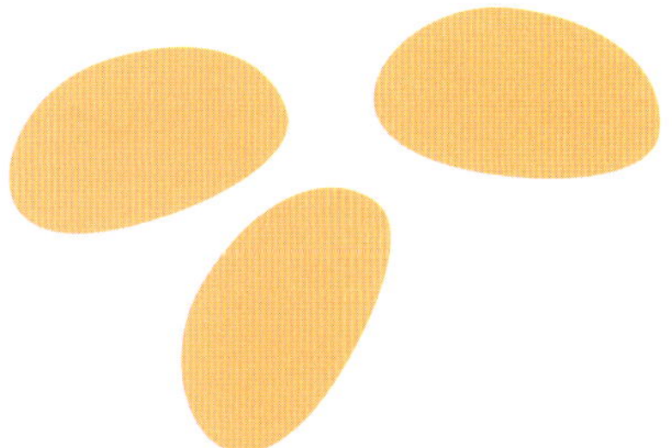

PROTEIN: 39 G NET CARBS: 22 G FAT: 41 G

Tuna, chickpea & caper salad

Tuna and chickpeas make a natural team – one from the sea, one from the pantry – both adding substance in different ways. The salty pop of capers and a sprinkle of parmesan round it out for an easy lunch or dinner that's more filling than it looks. Feel free to throw in any herbs you have on hand to add to this hearty salad.

- 95 g (3¼ oz) tinned tuna in oil, drained
- 100 g (3½ oz) tinned chickpeas (garbanzo beans), drained and rinsed
- ¼ red onion, finely sliced
- 2 tablespoons finely grated parmesan
- 70 g (2 cups) shredded iceberg lettuce
- 1 tablespoon baby capers
- 1 tablespoon chopped dill

RED WINE VINEGAR DRESSING

- 1 tablespoon red wine vinegar
- 2 tablespoons extra virgin olive oil

1. Place the salad ingredients in a bowl and toss lightly, then season to taste with salt and pepper.
2. Combine the dressing ingredients in a small bowl.
3. Pour the dressing over the salad just before serving and toss well to coat.

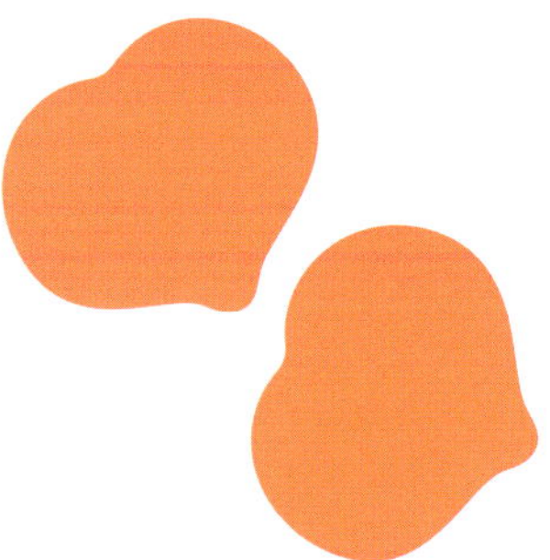

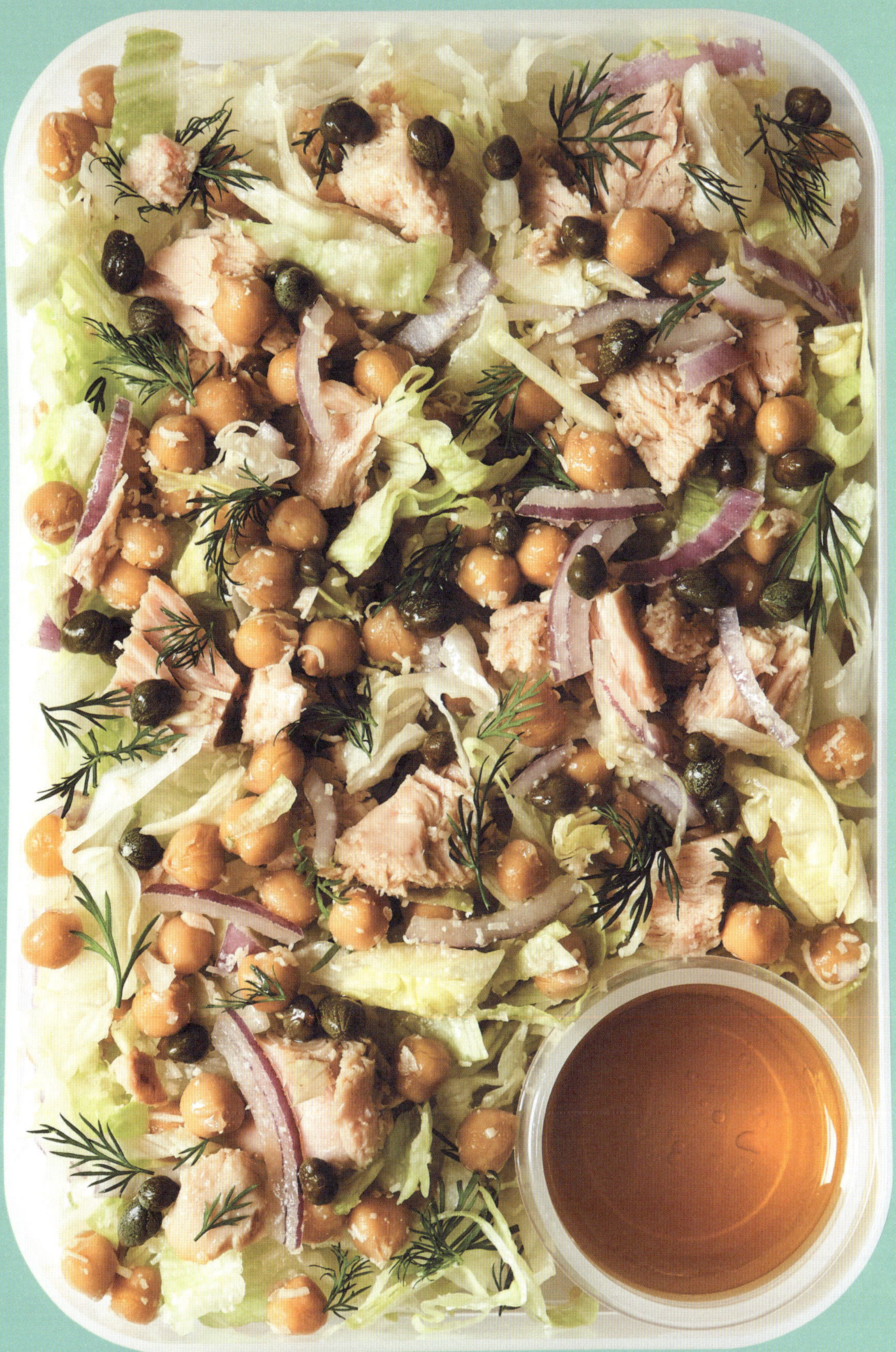

PROTEIN: 32 G   NET CARBS: 30 G   FAT: 25 G

Tuna noodles with soy-ginger dressing

Tinned tuna is such a quick and easy way to make your salads all the more satisfying. The tuna adds flavour and heft to this rice noodle salad, while spiralised cucumber and cabbage lighten it up, and the soy and ginger dressing pulls it all together.

- 1 short cucumber, spiralised
- 100 g (3½ oz) tinned tuna in chilli oil, drained
- 75 g (1 cup) finely sliced red cabbage
- 80 g (2¾ oz) wide rice noodles, prepared as per packet instructions
- 2 teaspoons toasted sesame seeds
- 1 teaspoon sliced red chilli

SOY-GINGER DRESSING

- 1 tablespoon sesame oil
- 2 teaspoons rice vinegar
- 1 teaspoon tamari or soy sauce
- ½ teaspoon minced ginger
- 1 small red chilli, sliced

1. Place the salad ingredients in a bowl and toss lightly.
2. Combine the dressing ingredients in a small bowl.
3. Pour the dressing over the salad just before serving and toss well to coat.

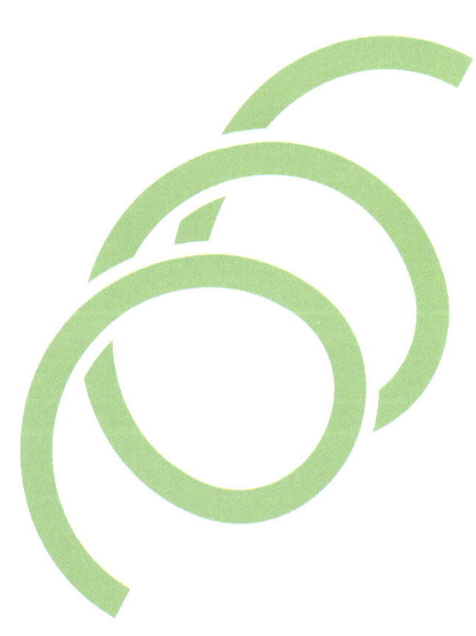

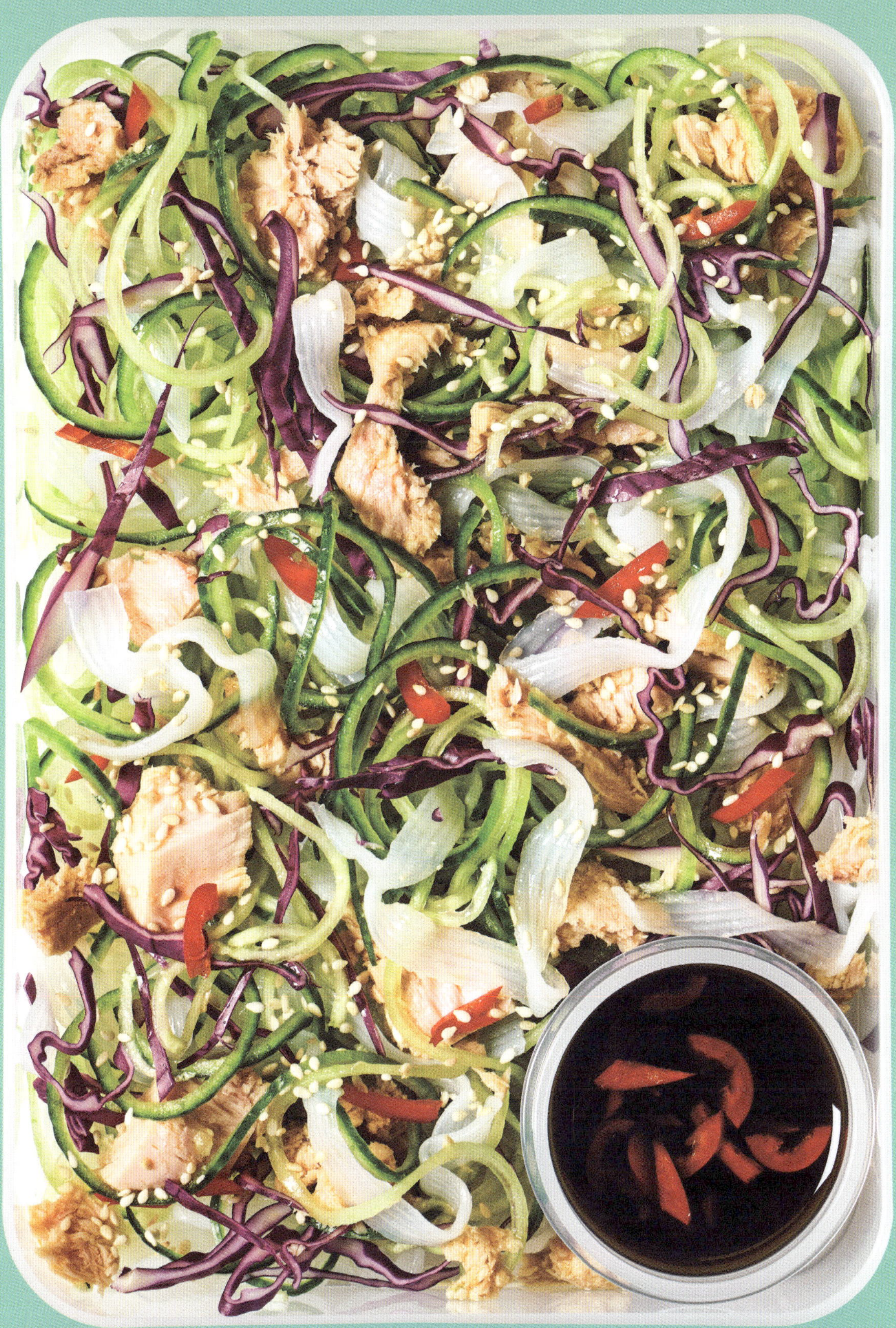

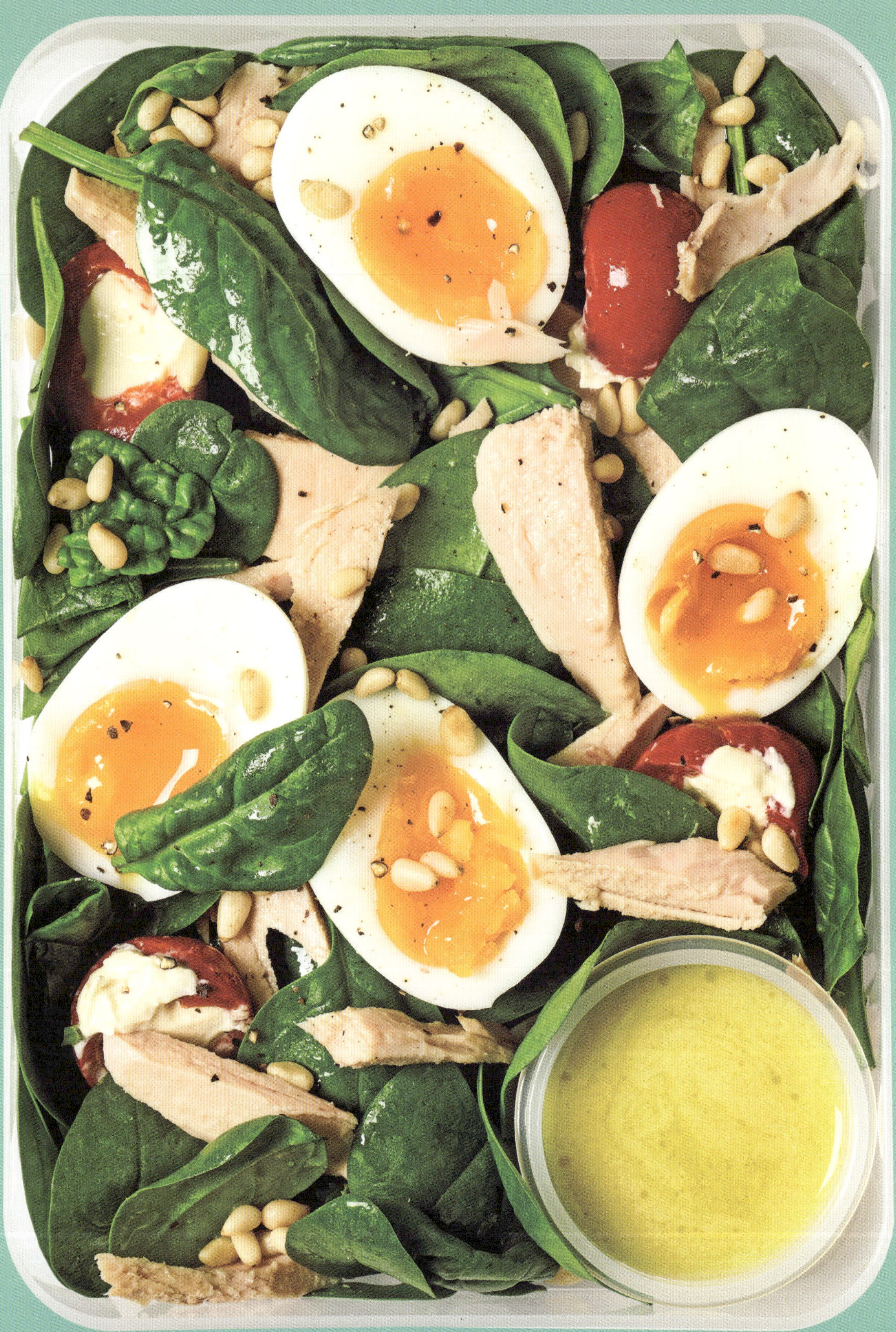

PROTEIN: 34 G NET CARBS: 9 G FAT: 49 G

Tuna & spinach salad

This simple salad is packed with protein and healthy fats to keep you full, with plenty of fibre to aid digestion. Dijonnaise is stocked in the condiment aisle of your supermarket and adds a gentle kick to this zesty dressing.

- 95 g (3¼ oz) tinned tuna in olive oil, drained
- 2 boiled eggs, halved
- 2 feta-stuffed baby peppers in olive oil, halved
- 75 g (1½ cups) baby spinach leaves
- 2 teaspoons toasted pine nuts

CREAMY LEMON VINAIGRETTE

- 1 tablespoon extra virgin olive oil
- 2 teaspoons lemon juice
- 1 teaspoon dijonnaise

1. Place the salad ingredients in a bowl and toss lightly.
2. In a small bowl, whisk the vinaigrette ingredients until smooth, then season to taste with salt and pepper.
3. Pour the vinaigrette over the salad just before serving and toss well to coat.

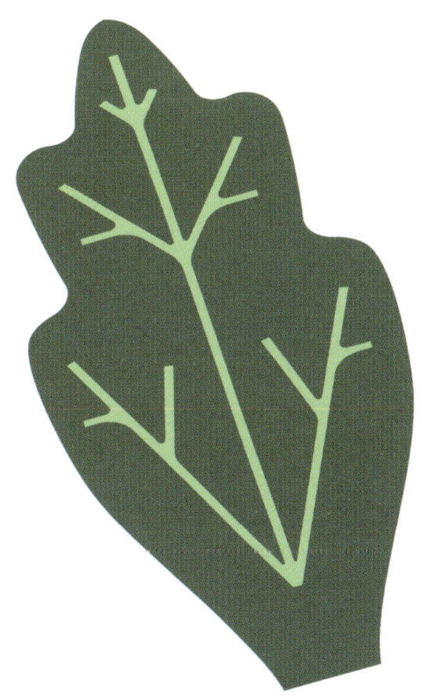

PROTEIN: 29 G NET CARBS: 17 G FAT: 22 G

Chilli & lime tuna noodle salad

Using the oil from a tin of chilli tuna means nothing goes to waste, and it gives this noodle salad extra depth. With spinach, celery and a hit of lime, it's a light but hearty dish that shows how much mileage you can get from one tin.

- 95 g (3¼ oz) tinned tuna in chilli oil, undrained
- 150 g (5½ oz) cooked ramen noodles, prepared as per packet instructions
- 30 g (⅔ cup) baby English spinach leaves
- 1 celery stalk, sliced
- lime wedges, to taste

1. Place the salad ingredients in a bowl, except the lime wedges, and toss lightly. Season to taste with freshly ground black pepper.
2. Squeeze the lime wedges over the salad just before serving and toss well to coat.

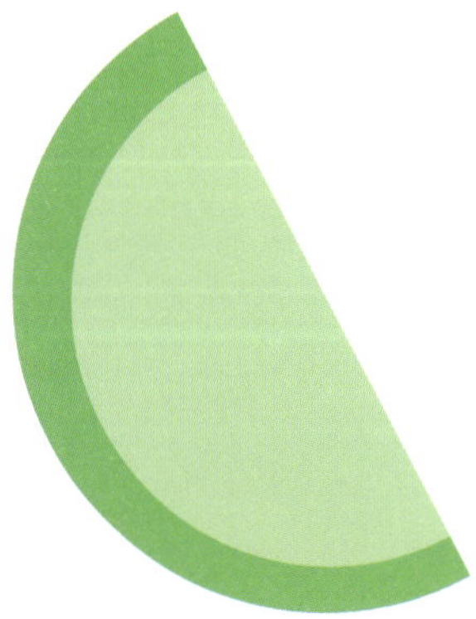

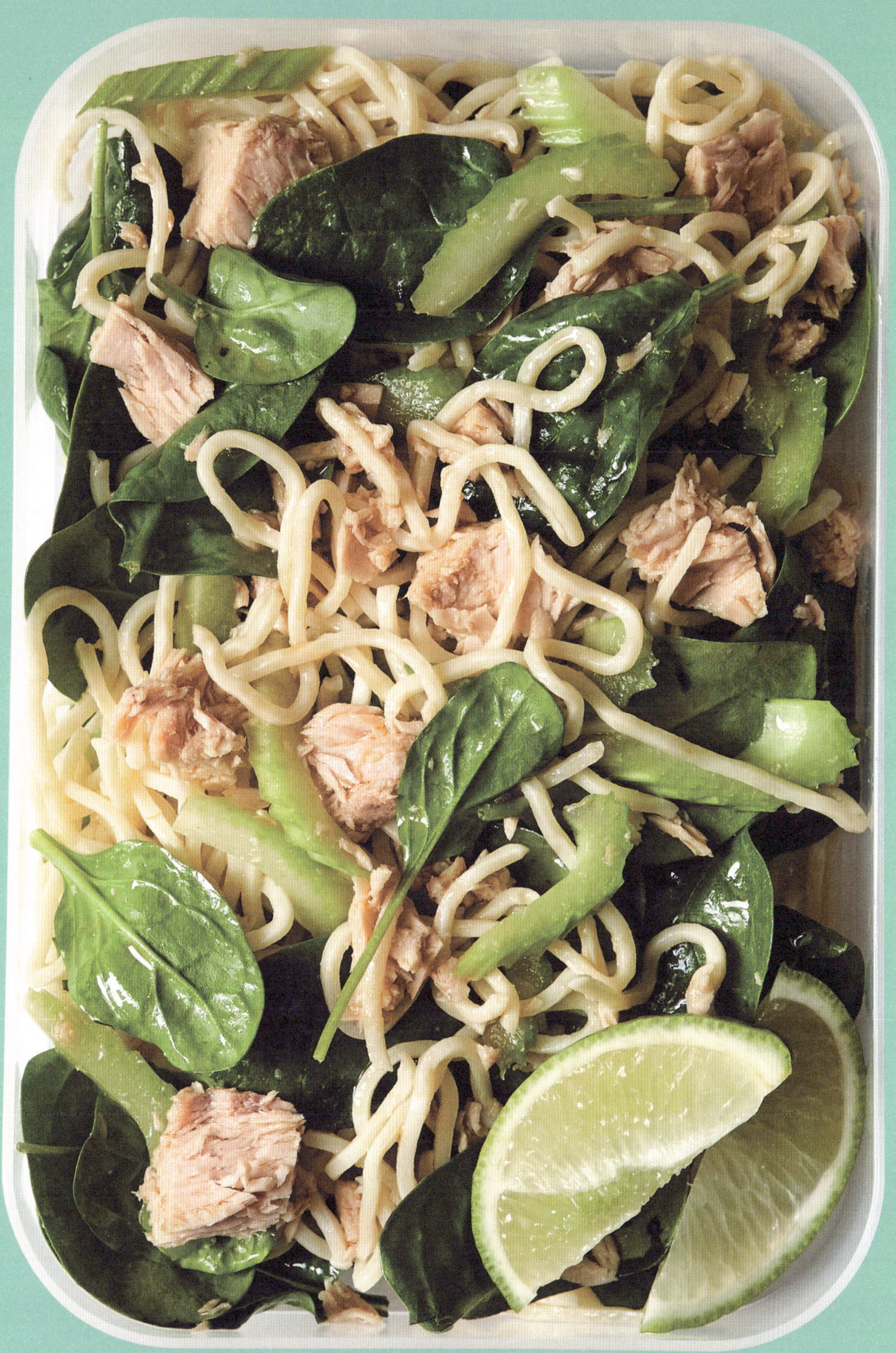

PROTEIN: 30 G NET CARBS: 11 G FAT: 9 G

Smoked trout salad

Smoked trout is a fabulous alternative to other more common tinned or smoked fish options. It's not only a great source of protein, but is also stacked with omega-3 fatty acids, vitamins and nutrients.

- 100 g (3½ oz) smoked trout slices
- 130 g (4½ oz) short cucumber, halved lengthways and sliced
- 60 g (2 oz) raw asparagus spears, woody ends trimmed, finely sliced
- 55 g (1½ cups) shredded iceberg lettuce
- 70 g (2½ oz) cherry tomatoes, halved
- 2-3 heirloom radishes, finely sliced

YOGHURT RANCH DRESSING

- 2 tablespoons high-protein Greek-style yoghurt
- 1 tablespoon blended cottage cheese (2% fat)
- 1 teaspoon apple cider vinegar
- 1 teaspoon chopped dill
- 1 teaspoon chopped chives
- 1 teaspoon chopped tarragon
- pinch of onion powder

1. Place the salad ingredients in a bowl and toss lightly.
2. Combine the dressing ingredients in a small bowl, then season to taste with salt and pepper.
3. Pour the dressing over the salad just before serving and toss well to coat.

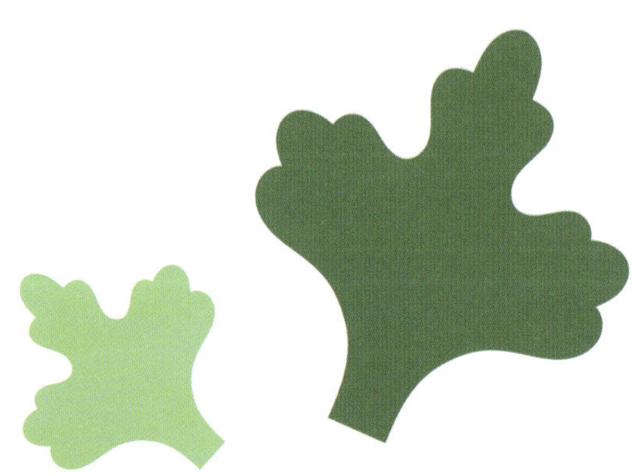

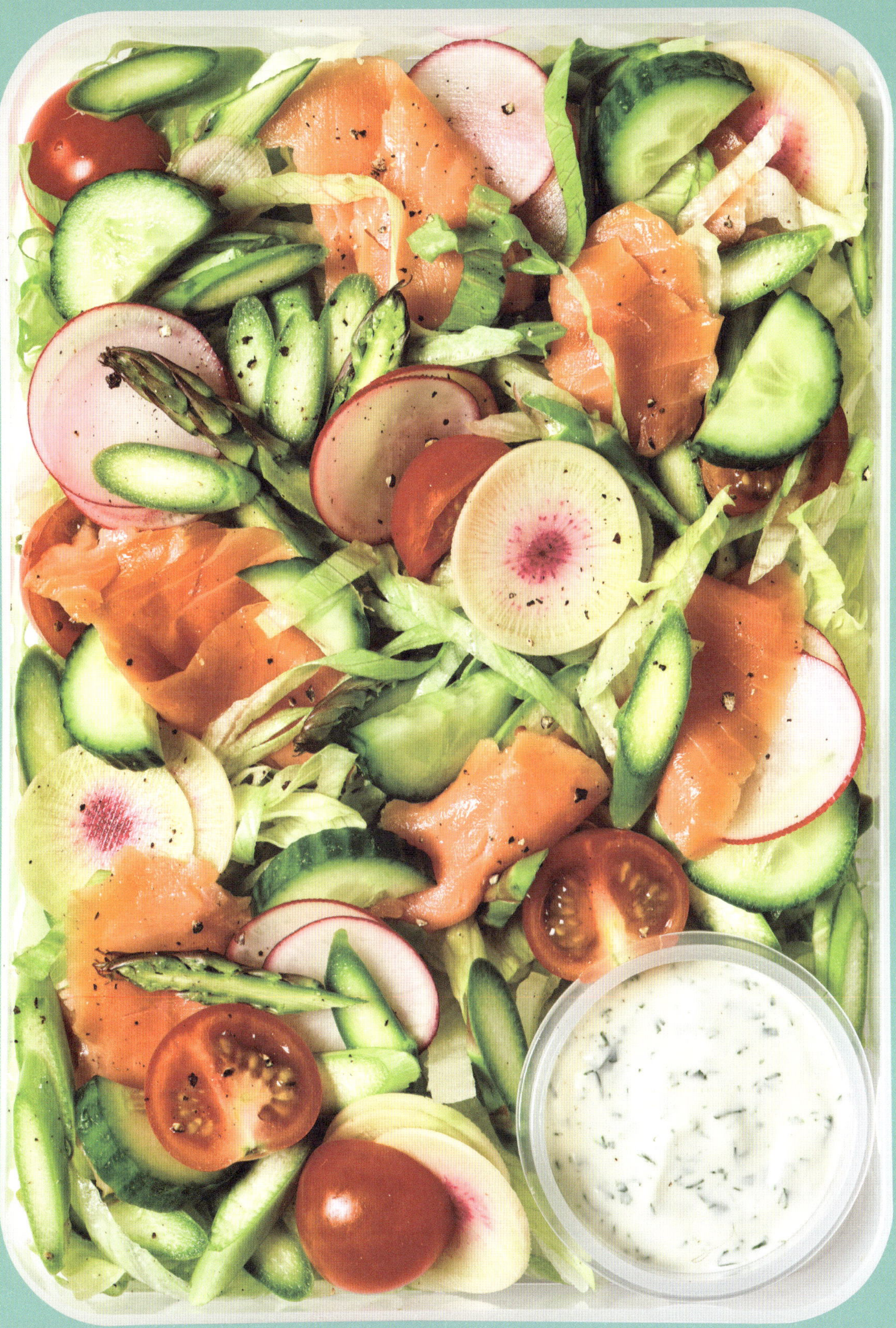

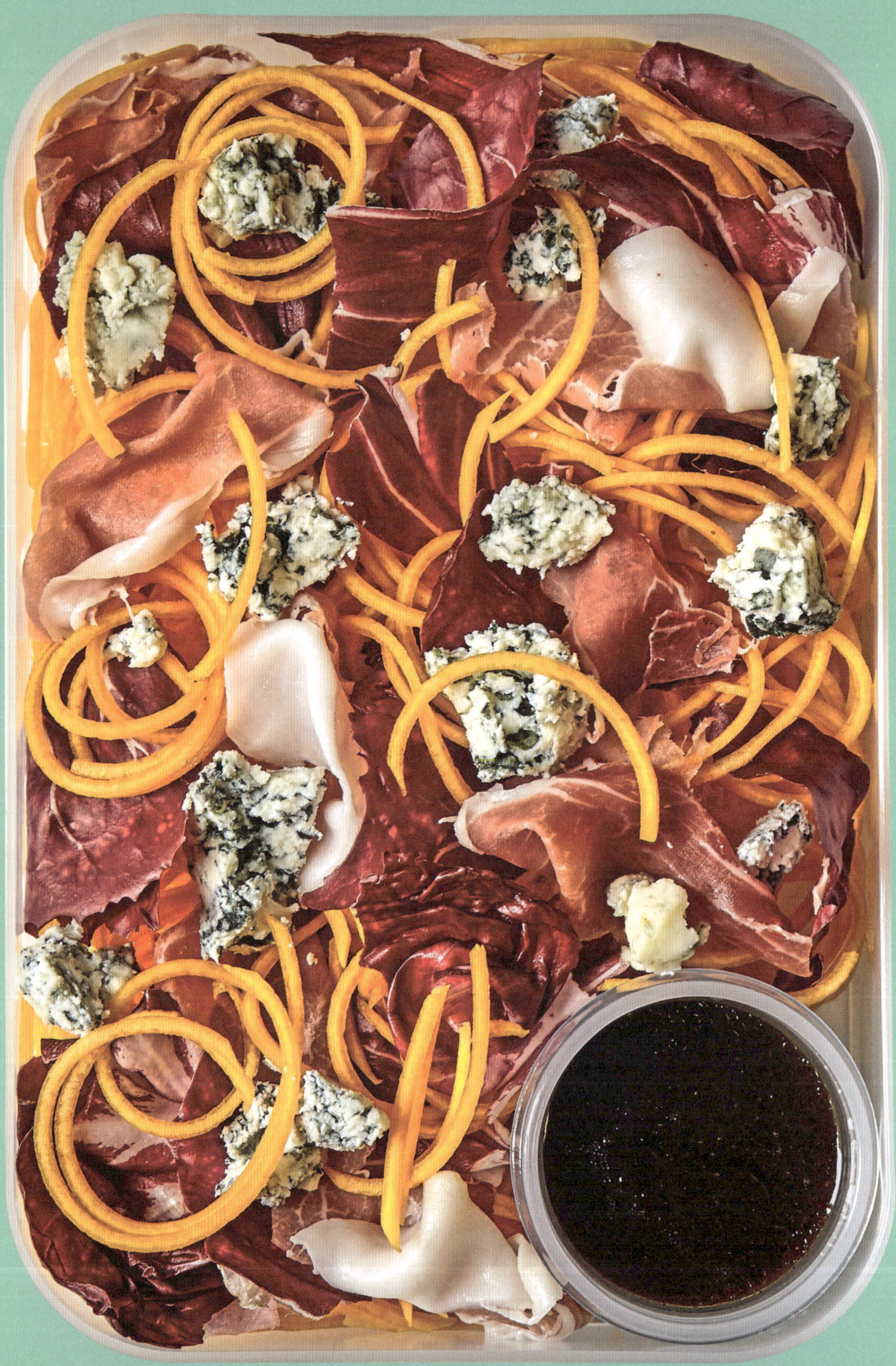

PROTEIN: 26 G NET CARBS: 24 G FAT: 49 G

Prosciutto, blue cheese and pumpkin salad

Pumpkin zoodles keep things light, while prosciutto and blue cheese add plenty of substance to this salad. It's a good example of how cured meats and strong cheeses can transform a vegetable-led dish into a main meal. If you have a good spiraliser, you can spiralise many different fruits and vegetables, including pumpkin for the zoodles used in this recipe. Alternatively, seek out pre-spiralised vegetables for an even quicker salad.

- 250 g (9 oz) pumpkin (winter squash) zoodles, blanched, refreshed and cooled
- 5 prosciutto slices, torn
- 30 g (1 cup) chopped radicchio
- 60 g (2 oz) blue cheese, crumbled

BALSAMIC-DIJON DRESSING

- 2 tablespoons extra virgin olive oil
- 1 tablespoon balsamic vinegar
- 1 teaspoon dijon mustard
- 1 teaspoon honey

1. Place the salad ingredients in a bowl and toss lightly.
2. Combine the dressing ingredients in a small bowl.
3. Pour the dressing over the salad just before serving and toss well to coat.

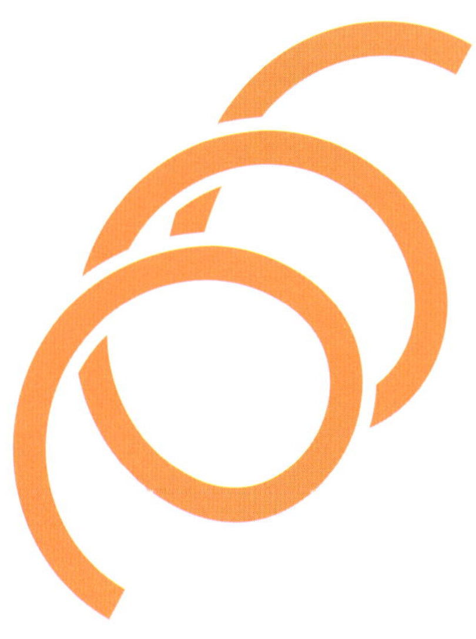

PROTEIN: 36 G NET CARBS: 16 G FAT: 26 G

Prawn cabbage salad

Prawns are an easy way to add substance without heaviness, especially when paired with crunchy high-fibre cabbage. The tahini dressing is sweet and salty, with added umami from the miso paste. If you're not a big fan of prawns feel free to substitute them for cooked chicken or tofu.

- 130 g (¾ cup) chopped cucumber
- 100 g (3½ oz) cooked peeled prawns (shrimp), deveined and sliced
- 75 g (1 cup) shredded red cabbage
- small handful of mint leaves
- small handful of coriander (cilantro) leaves
- 2 tablespoons chopped roasted salted almonds
- 2 teaspoons toasted sesame seeds

TAHINI, GINGER & MISO DRESSING

- 4 teaspoons tahini
- 1 tablespoon orange juice
- 1 tablespoon water
- 1 teaspoon white (shiro) miso paste
- ½ teaspoon minced ginger

1. Place the salad ingredients in a bowl and toss lightly.
2. In a small bowl, whisk the dressing ingredients until smooth.
3. Pour the dressing over the salad just before serving and toss well to coat.

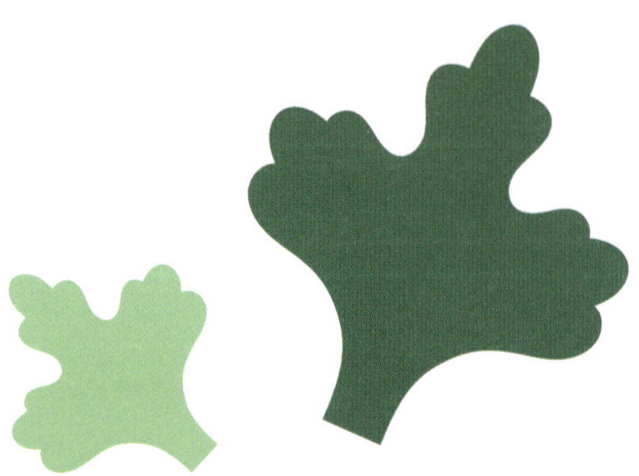

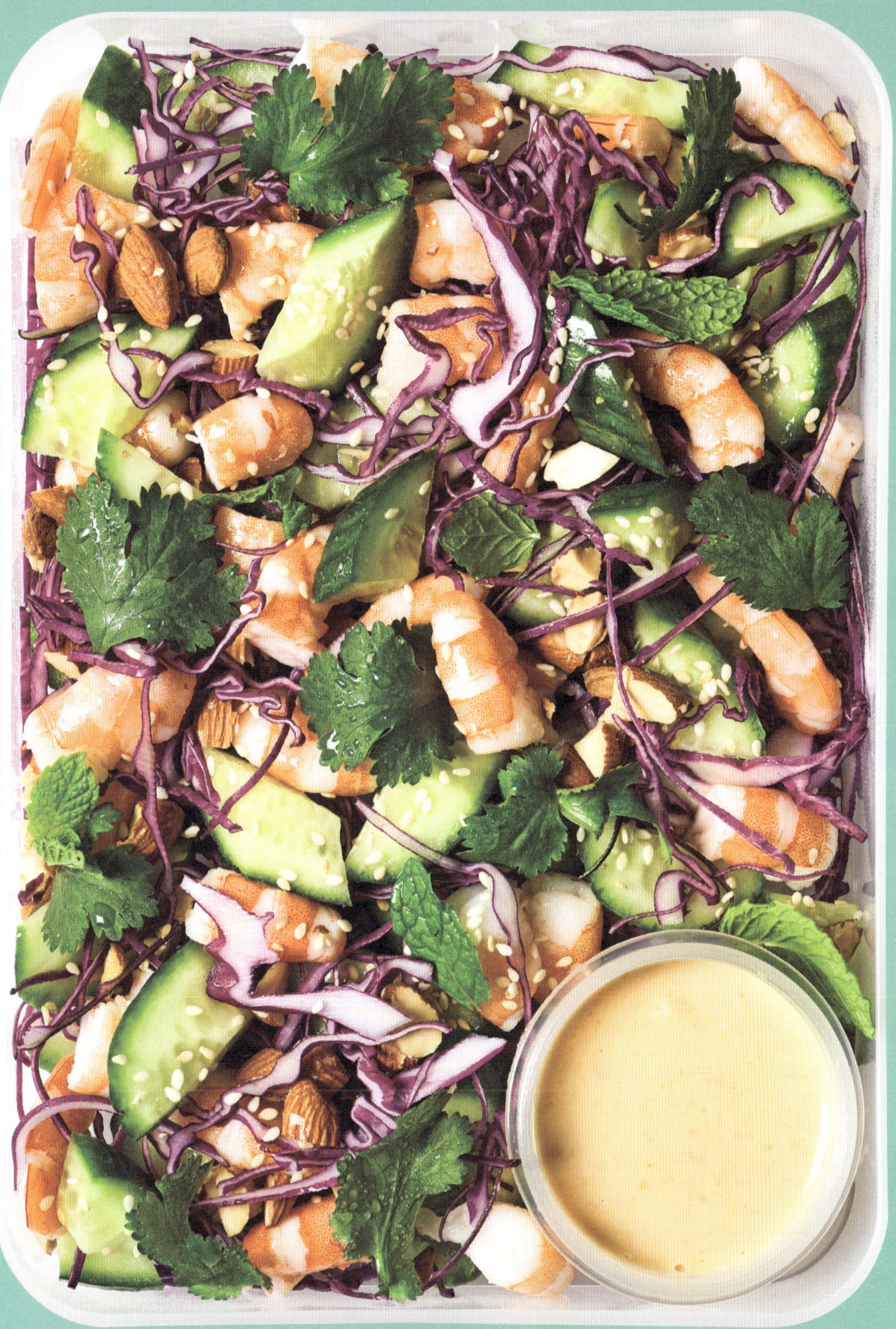

PROTEIN: 40 G NET CARBS: 13 G FAT: 37 G

Prawn cocktail salad

This deconstructed take on the retro favourite proves how versatile prawns can be. Avocado keeps it creamy, lettuce adds crunch, and the classic Marie-Rose dressing ties it together – all in minutes.

- 1 avocado, diced
- juice of ½ lemon
- 150 g (5½ oz) cooked peeled prawns (shrimp), deveined
- 35 g (1 cup) shredded iceberg lettuce
- 1 short cucumber, chopped

MARIE-ROSE DRESSING

- 1½ tablespoons whole-egg mayonnaise
- 1 tablespoon tomato ketchup
- 1 tablespoon lemon juice
- dash of Tabasco sauce, to taste

1. Place the avocado in a bowl and gently toss in the lemon juice. Add the remaining salad ingredients and toss lightly. Season to taste with salt and pepper.
2. Combine the dressing ingredients in a small bowl.
3. Pour the dressing over the salad just before serving and toss well to coat.

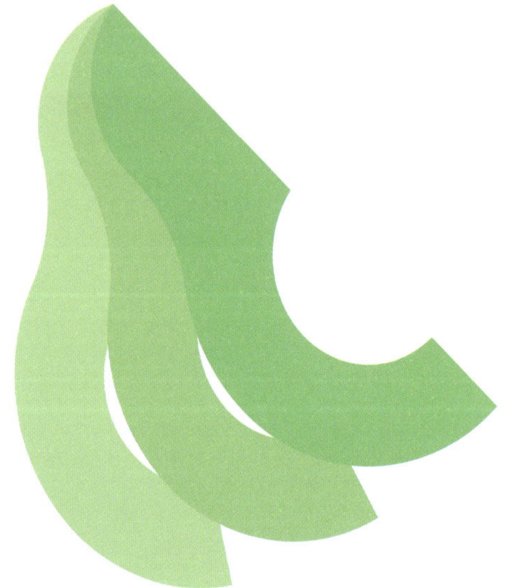

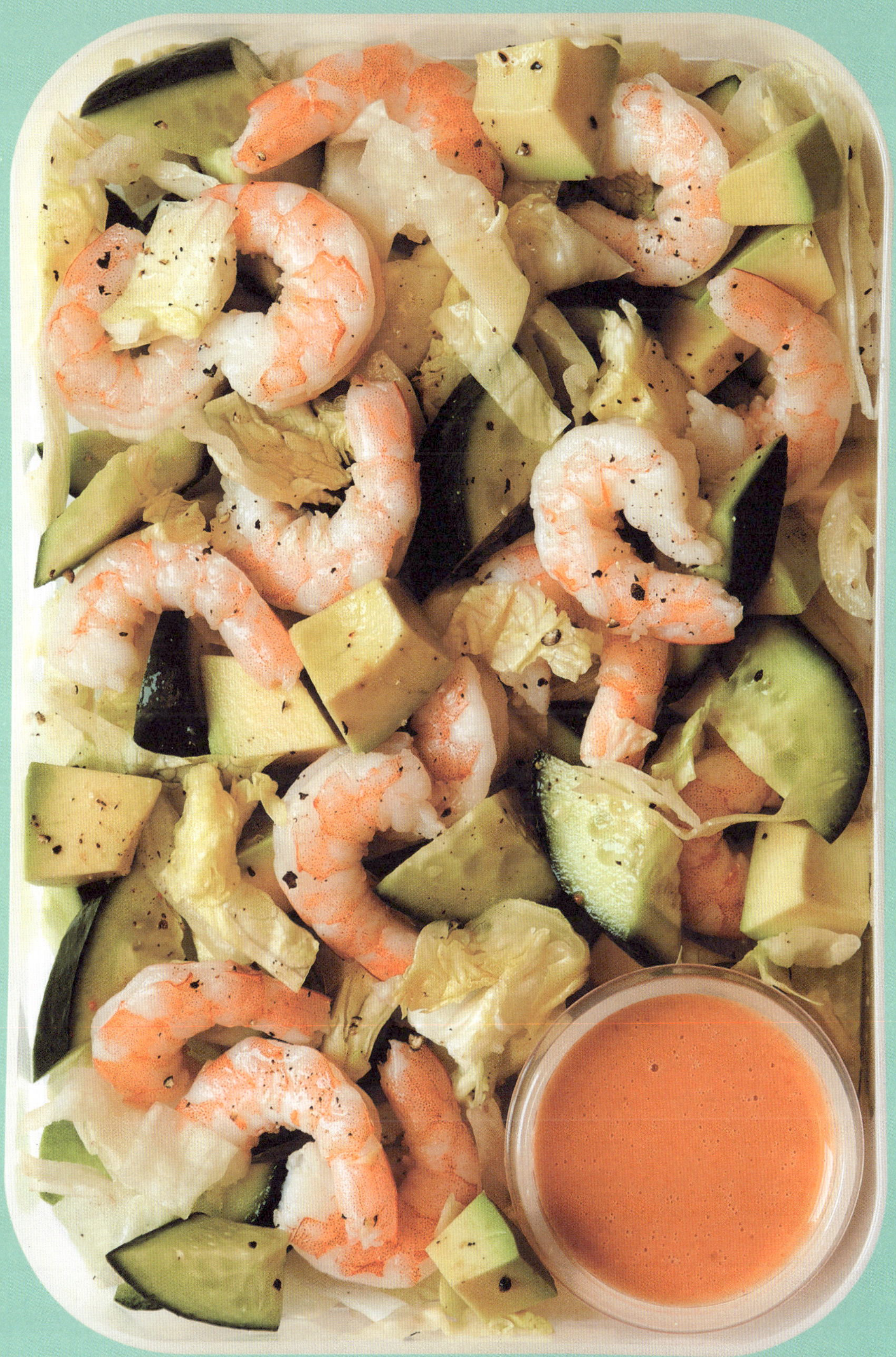

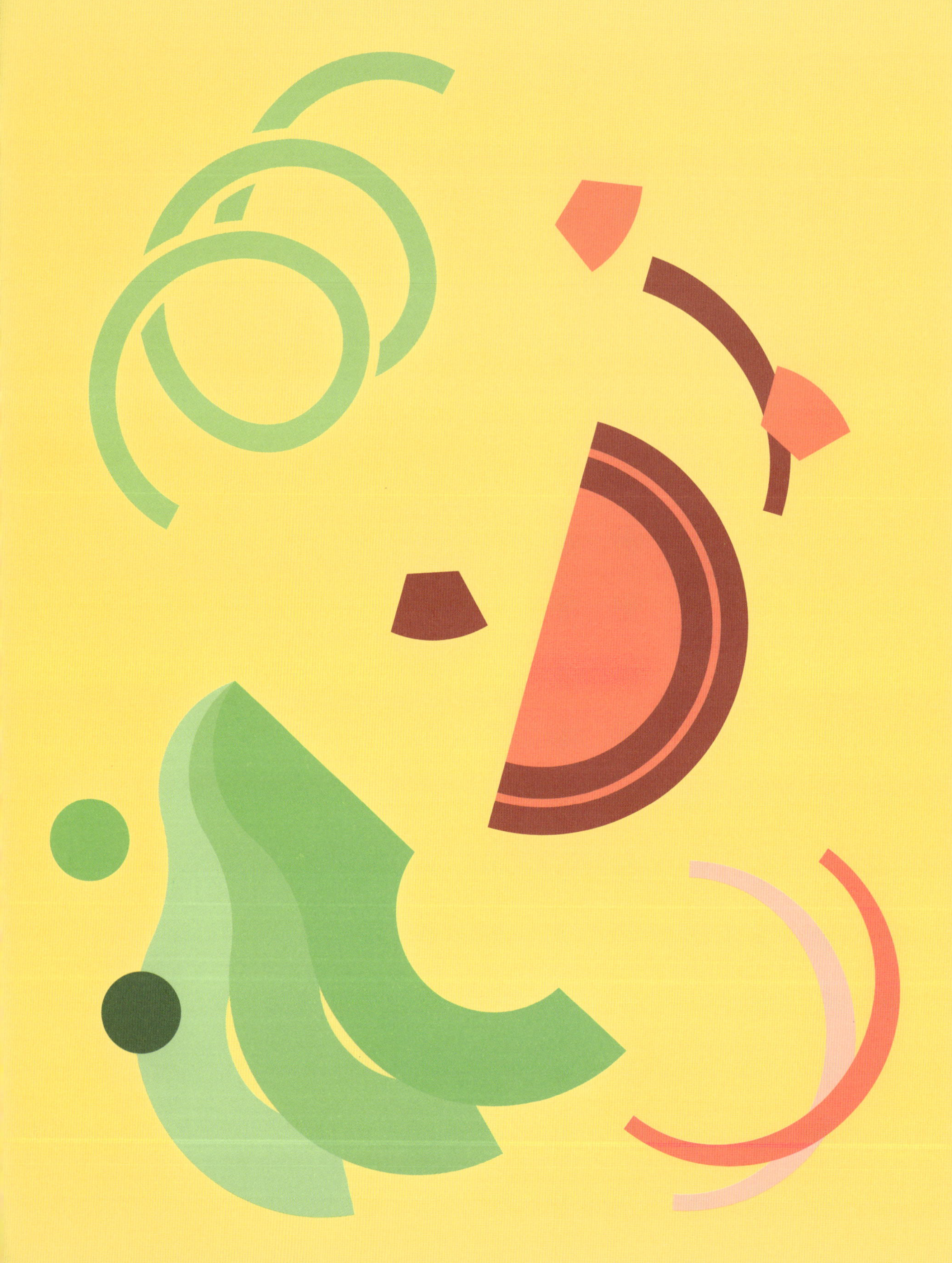

light &

low carb

PROTEIN: 47 G NET CARBS: 4 G FAT: 46 G

Chicken, asparagus & brie salad

Chicken breast and brie make a surprisingly good pair – one super lean, the other rich and creamy, and both high in protein! The asparagus adds freshness, while almonds bring crunch and a little extra staying power. It's a good example of how dairy and nuts can turn a simple salad into a full meal.

- 100 g (3½ oz) cooked chicken breast, sliced
- 50 g (1¾ oz) raw asparagus spears, woody ends trimmed, finely sliced
- 50 g (1¾ oz) brie, sliced
- 30 g (1 cup) rocket (arugula) leaves
- 2 tablespoons toasted flaked almonds

LEMON-CHIVE VINAIGRETTE

- 1½ tablespoons extra virgin olive oil
- 2 teaspoons chopped chives
- 2 teaspoons lemon juice
- pinch of lemon zest
- 1 teaspoon dijon mustard

1. Place the salad ingredients in a bowl and toss lightly.
2. Combine the vinaigrette ingredients in a small bowl, then season to taste with salt and pepper.
3. Pour the vinaigrette over the salad just before serving and toss well to coat.

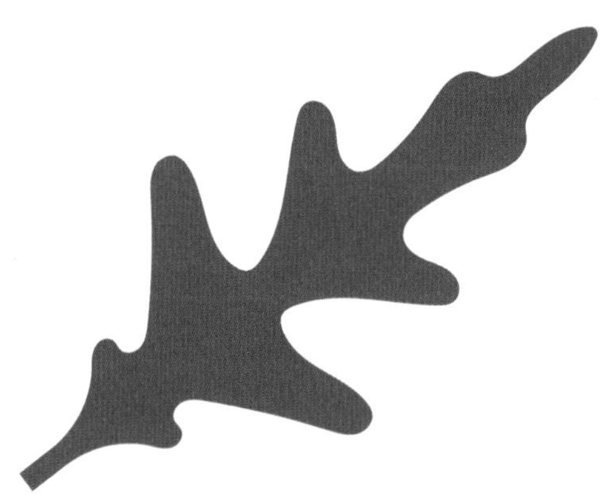

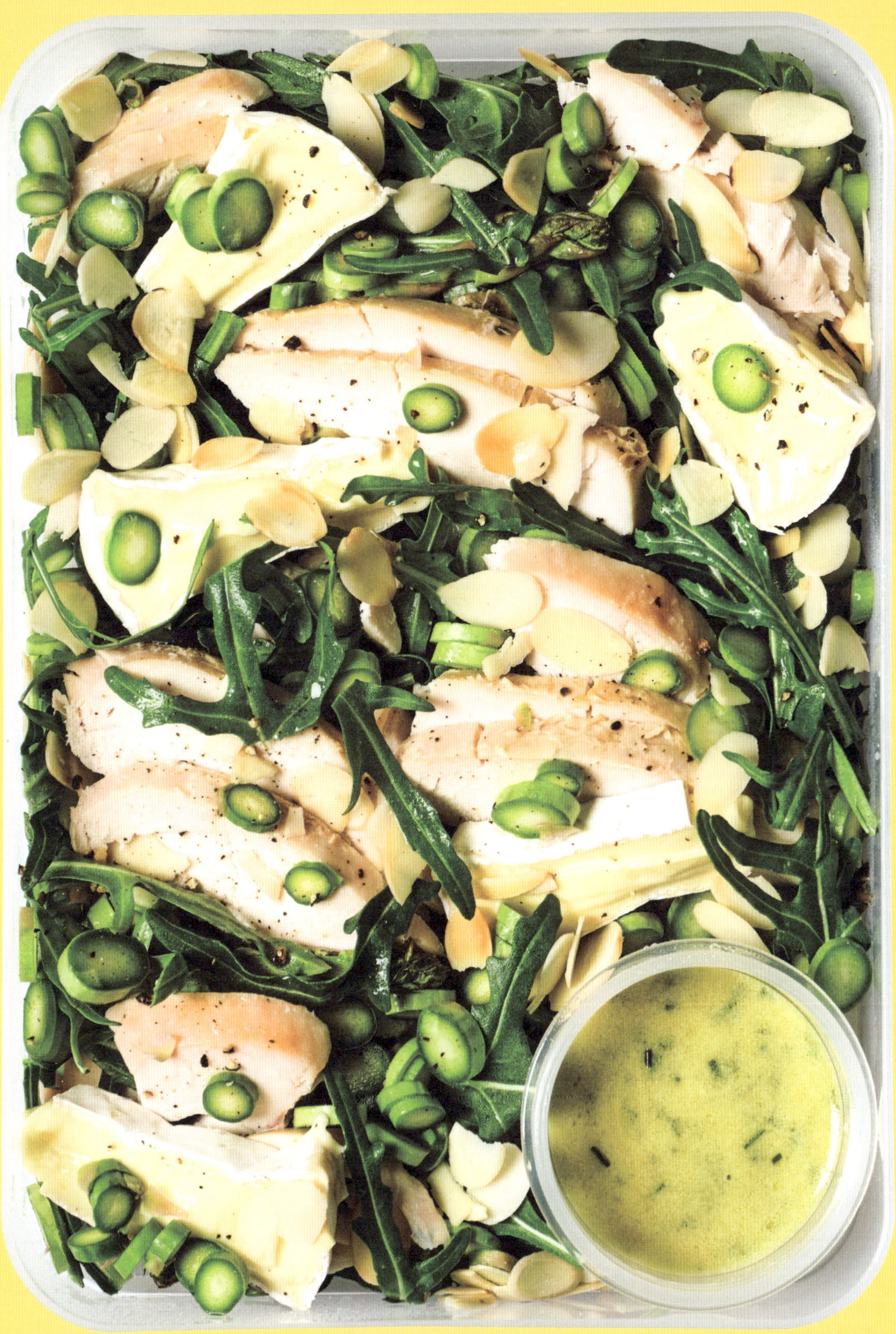

PROTEIN: 37 G NET CARBS: 5 G FAT: 53 G

Smoked chicken, pecan & watercress salad

Smoked chicken is an easy way to add flavour and depth without much effort. Here it's matched with tangy goat's cheese and peppery watercress, with pecans adding a nutty crunch. Each ingredient works differently, but together they create a hearty balance.

- 120 g (4½ oz) smoked chicken breast, sliced
- 50 g (⅓ cup) shaved fennel, plus a few fronds
- 40 g (1½ oz) goat's cheese, crumbled
- 30 g (1 cup) watercress leaves
- 2 tablespoons roughly chopped pecans

WHOLEGRAIN MUSTARD VINAIGRETTE

- 2 tablespoons extra virgin olive oil
- 1 tablespoon lemon juice
- 1 teaspoon wholegrain mustard

1. Place the salad ingredients in a bowl and toss lightly.
2. Combine the vinaigrette ingredients in a small bowl, then season to taste with salt and pepper.
3. Pour the vinaigrette over the salad just before serving and toss well to coat.

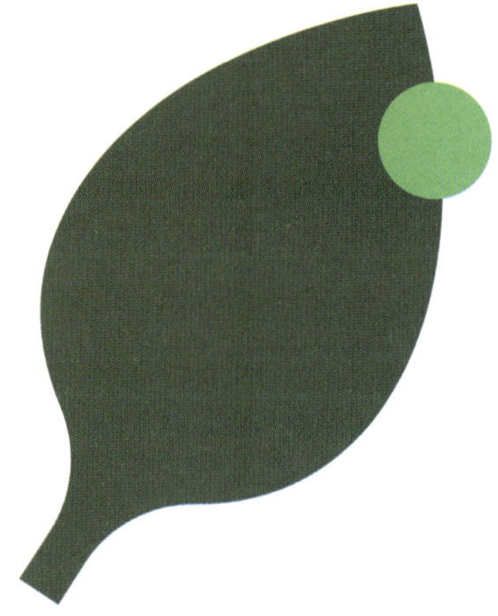

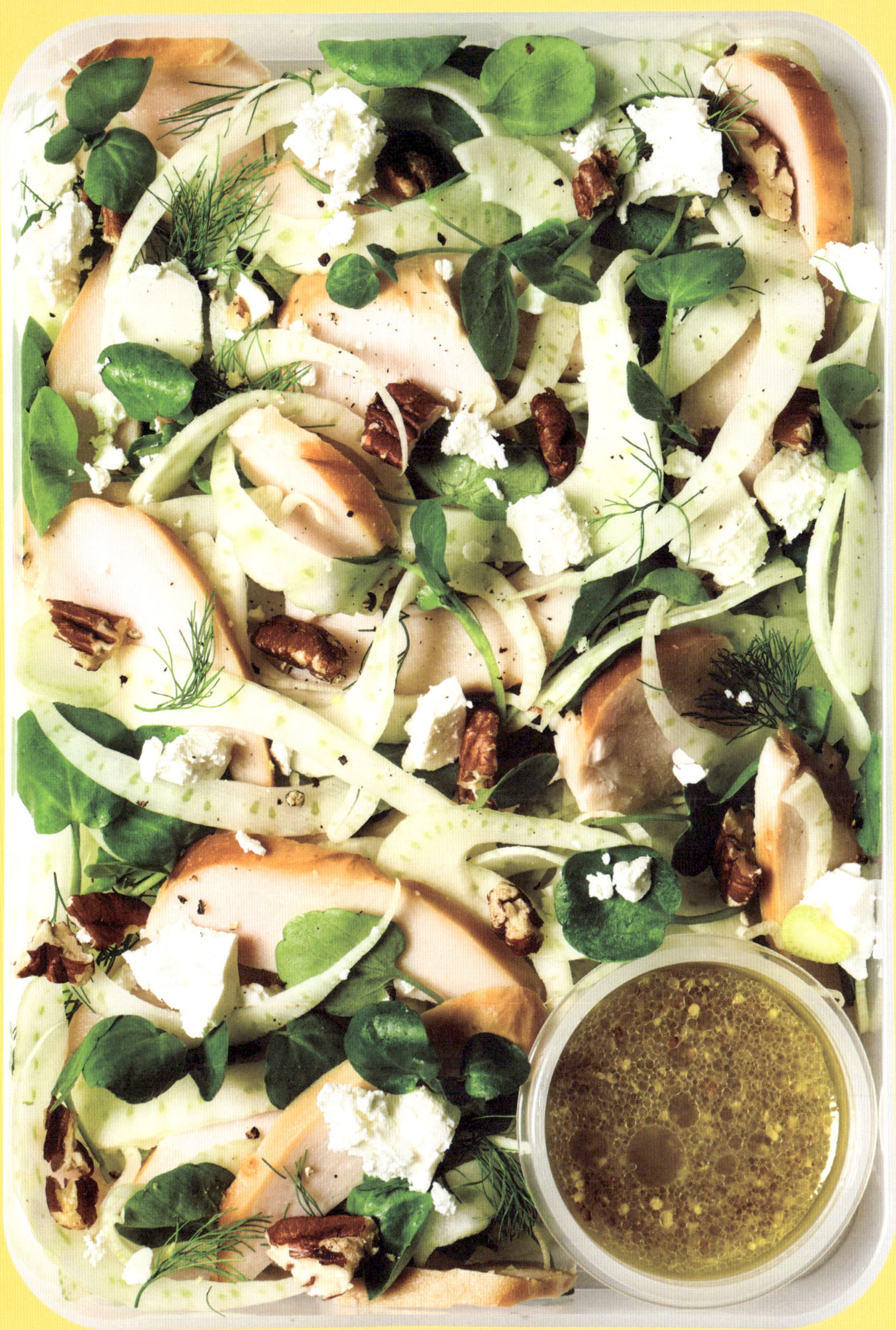

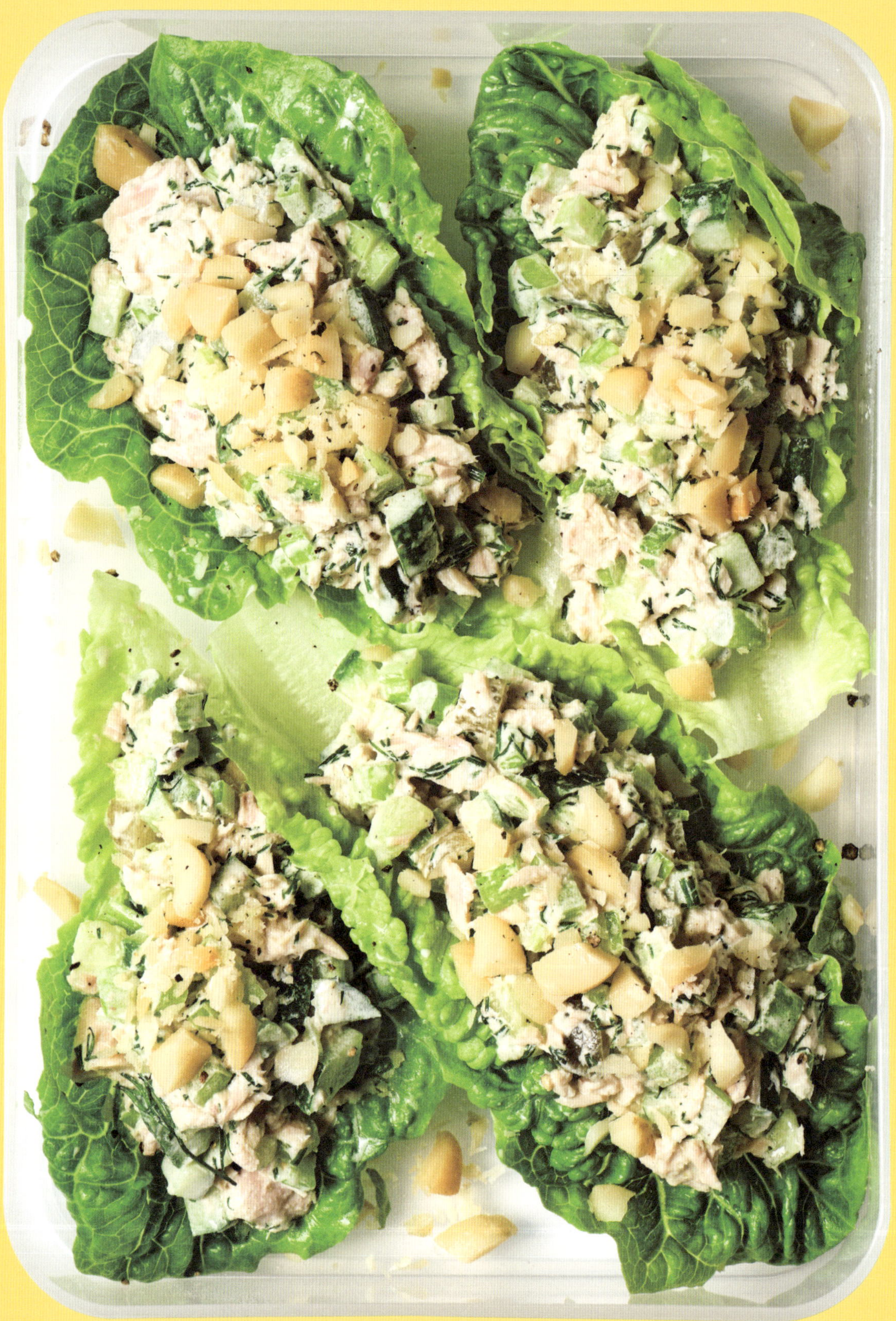

PROTEIN: 32 G   NET CARBS: 7 G   FAT: 14 G

Creamy, crunchy tuna salad

This salad shows how texture and substance can go hand in hand. Tuna and cottage cheese keep it filling, while chopped macadamias add crunch and healthy fats. Serving it in lettuce cups makes it light but satisfying.

- 100 g (3½ oz) tinned tuna in olive oil, drained
- 1 celery stalk, diced
- 60 g (⅓ cup) diced short cucumber
- 2 tablespoons blended cottage cheese (2% fat)
- 1½ teaspoons chopped dill pickle
- 1½ teaspoons chopped chives
- 1½ teaspoons chopped dill
- 2 teaspoons lemon juice
- 4 cos (romaine) lettuce leaves
- 1 tablespoon chopped toasted macadamia nuts

1. In a bowl, mix together all the ingredients except the lettuce leaves and macadamias. Season to taste with salt and pepper.
2. To serve, spoon the tuna mixture into the lettuce leaves, then scatter over the toasted macadamia nuts.

PROTEIN: 26 G NET CARBS: 6 G FAT: 36 G

Tuna & fennel salad

Tuna and fennel are a natural combination – the fish brings body, the fennel freshness and crunch. Adding almonds gives another layer of substance, proving that even a light, crisp salad can feel like a meal. Using a mandoline will give you perfectly uniform, feather-thin shavings of fennel – just be careful of your fingers!

125 g (4½ oz) tinned tuna slices in olive oil, drained

1 celery stalk, finely sliced

50 g (⅓ cup) shaved fennel, plus a few fronds

30 g (1 cup) shredded radicchio leaves

2 tablespoons toasted flaked almonds

LEMON VINAIGRETTE

1½ tablespoons extra virgin olive oil

1 tablespoon lemon juice

1. Place the salad ingredients in a bowl and toss lightly.
2. Combine the vinaigrette ingredients in a small bowl, then season to taste with salt and pepper.
3. Pour the vinaigrette over the salad just before serving and toss well to coat.

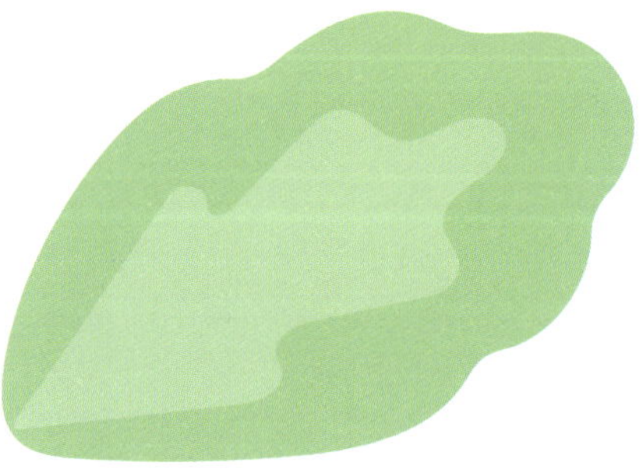

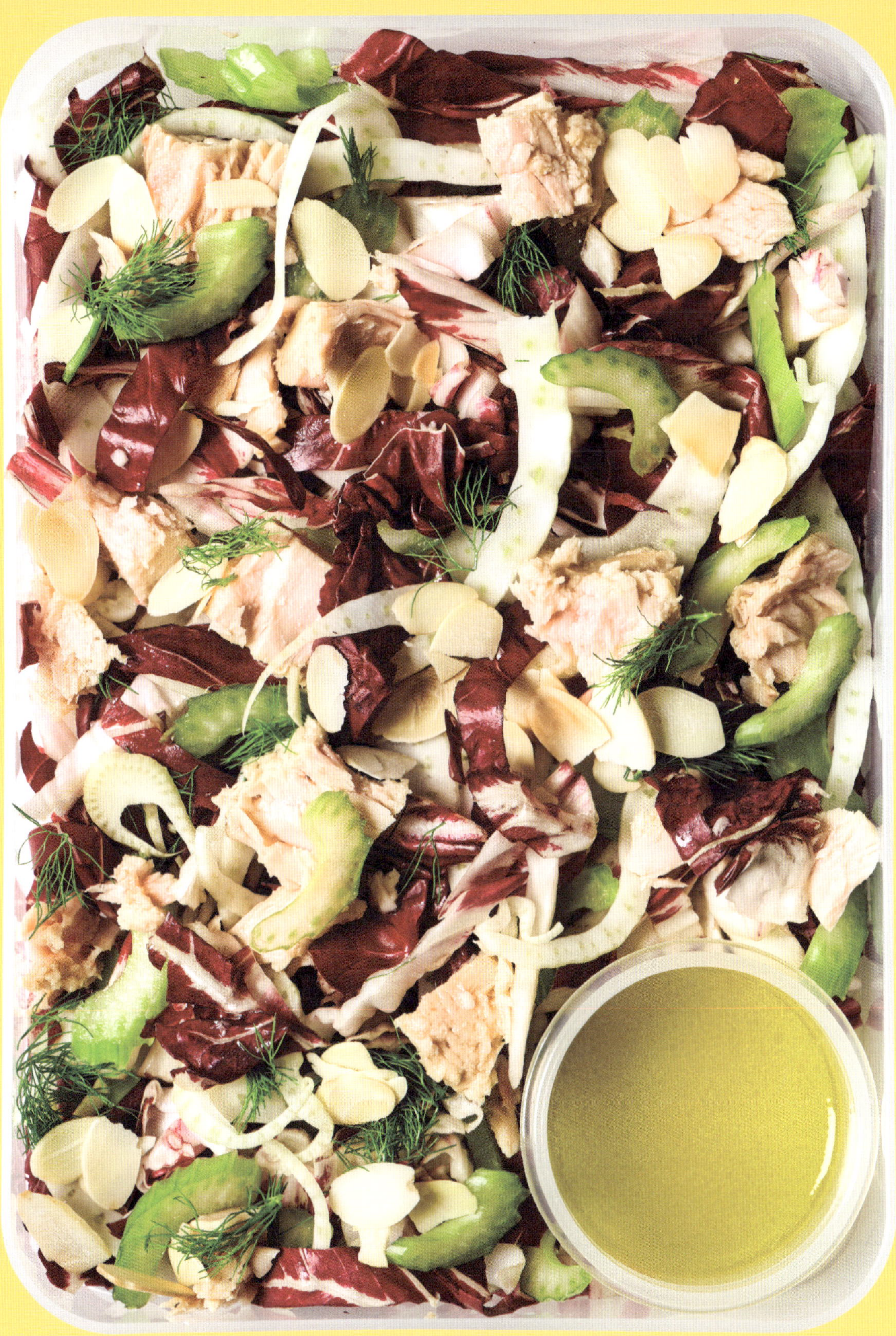

PROTEIN: 30 G NET CARBS: 10 G FAT: 37 G

Tuna poke with cauliflower rice

Swapping rice for cauliflower rice makes this poke bowl lighter but still filling. Raw tuna is the centrepiece, while avocado and sesame seeds add richness. It's a great example of how different ingredients – from seafood to vegetables – can contribute to making a dish more sustaining.

- 150 g (1½ cups) cauliflower rice
- 100 g (3½ oz) raw sashimi-grade tuna, diced
- ½ avocado, diced
- ½ short cucumber, diced
- 2 radishes, finely sliced
- 1 spring onion (scallion), sliced
- ½ teaspoon toasted sesame seeds

SPICY SRIRACHA MAYO

- 2½ tablespoons mayonnaise
- 2 teaspoons rice vinegar or lime juice
- 1 teaspoon sriracha chilli sauce

1. Place the cauliflower rice in a bowl and top with the remaining salad ingredients.
2. Combine the sriracha mayo ingredients in a small bowl.
3. Spoon the sriracha mayo over the salad just before serving and toss well to coat.

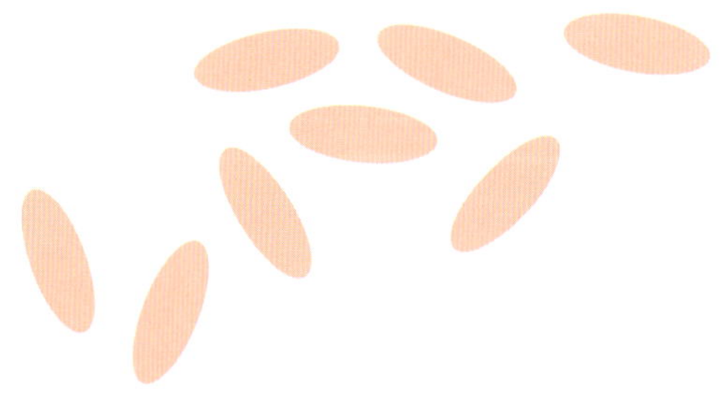

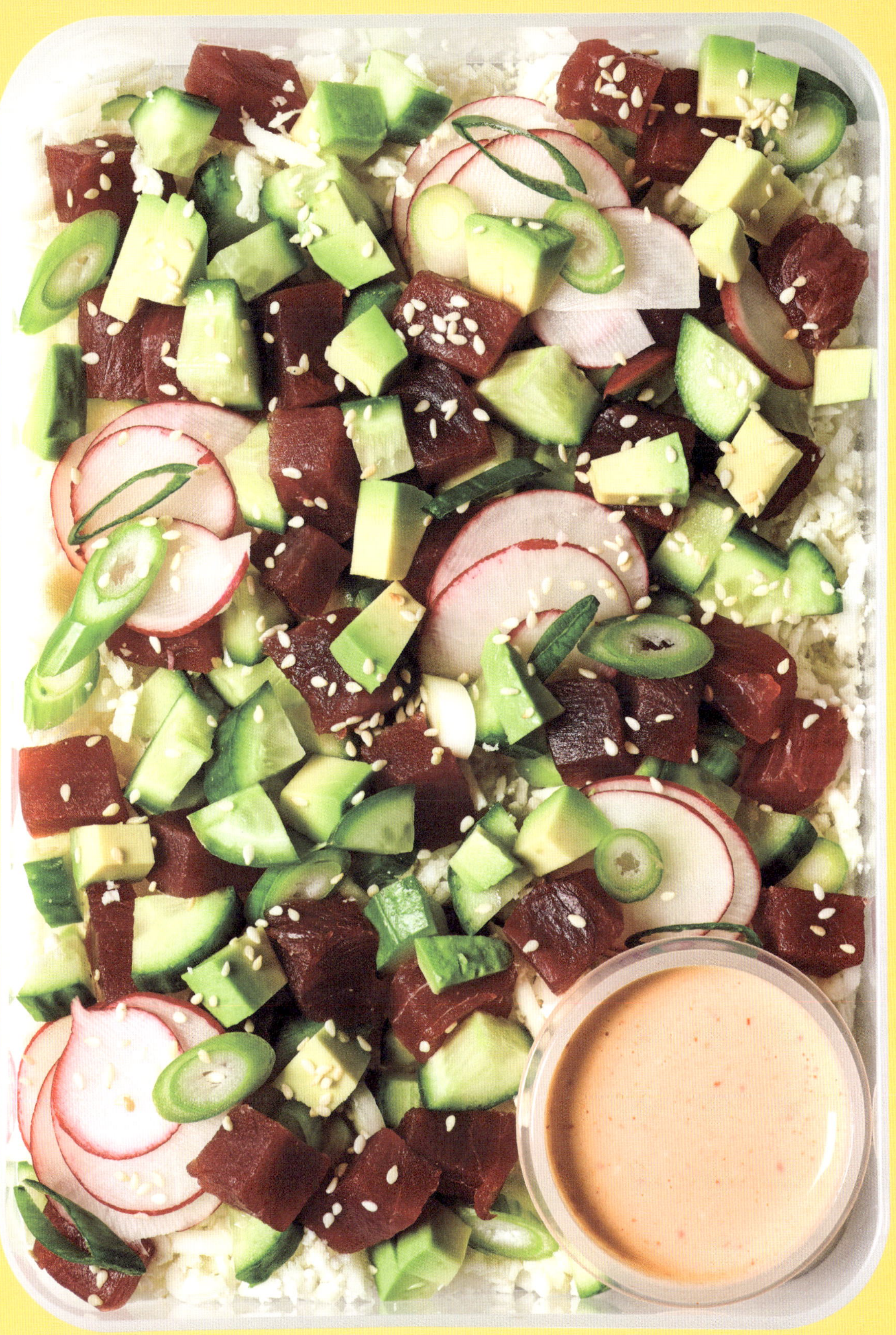

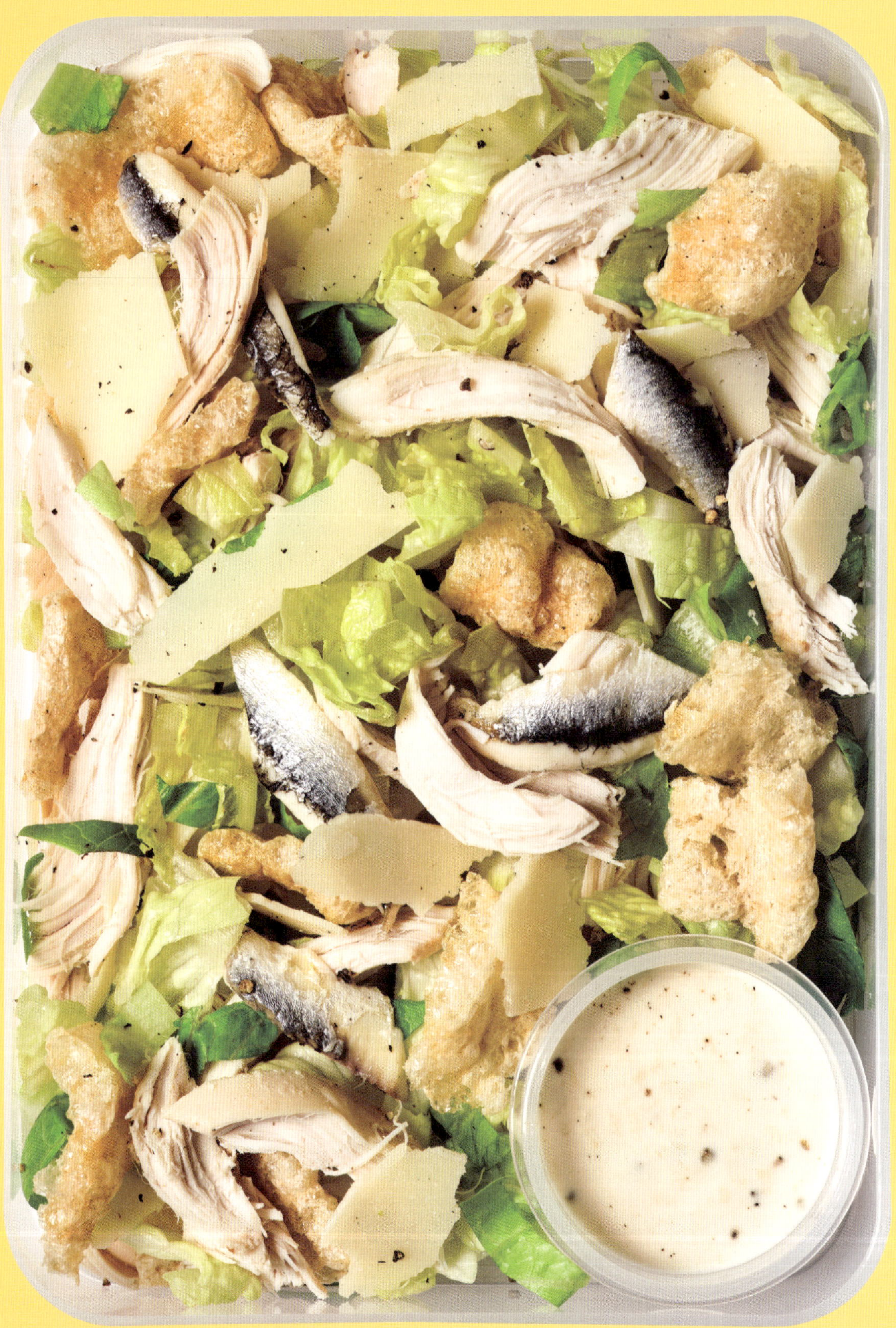

PROTEIN: 64 G NET CARBS: 6 G FAT: 24 G

Chicken Caesar salad

This version of the Caesar salad keeps all the familiar flavours but leans on chicken as the main element. Pork rinds (also called chicharrones or pork crackle) takes the place of bacon for crunch, while yoghurt in the dressing adds creaminess without heaviness.

110 g (¾ cup) shredded cooked chicken

70 g (2 cups) chopped cos (romaine) lettuce

30 g (1 oz) shaved parmesan

20 g (¾ oz) crunchy pork rinds, crumbled

2-3 white anchovy fillets in oil, drained and sliced

CREAMY CAESAR DRESSING

2 tablespoons high-protein Greek-style yoghurt

1 tablespoon finely grated parmesan

2 teaspoons lemon juice

½ teaspoon Worcestershire sauce

¼ teaspoon minced garlic

1. Place the salad ingredients in a bowl and toss lightly.
2. Combine the dressing ingredients in a small bowl, then season to taste with salt and pepper.
3. Pour the dressing over the salad just before serving and toss well to coat.

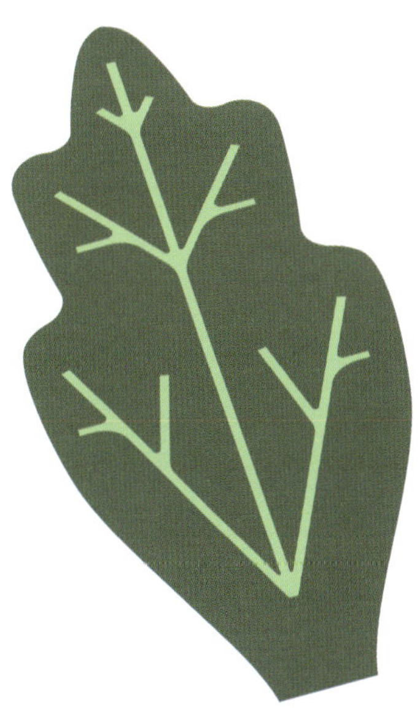

Sardine niçoise

Sardines are an underappreciated source of protein and work beautifully in place of tuna here. Paired with olives, cucumber and rocket, they bring a salty richness that makes this a sturdy salad with plenty of character. They're also full of omega-3 fatty acids, which have been linked to improved brain and heart health.

- 110 g (4 oz) tinned sardines in oil, drained
- 3 white anchovy fillets in olive oil
- ½ short cucumber, cut into chunks
- 100 g (3½ oz) cherry tomatoes, halved
- 30 g (¼ cup) pitted marinated olives
- 4 caper berries, sliced
- 20 g (⅔ cup) rocket (arugula) leaves
- lemon wedge, to serve

SIMPLE LEMON DRESSING

- 1 tablespoon extra virgin olive oil
- 2 teaspoons lemon juice

1. Place all the salad ingredients in a bowl, except the lemon wedge, and toss lightly.
2. Combine the dressing ingredients in a small bowl, then season to taste with salt and pepper.
3. Pour the dressing over the salad just before serving and toss well to coat, then squeeze over the lemon.

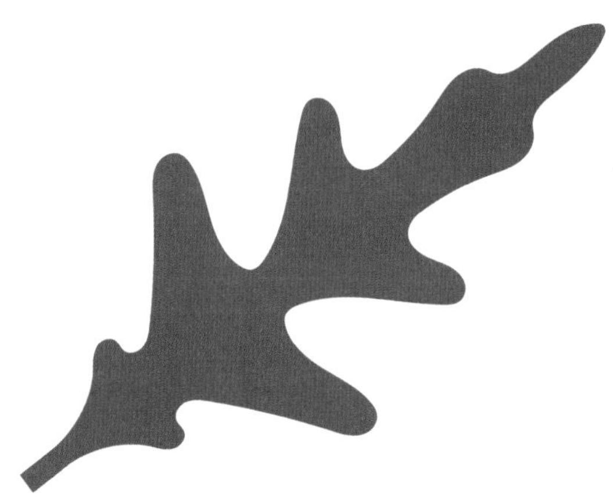

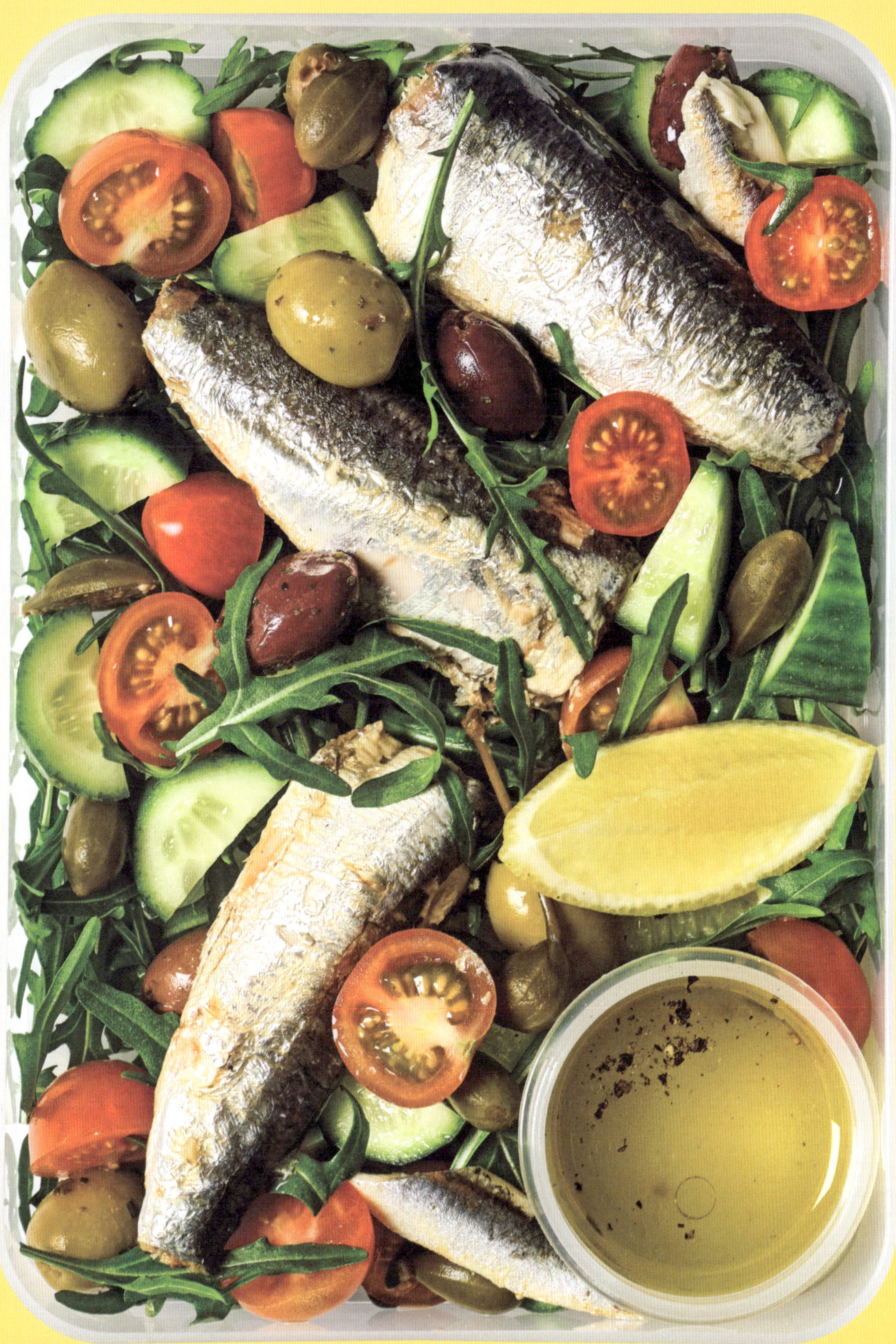

PROTEIN: 41 G NET CARBS: 7 G FAT: 37 G

Ham & cheese salad

This is basically a sandwich without the bread – ham, cheese and eggs all working together to keep this salad super filling. The lettuce and spring onion lighten it up, while the creamy dressing ties it back to its deli-counter roots. Eggs are a satisfying high-protein, low-carb addition to your salads, with two large hard-boiled eggs containing around 13 grams protein, 11 grams fat and just over 1 gram of carbs.

2 hard-boiled eggs, quartered

80 g (2¾ oz) shaved ham, sliced

50 g (⅓ cup) grated smoked mozzarella

55 g (1½ cups) chopped cos (romaine) lettuce

1 spring onion (scallion), sliced

CREAMY ITALIAN DRESSING

2 teaspoons blended cottage cheese (2% fat)

2 teaspoons extra virgin olive oil

1 teaspoon balsamic vinegar

½ teaspoon dried Italian herbs

¼ teaspoon minced garlic

1. Place the salad ingredients in a bowl and toss lightly, then season to taste with salt and pepper.
2. Combine the dressing ingredients in a small bowl.
3. Pour the dressing over the salad just before serving and toss well to coat.

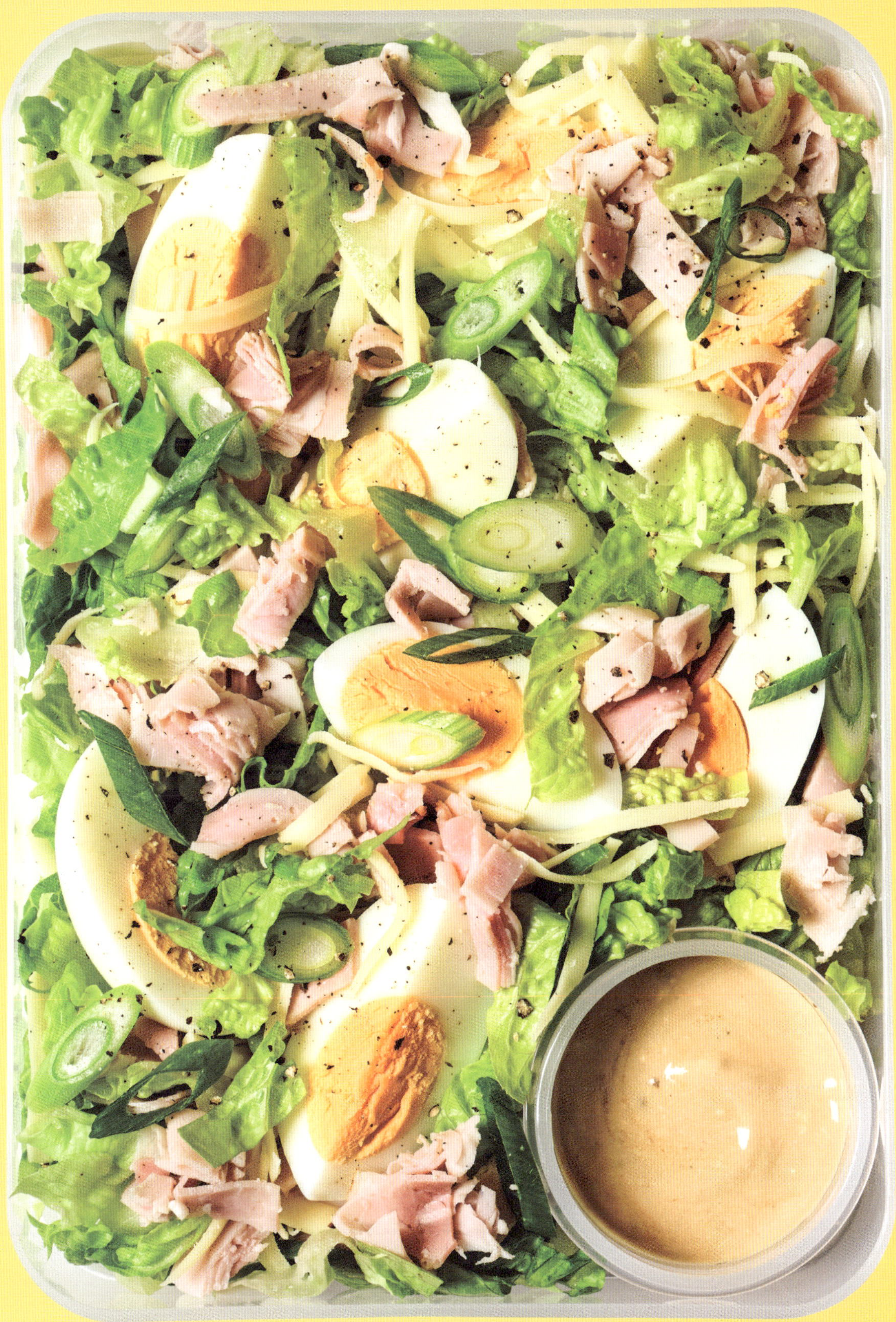

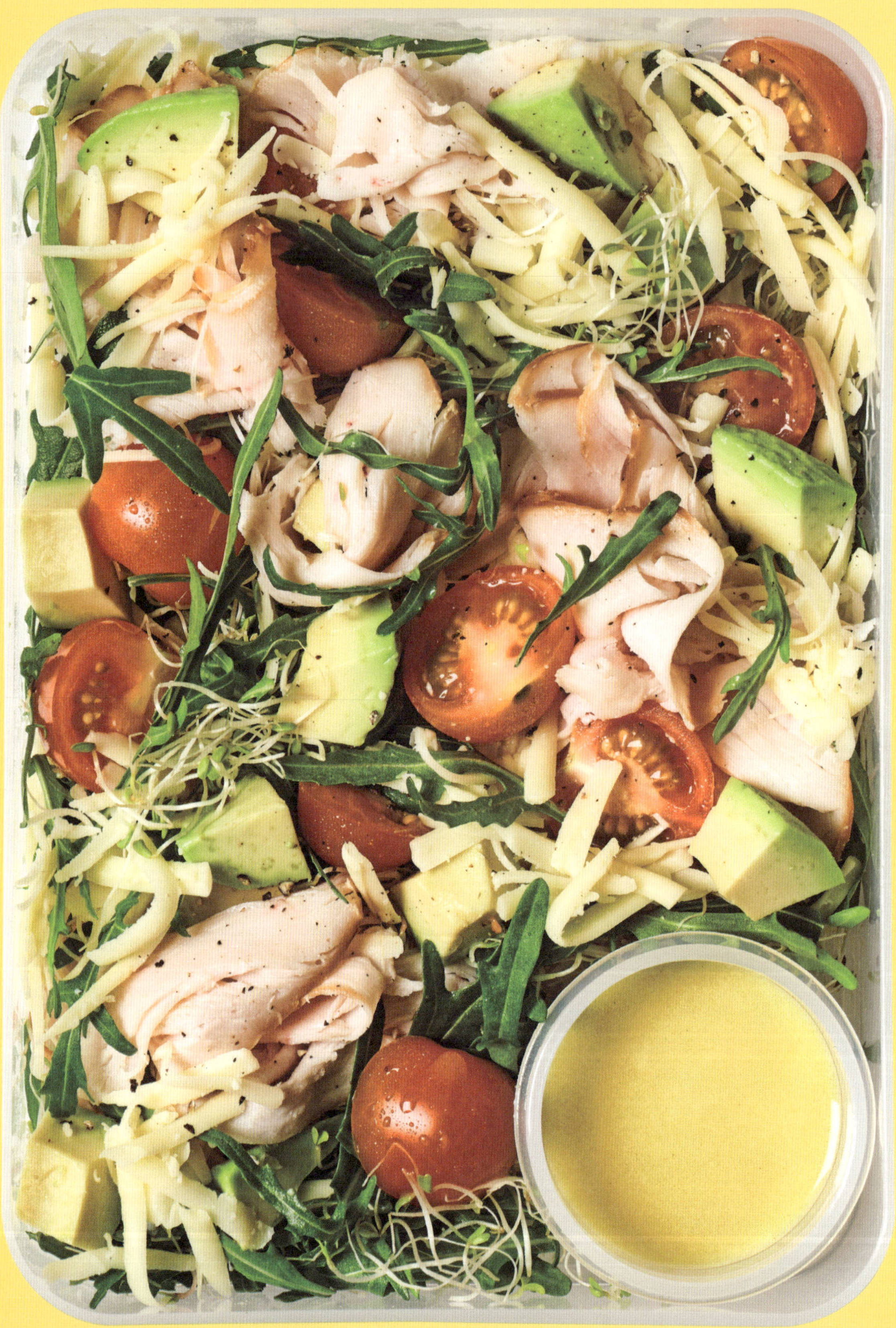

PROTEIN: 29 G NET CARBS: 7 G FAT: 38 G

Turkey salad

Turkey and Swiss cheese are the backbone of this simple salad. Adding avocado and sprouts makes it fresher and all the more satisfying. This simple salad shows that lean deli meats can still anchor a main meal.

- 80 g (2¾ oz) shaved turkey
- 50 g (1¾ oz) Swiss cheese, shredded
- ¼ avocado, diced
- 85 g (3 oz) cherry tomatoes, halved
- 30 g (1 cup) rocket (arugula) leaves
- 40 g (⅔ cup) alfalfa sprouts

DIJON & CHAMPAGNE VINEGAR DRESSING

- 1 tablespoon extra virgin olive oil
- 2 teaspoons finely diced shallot or red onion
- 2 teaspoons champagne vinegar
- 1 teaspoon dijon mustard

1. Place the salad ingredients in a bowl and toss lightly, then season to taste with salt and pepper.
2. Combine the dressing ingredients in a small bowl.
3. Pour the dressing over the salad just before serving and toss well to coat.

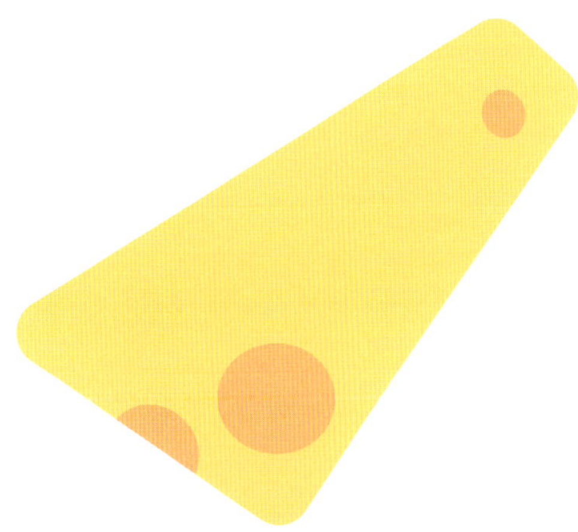

PROTEIN: 36 G   NET CARBS: 8 G   FAT: 5 G

Chicken ranch salad

The appeal of ranch dressing lies in its creaminess and herbal lift. Here, Greek-style yoghurt underpins the dressing, while chicken is the core of the meal. The addition of fresh cherry tomatoes, crisp cos lettuce and peppery radishes keeps the balance in check.

- 100 g (2/3 cup) shredded cooked chicken
- 3 radishes, sliced
- 85 g (3 oz) heirloom cherry tomatoes, halved
- 55 g (1½ cups) chopped cos (romaine) lettuce
- 40 g (¼ cup) grated carrot

RANCH DRESSING

- 2 tablespoons high-protein Greek-style yoghurt
- 1 tablespoon buttermilk
- 1 tablespoon mixed chopped herbs, such as dill, chives and parsley

1. Place the salad ingredients in a bowl and toss lightly, then season to taste with salt and pepper.
2. Combine the dressing ingredients in a small bowl.
3. Pour the dressing over the salad just before serving and toss well to coat.

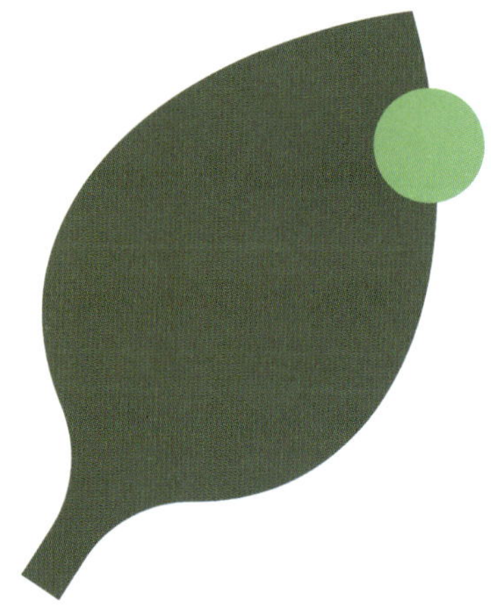

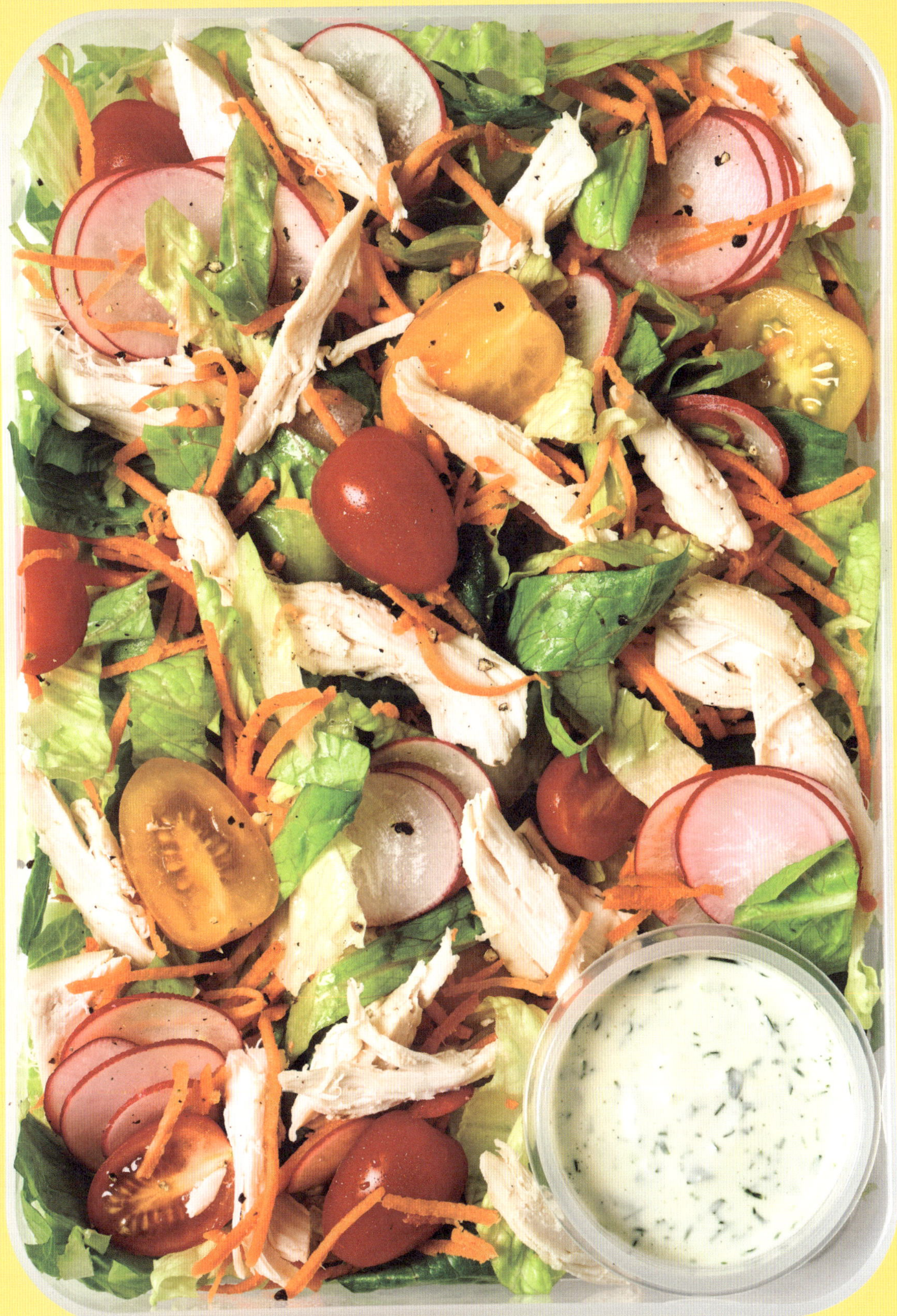

PROTEIN: 27 G NET CARBS: 7 G FAT: 19 G

Sashimi tuna salad

Sashimi-grade tuna gives this salad a luxe feel. Shirataki noodles provide texture without heaviness, and the combination of fresh herbs and nori crisps makes the salad both filling and light. Be sure to get your hands on some fresh sashimi-grade tuna from your fishmonger or seafood market for this recipe.

- 100 g (3½ oz) raw sashimi-grade tuna, finely sliced
- ½ short cucumber, halved lengthways and sliced
- 70 g (2½ oz) shirataki noodles, prepared as per packet instructions
- 3 radishes, finely sliced
- handful of Asian herbs, such as Thai basil, Vietnamese mint and coriander (cilantro)
- 4 store-bought nori seaweed crisps, sliced

GINGER DRESSING

- 1 tablespoon finely diced shallot
- 1 tablespoon tamari
- 1 tablespoon sesame oil
- 2 teaspoons rice vinegar
- 1 teaspoon minced ginger

1. Place the salad ingredients in a bowl and toss lightly.
2. Combine the dressing ingredients in a small bowl.
3. Pour the dressing over the salad just before serving and toss well to coat.

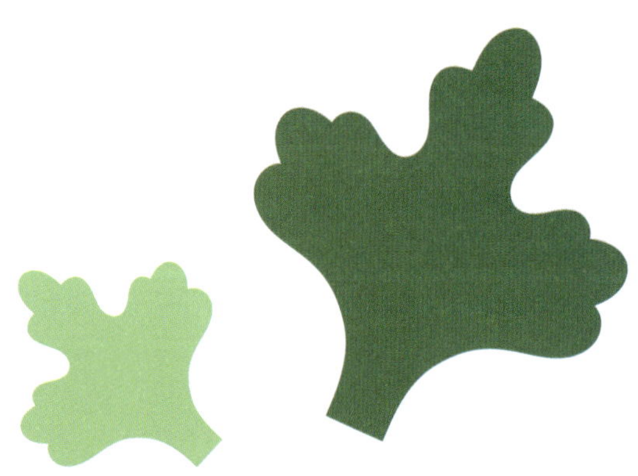

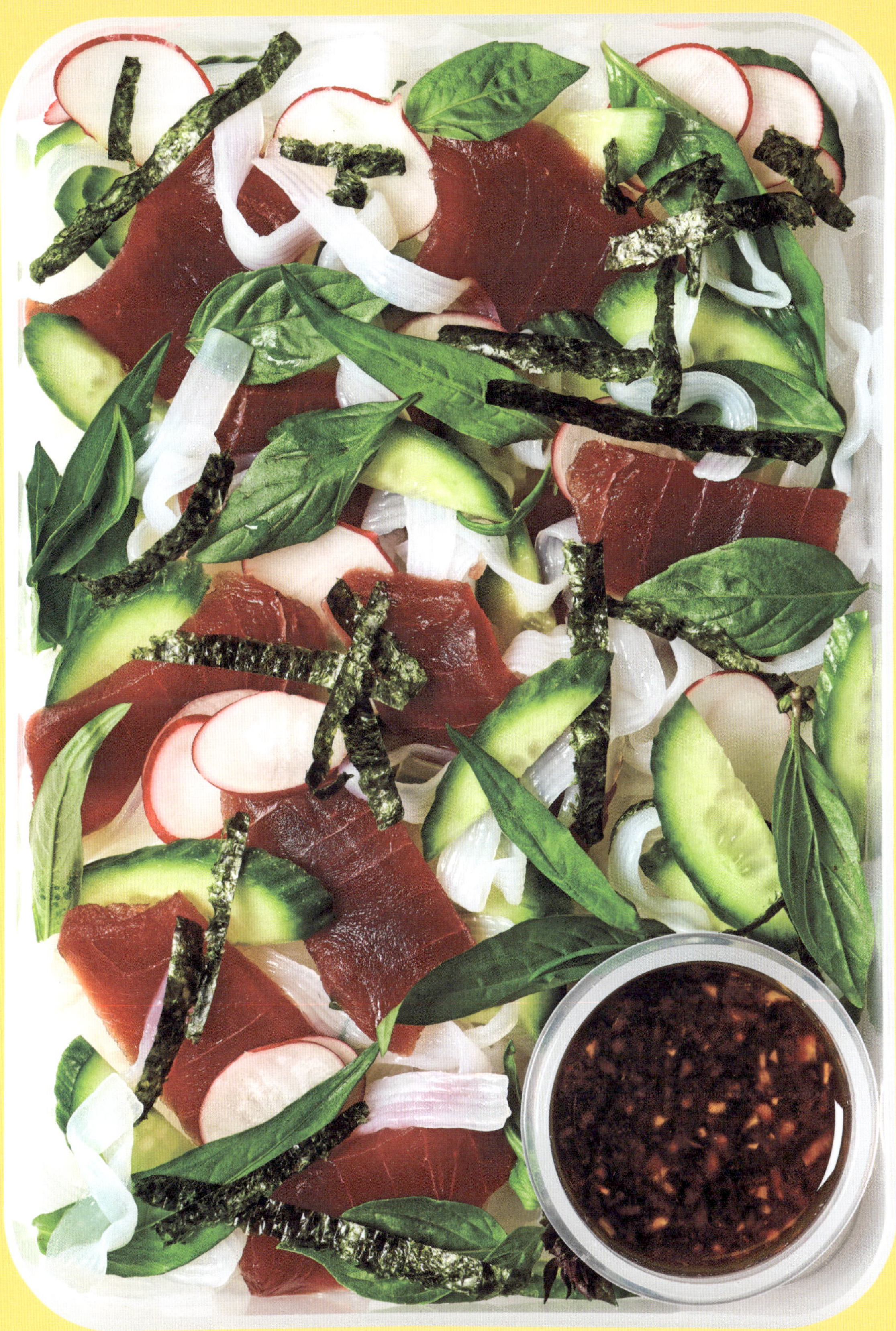

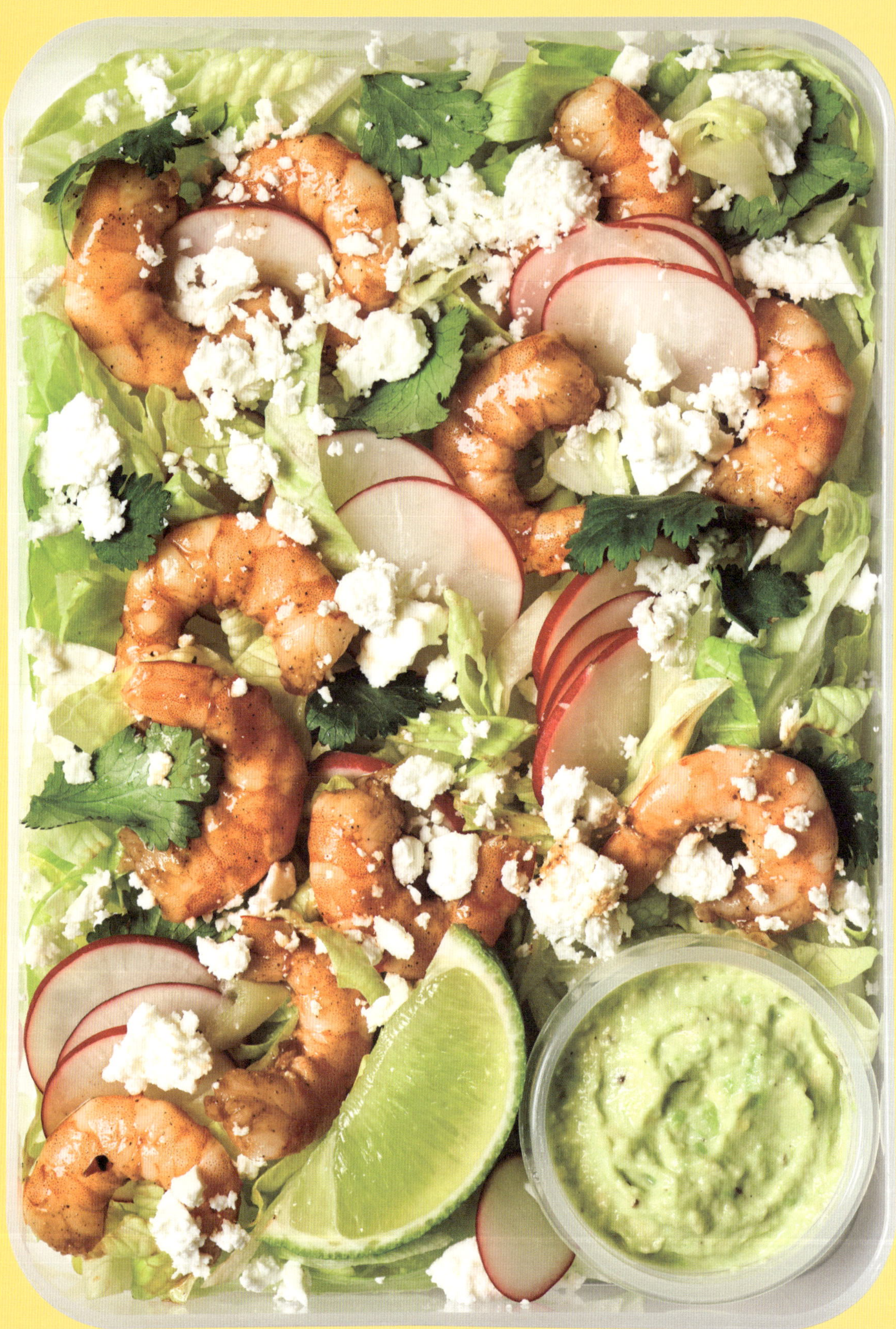

PROTEIN: 35 G NET CARBS: 8 G FAT: 14 G

Chipotle prawn salad

Prawns form the centre of this salad, dressed in smoky chipotle sauce. Queso fresco is a Mexican fresh cheese sold in some delicatessens, but if you can't find it you can just use a mild feta instead.

- 100 g (3½ oz) cooked peeled prawns (shrimp), deveined
- 1-2 teaspoons chipotle sauce, or to taste
- 3 radishes, finely sliced
- 70 g (2 cups) chopped cos (romaine) lettuce
- 45 g (1½ oz) queso fresco or mild feta, crumbled
- small handful of coriander (cilantro) leaves
- lime wedge, to serve

GUACAMOLE-LIME DRESSING

- 2 tablespoons store-bought guacamole
- 1 tablespoon lime juice
- 1 tablespoon high-protein Greek-style yoghurt

1. Place the prawns in a small bowl with the chipotle sauce and toss well to coat.
2. Place the radish, lettuce, queso fresco and coriander in a bowl and toss lightly, then top with the prawns.
3. In a small bowl, whisk the dressing ingredients until smooth.
4. Squeeze the lime wedge over the salad just before serving. Dollop the dressing over and toss well to combine.

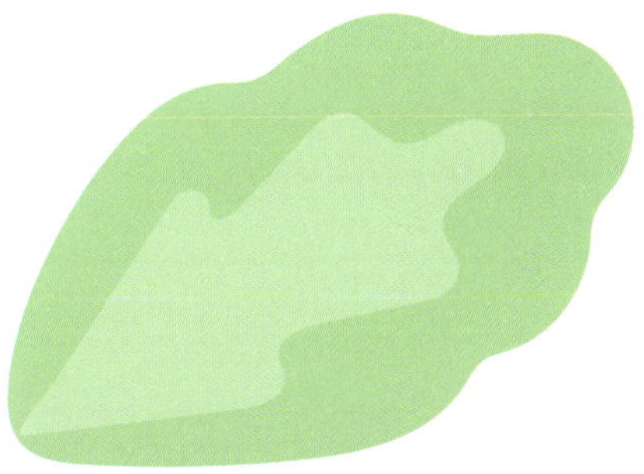

PROTEIN: 41 G NET CARBS: 8 G FAT: 26 G

Prawn asparagus salad

Pairing prawns with finely sliced asparagus delivers freshness with a firm, satisfying bite. Parmesan and almond flakes introduce a nutty note, while lemon zest lifts the whole dish. You can blanch the asparagus spears before slicing them, but they are wonderful raw – especially in peak season.

100 g (3½ oz) cooked peeled prawns (shrimp), deveined

100 g (3½ oz) raw asparagus spears, woody ends trimmed, finely sliced lengthways

50 g (1⅔ cups) watercress leaves

30 g (1 oz) shaved parmesan

1 tablespoon toasted almond flakes

pinch of lemon zest

CREAMY DIJONNAISE DRESSING

2 tablespoons dijonnaise

1 tablespoon lemon juice

1 tablespoon chopped chives

1. Place the salad ingredients in a bowl and toss lightly.
2. Combine the dressing ingredients in a small bowl, then season to taste with salt and pepper.
3. Pour the dressing over the salad just before serving and toss well to coat.

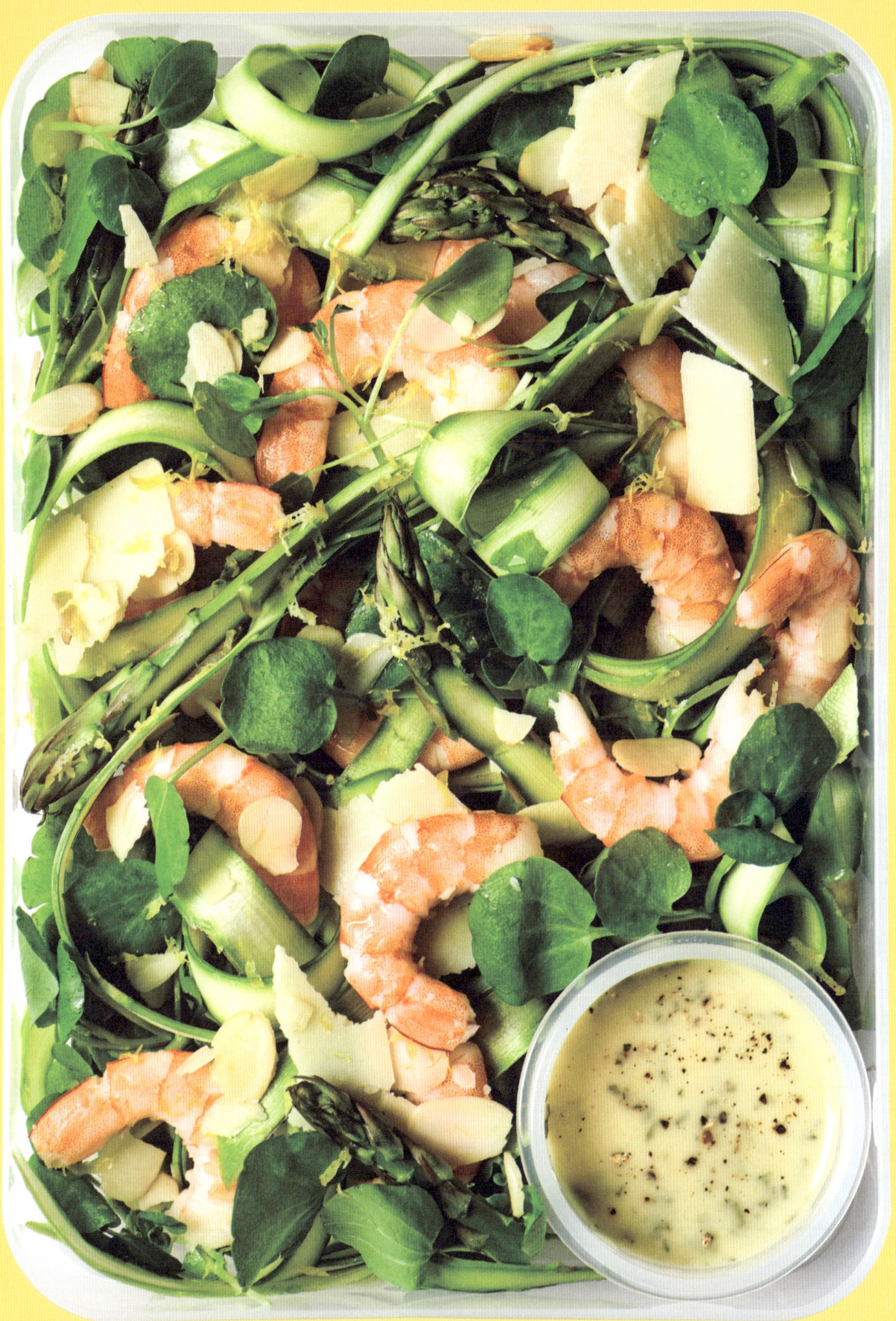

PROTEIN: 39 G NET CARBS: 9 G FAT: 38 G

Zesty Thai-style beef & shirataki salad

Roast beef brings heft to this light salad, with shirataki noodles absorbing the aromatic lime and chilli dressing, and fresh herbs and peanuts adding contrast in both flavour and texture. You can either use left-over roast beef or simply get some from your supermarket deli counter.

- 125 g (4½ oz) shirataki noodles, prepared as per packet instructions
- 125 g (4½ oz) sliced roast beef
- 75 g (1 cup) finely sliced red cabbage
- ¼ red bell pepper (capsicum), sliced
- small handful of Vietnamese mint leaves
- small handful of coriander (cilantro) leaves
- 1 tablespoon chopped roasted peanuts

LIME-CHILLI DRESSING

- 1 tablespoon toasted sesame oil
- 2 teaspoons lime juice
- pinch of lime zest
- 1 teaspoon fish sauce
- 1 teaspoon soy sauce
- ½ teaspoon chilli sambal or fresh chopped chilli

1. Place the salad ingredients in a bowl and toss lightly.
2. Combine the dressing ingredients in a small bowl.
3. Pour the dressing over the salad just before serving and toss well to coat.

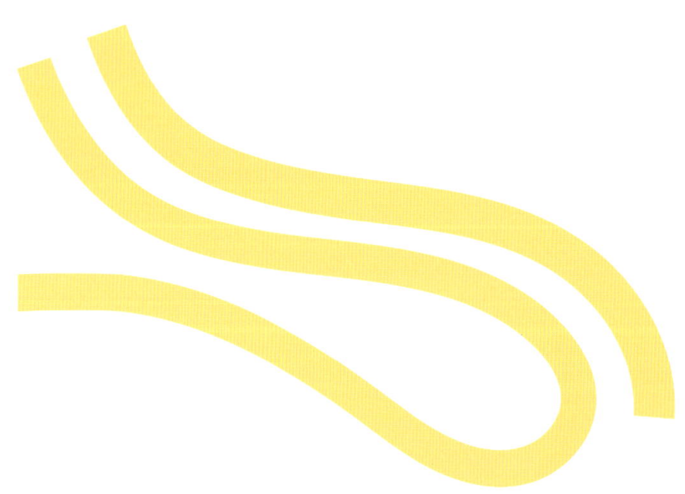

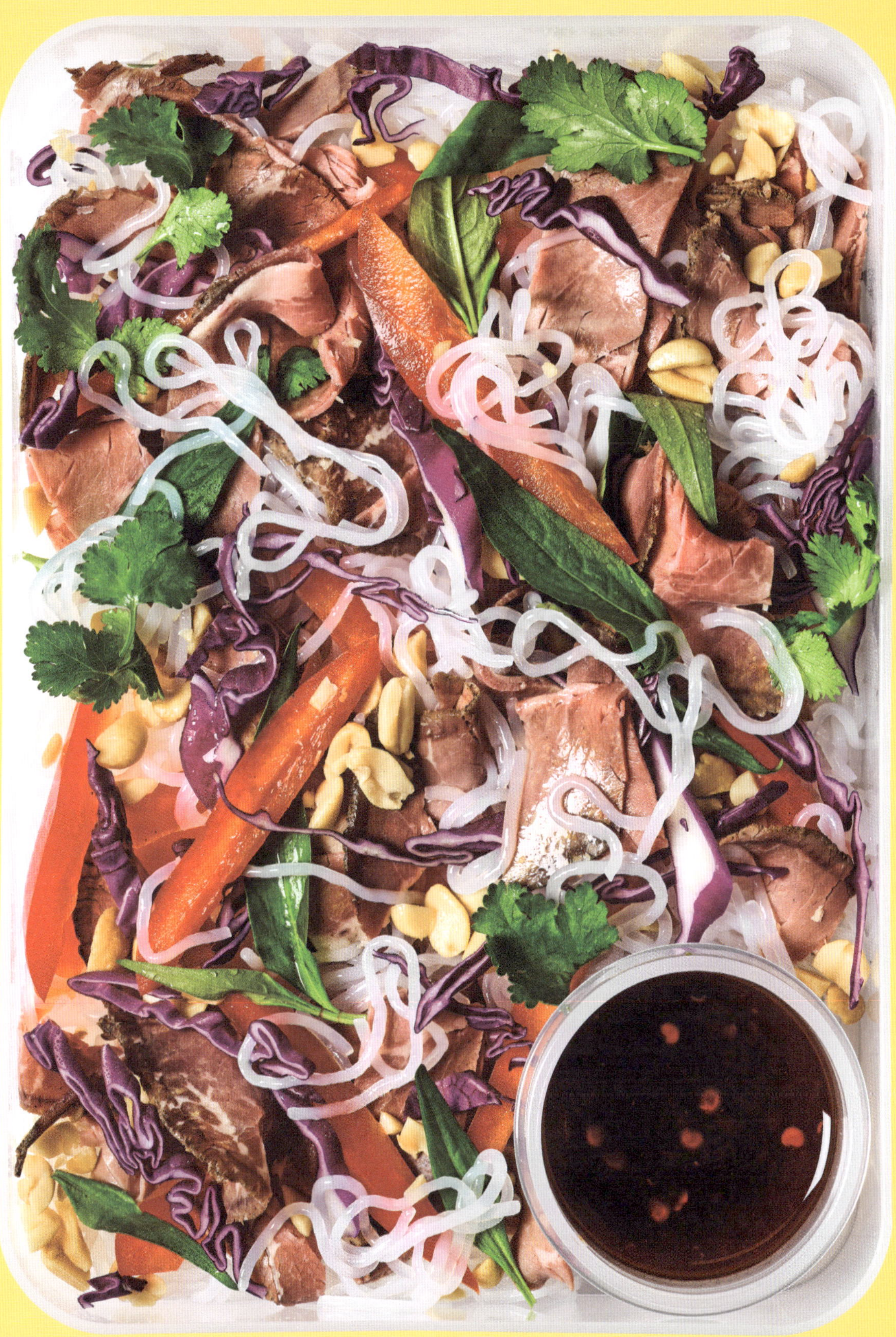

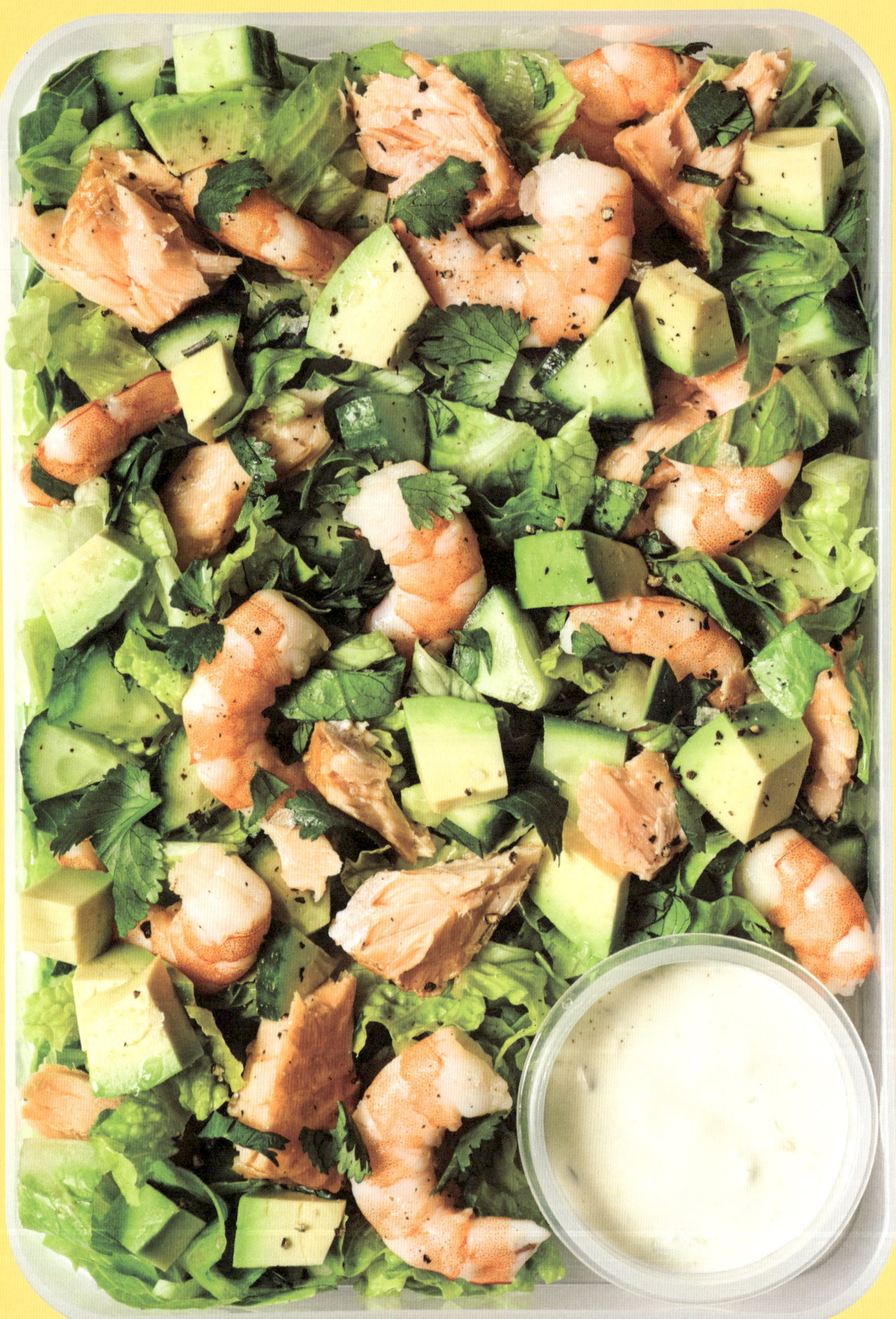

PROTEIN: 56 G NET CARBS: 8 G FAT: 20 G

Prawn & flaked salmon salad

Two seafood elements – prawns and hot-smoked salmon – make this salad particularly substantial. Avocado and cucumber add freshness, while yoghurt in the dressing keeps it creamy without being heavy. You can swap the hot-smoked salmon for left-over cooked salmon if you prefer, or omit it altogether and double the prawns.

- ½ avocado, diced
- 100 g (3½ oz) short cucumber, diced
- 120 g (2½ oz) cooked peeled prawns (shrimp), deveined
- 75 g (2¾ oz) hot-smoked salmon, flaked
- 55 g (1½ cups) chopped cos (romaine) lettuce
- 2 tablespoons chopped coriander (cilantro) leaves

CREAMY LIME-JALAPEÑO DRESSING

- 2 tablespoons high-protein Greek-style yoghurt
- 1 tablespoon lime juice
- pinch of lime zest
- 1 teaspoon chopped pickled jalapeño

1. Place the salad ingredients in a bowl and toss lightly, then season to taste with salt and pepper.
2. Combine the dressing ingredients in a small bowl.
3. Pour the dressing over the salad just before serving and toss well to coat.

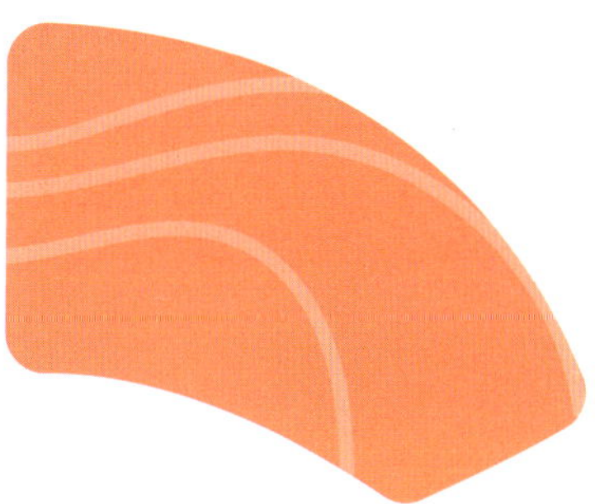

PROTEIN: 48 G NET CARBS: 8 G FAT: 37 G

Chicken caprese

The Italian caprese salad is a universal favourite for a reason, and adding some left-over roasted or poached chicken is an easy way to pump up the protein even further. Burrata is an Italian fresh cheese made from mozzarella that is filled with cream. You'll find it in most supermarkets, or it can be substituted with bocconcini.

- 2 tomatoes, sliced
- 120 g (4½ oz) cooked chicken breast, sliced
- 50 g (1¾ oz) burrata, torn
- 30 g (1 cup) mixed salad greens
- small handful of basil leaves

BALSAMIC-SHALLOT VINAIGRETTE

- 1½ tablespoons extra virgin olive oil
- 2 teaspoons red wine vinegar
- 1 teaspoon balsamic vinegar
- 1 teaspoon finely chopped shallot

1. Place the salad ingredients in a bowl and toss lightly, then season to taste with salt and pepper.
2. Combine the vinaigrette ingredients in a small bowl.
3. Pour the vinaigrette over the salad just before serving and toss well to coat.

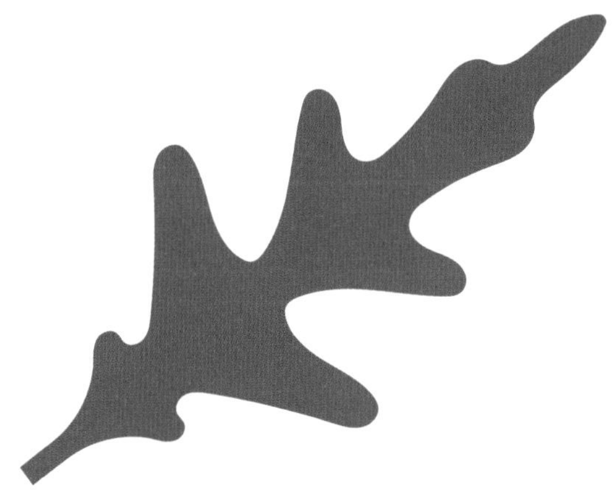

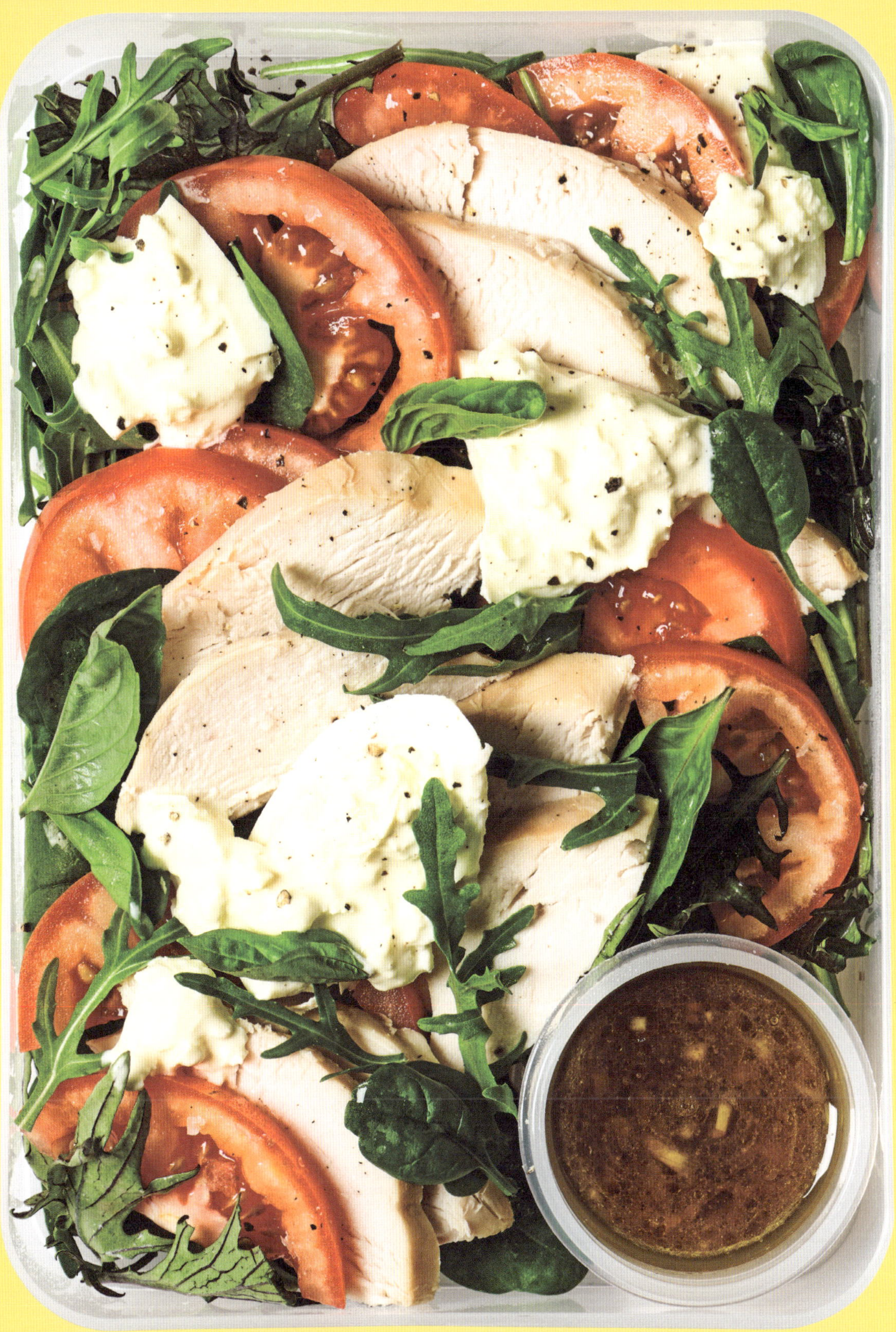

PROTEIN: 38 G NET CARBS: 4 G FAT: 10 G

Curried chicken salad

A generous pinch of curry powder transforms this chicken salad into a flavour-packed lunchtime staple. Using Greek-style yoghurt instead of mayonnaise to bind the chicken salad is a great way to increase your protein and ensure you're getting plenty of healthy fats.

- 2 tablespoons high-protein Greek-style yoghurt
- 1 teaspoon apple cider vinegar
- ½ teaspoon curry powder
- 110 g (¾ cup) shredded cooked chicken
- 1 celery stalk, sliced
- 30 g (1 cup) sliced radicchio leaves
- 1 tablespoon chopped pecans
- 1 tablespoon finely diced red onion

1. In a bowl, whisk together the yoghurt, vinegar and curry powder.
2. Add the chicken, toss to coat and season to taste with salt and pepper.
3. To serve, place the remaining ingredients in a bowl, toss lightly and top with the curried chicken.

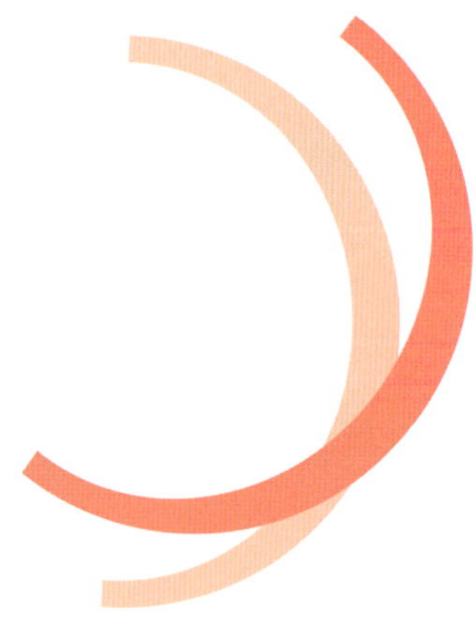

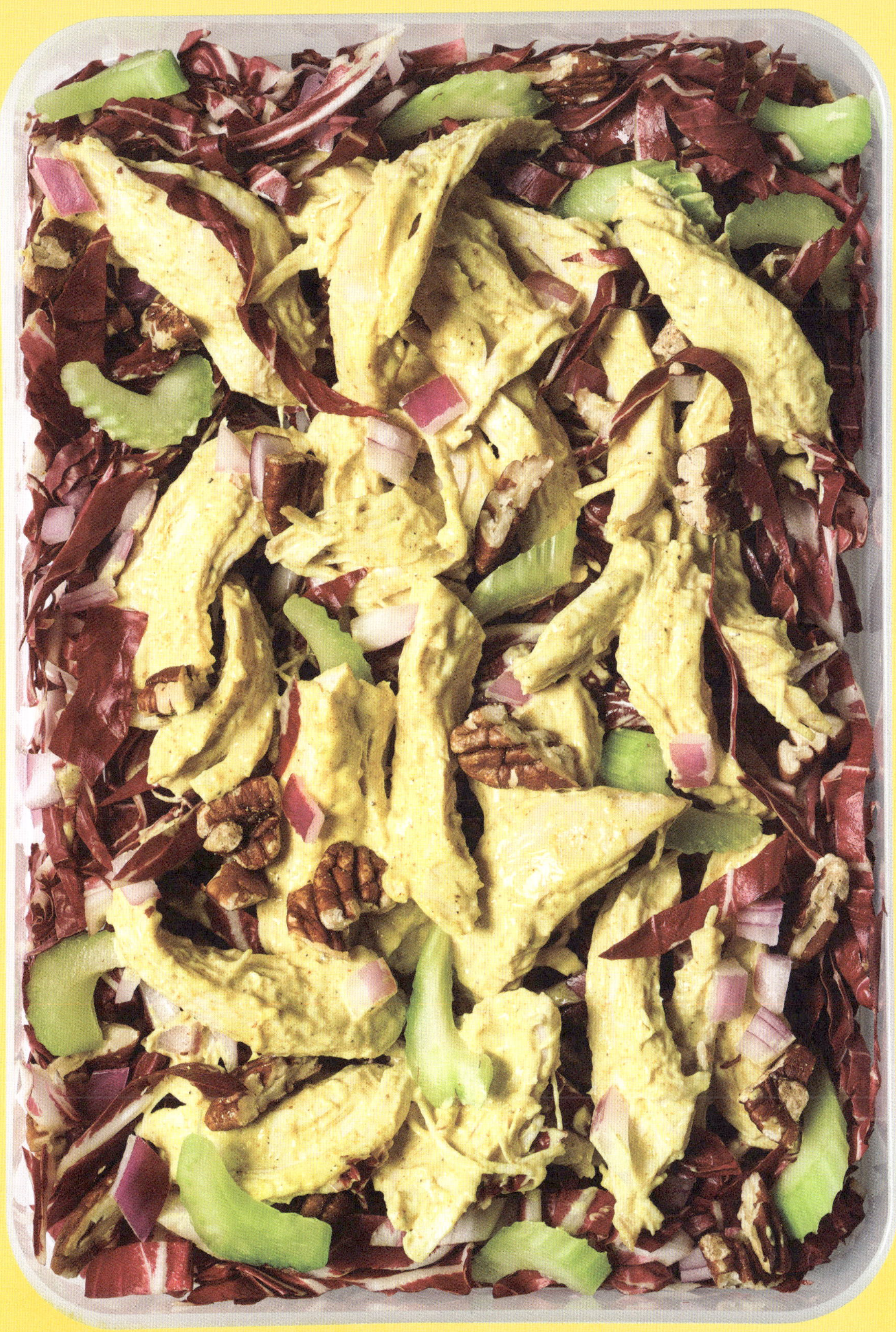

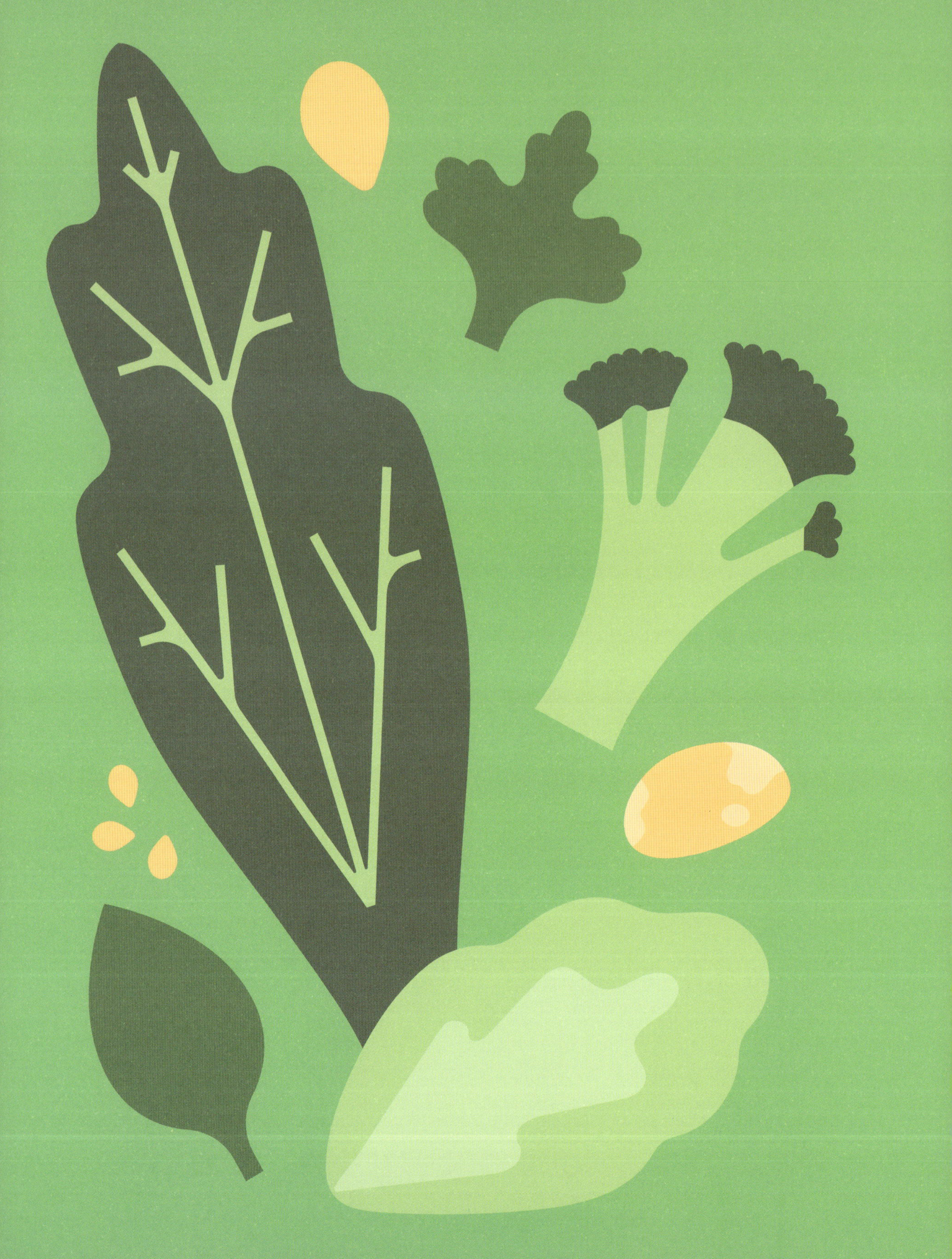

leafy &

loaded

PROTEIN: 38 G NET CARBS: 29 G FAT: 14 G

Vietnamese-style chicken coleslaw

This dish is a good example of how adding a modest amount of meat to a generous base of vegetables creates a meal that feels both light and satisfying.

- 100 g (⅔ cup) shredded cooked chicken
- 60 g (2 oz) shredded carrot
- 75 g (1 cup) shredded white cabbage
- 40 g (1½ oz) bean sprouts
- small handful of mint leaves, chopped
- small handful of coriander (cilantro) leaves, chopped
- 1 tablespoon chopped roasted peanuts
- 1 tablespoon crispy-fried shallots

NUOC CHAM DRESSING

- 1 tablespoon fish sauce
- 1½ tablespoons lime juice
- 2 teaspoons rice vinegar
- 1 teaspoon caster (superfine) sugar
- ½ red bird's eye chilli, deseeded and finely sliced
- ½ teaspoon minced garlic

1. Place the salad ingredients in a bowl, except the peanuts and fried shallots, and toss lightly.
2. Combine the dressing ingredients in a small bowl.
3. Pour the dressing over the salad just before serving and toss through the peanuts and fried shallots.

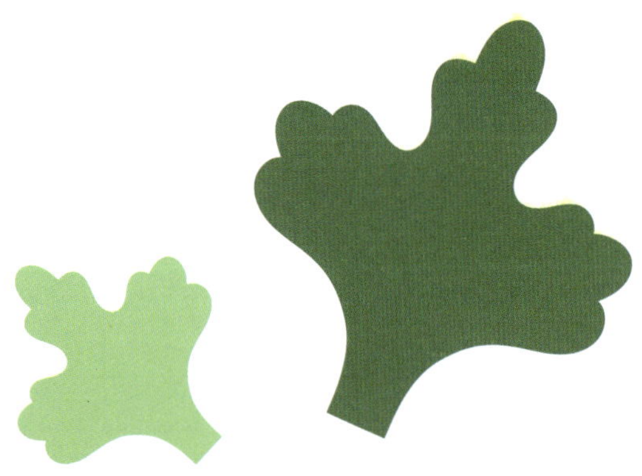

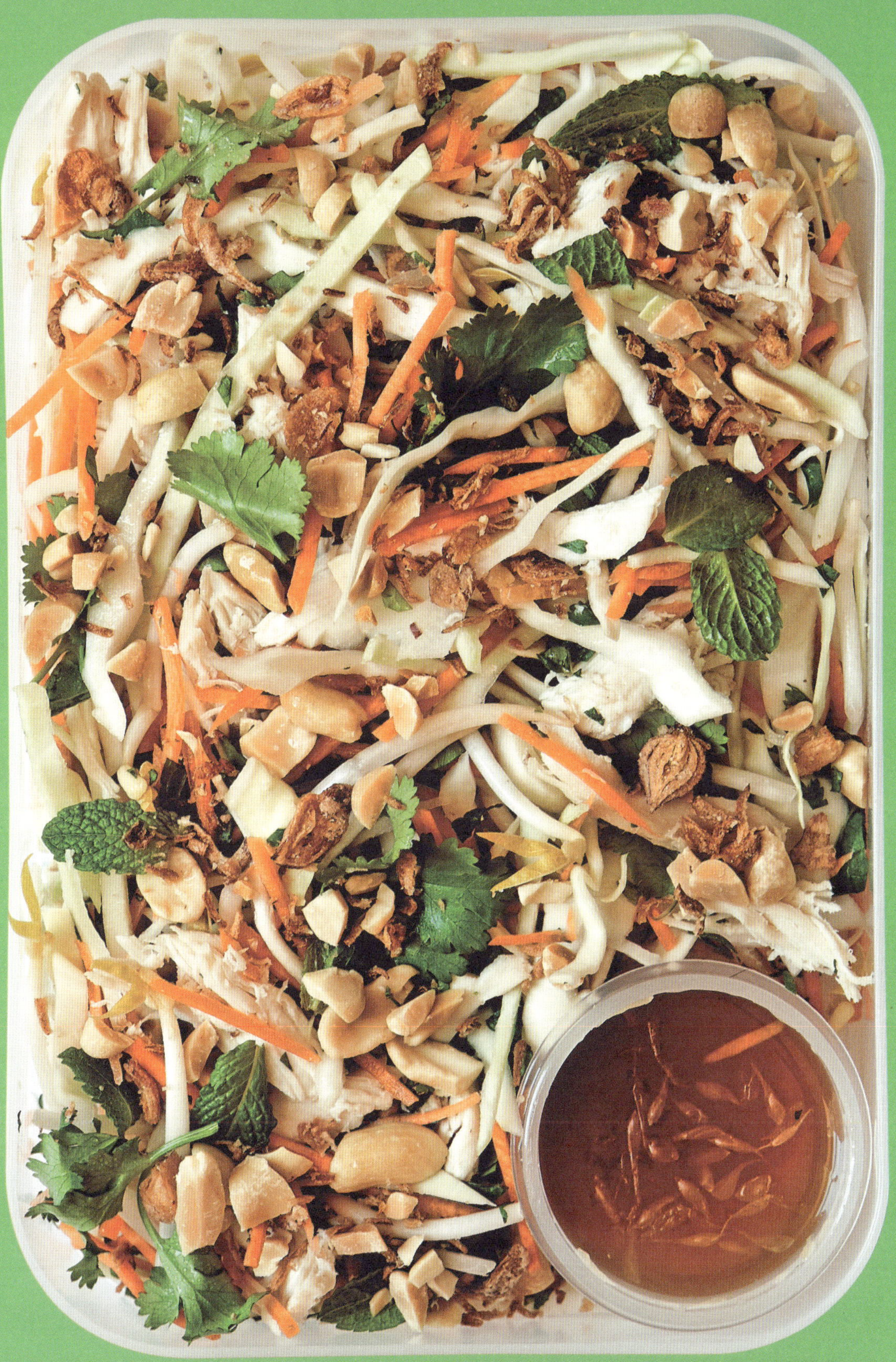

PROTEIN: 25 G NET CARBS: 73 G FAT: 32 G

Tuna, cannellini bean, goji berry & kale salad

Tuna and cannellini beans combine to give this salad a satiating base. Goji berries bring sweetness, while parmesan and kale respectively add a savoury and leafy counterpoint. Use baby kale for this recipe, as the larger leaves can be a little tough and bitter to eat raw. If unavailable, you can substitute your favourite green leafy vegetable, such as spinach leaves.

- 100 g (3½ oz) tinned cannellini beans, drained and rinsed
- 95 g (3¼ oz) tinned tuna in oil, drained
- 3 tablespoons goji berries
- 2 tablespoons grated parmesan
- 50 g (1¼ cups) baby kale leaves

CIDER VINEGAR DRESSING

- 1½ tablespoons apple cider vinegar
- ½ teaspoon dijon mustard
- ½ teaspoon honey
- 2 tablespoons extra virgin olive oil

1. Place the salad ingredients in a bowl and toss lightly, then season to taste with salt and pepper.
2. Combine the dressing ingredients in a small bowl.
3. Pour the dressing over the salad just before serving and toss well to coat.

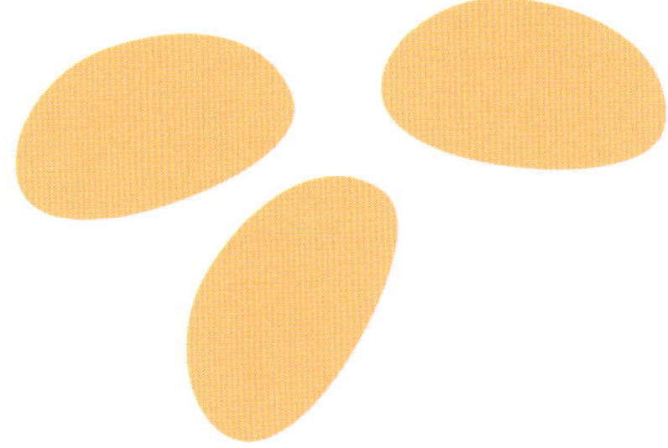

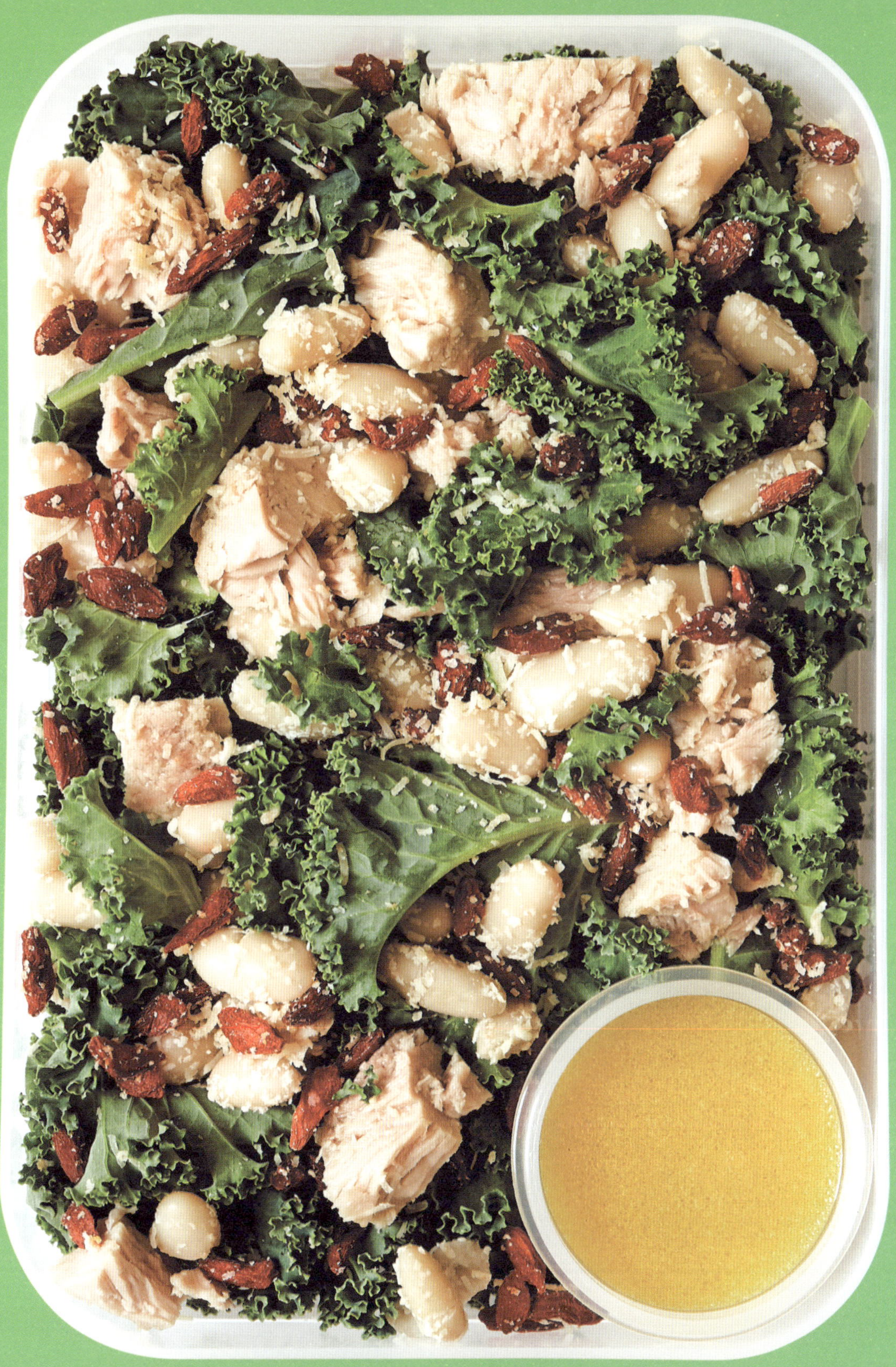

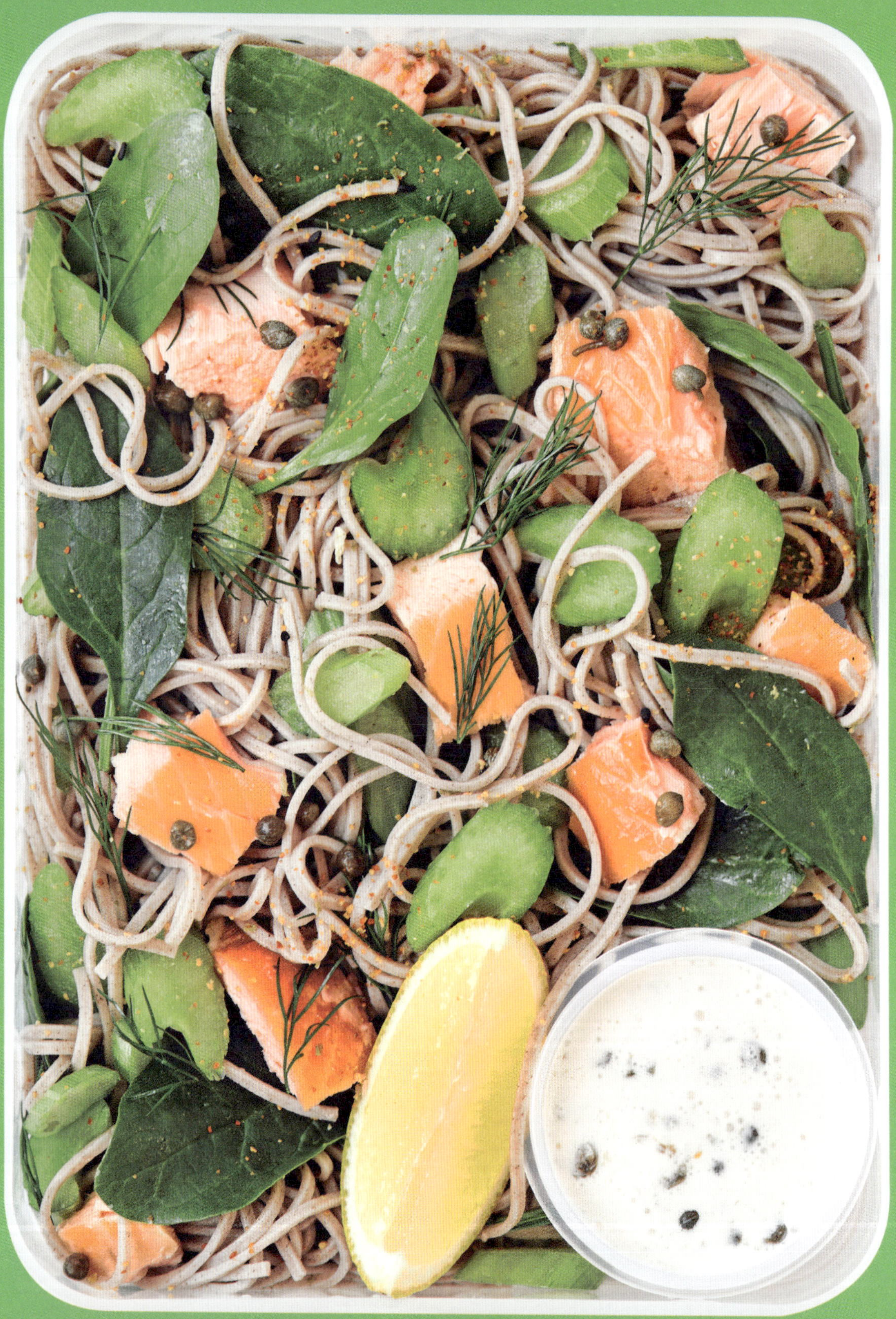

PROTEIN: 33 G NET CARBS: 37 G FAT: 6 G

Soba noodles with salmon, capers, spinach & dill

Hot-smoked salmon is such a decadent protein hero in this salad. Capers and dill provide sharpness, and the yoghurt–horseradish dressing adds creaminess with a spike of heat. The soba noodles ensure it feels like a meal in its own right.

180 g (6½ oz) cooked soba noodles, prepared as per packet instructions

100 g (3½ oz) hot-smoked salmon, flaked

1 small celery stalk, sliced

1 tablespoon chopped dill

2 teaspoons baby capers

30 g (⅔ cup) baby spinach leaves

sprinkle of shichimi togarashi (Japanese seven-flavour seasoning)

lemon wedge, to serve

CREAMY HORSERADISH DRESSING

3 tablespoons high-protein Greek-style yoghurt

2 teaspoons lemon juice

1½ teaspoons prepared horseradish

1 teaspoon baby capers, chopped

1. Toss the salad ingredients together in a bowl and season with salt and pepper to taste.
2. Combine the dressing ingredients in a small bowl.
3. Pour the dressing over the salad just before serving and toss well.

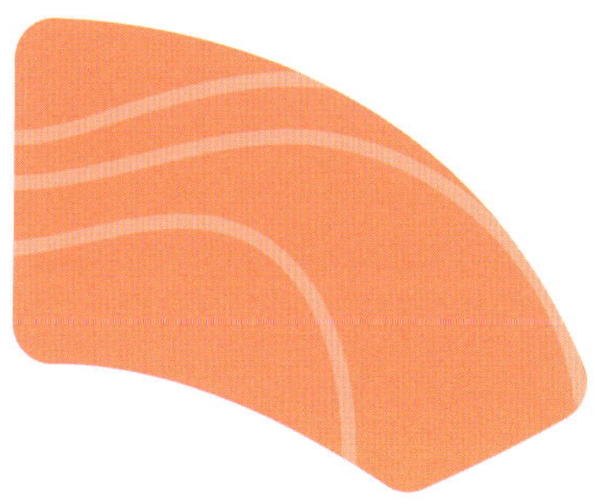

PROTEIN: 39 G   NET CARBS: 38 G   FAT: 37 G

Salmoriglio soba noodles with tuna & fennel

Here, tuna is tossed through noodles with fennel, olives and rocket, and brought together with a zesty salmoriglio dressing – a southern Mediterranean sauce that is most often served with fish. The combination of fish and beans or pulses is very common in Mediterranean cultures – this recipe shows how well it works in a salad.

- 180 g (6½ oz) cooked soba noodles, prepared as per packet instructions
- 95 g (3¼ oz) tinned tuna in olive oil, drained
- ½ baby fennel bulb, finely sliced, plus some fennel fronds
- 40 g (⅓ cup) pitted green olives
- 30 g (1 cup) rocket (arugula) leaves
- 2 teaspoons baby capers

SALMORIGLIO DRESSING

- 5 teaspoons extra virgin olive oil
- 1 tablespoon lemon juice
- ½ teaspoon lemon zest
- ½ teaspoon chopped parsley
- ½ teaspoon chopped oregano
- ½ small garlic clove, minced

1. Place the salad ingredients in a bowl and toss lightly.
2. Combine the dressing ingredients in a small bowl.
3. Pour the dressing over the salad just before serving and toss well to coat.

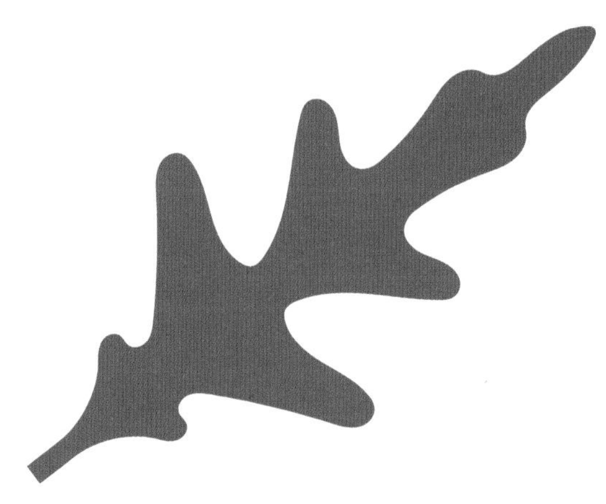

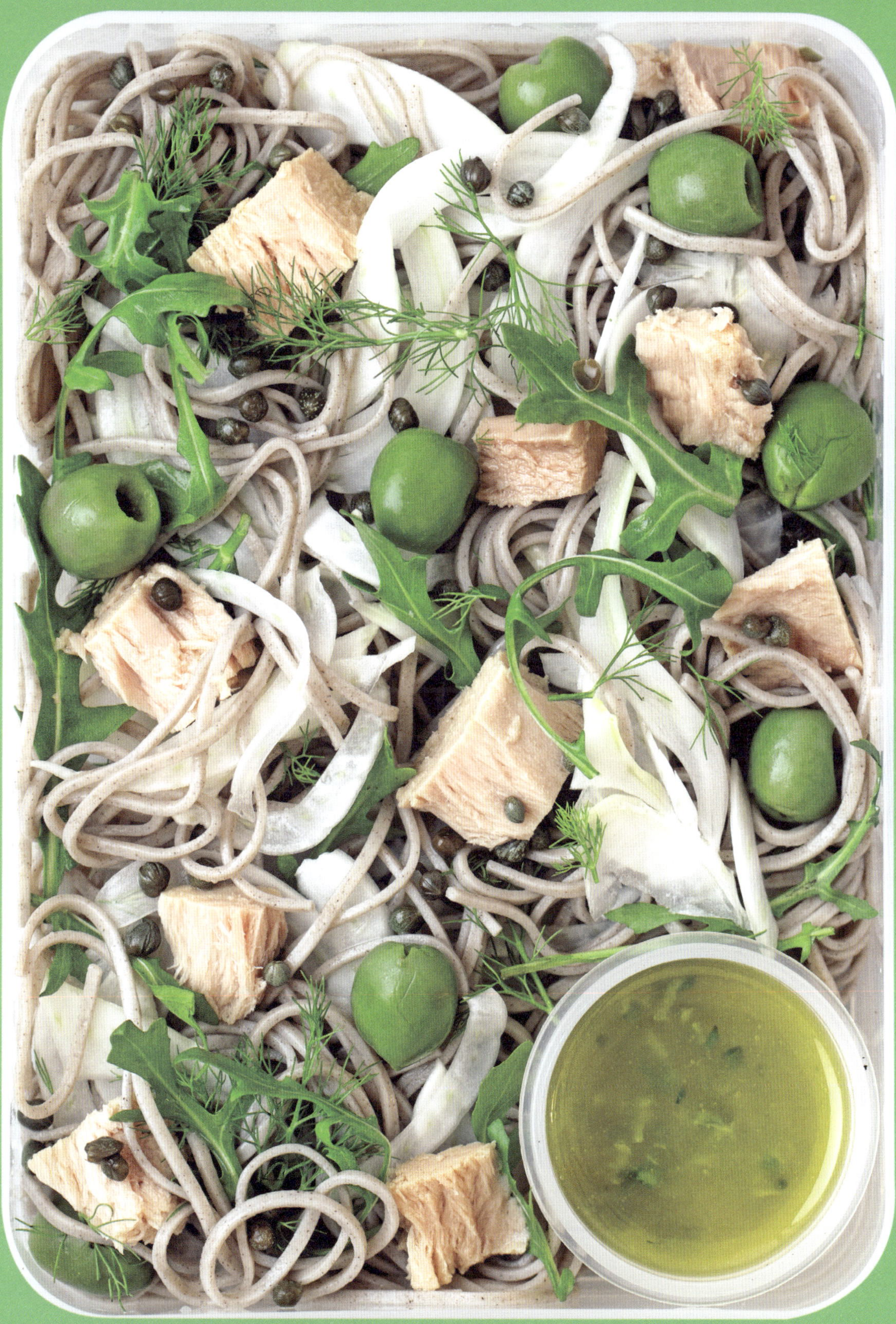

PROTEIN: 51 G NET CARBS: 43 G FAT: 55 G

Chicken, ramen, kale & orange salad

This delicious salad combines noodles, chicken and kale with orange slices – for an unexpected sweet touch! An orange, honey and ginger dressing balances it out alongside a sprinkling of nuts and seeds. If you like, swap the kale for rocket (arugula) or baby spinach leaves.

- 180 g (6½ oz) cooked ramen noodles, prepared as per packet instructions
- 100 g (⅔ cup) shredded cooked chicken
- 30 g (⅔ cup) finely shredded kale
- 1 orange, peeled and segmented
- 35 g (¼ cup) roasted hazelnuts
- 30 g (¼ cup) pumpkin seeds

ORANGE, HONEY & GINGER DRESSING

- 1 tablespoon orange juice
- 2 teaspoons extra virgin olive oil
- 1½ teaspoons balsamic vinegar
- ½ teaspoon honey
- 1 teaspoon minced ginger

1. Place the salad ingredients in a bowl and toss lightly.
2. Combine the dressing ingredients in a small bowl, then season to taste with salt and pepper.
3. Pour the dressing over the salad just before serving and toss well to coat.

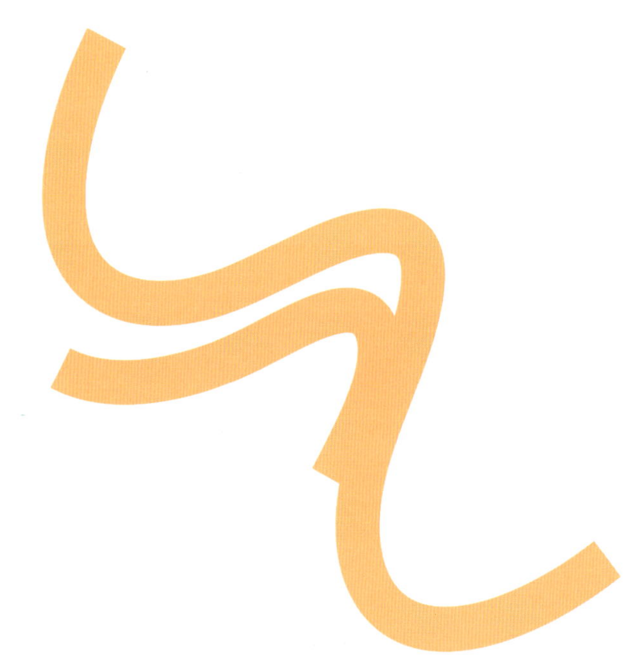

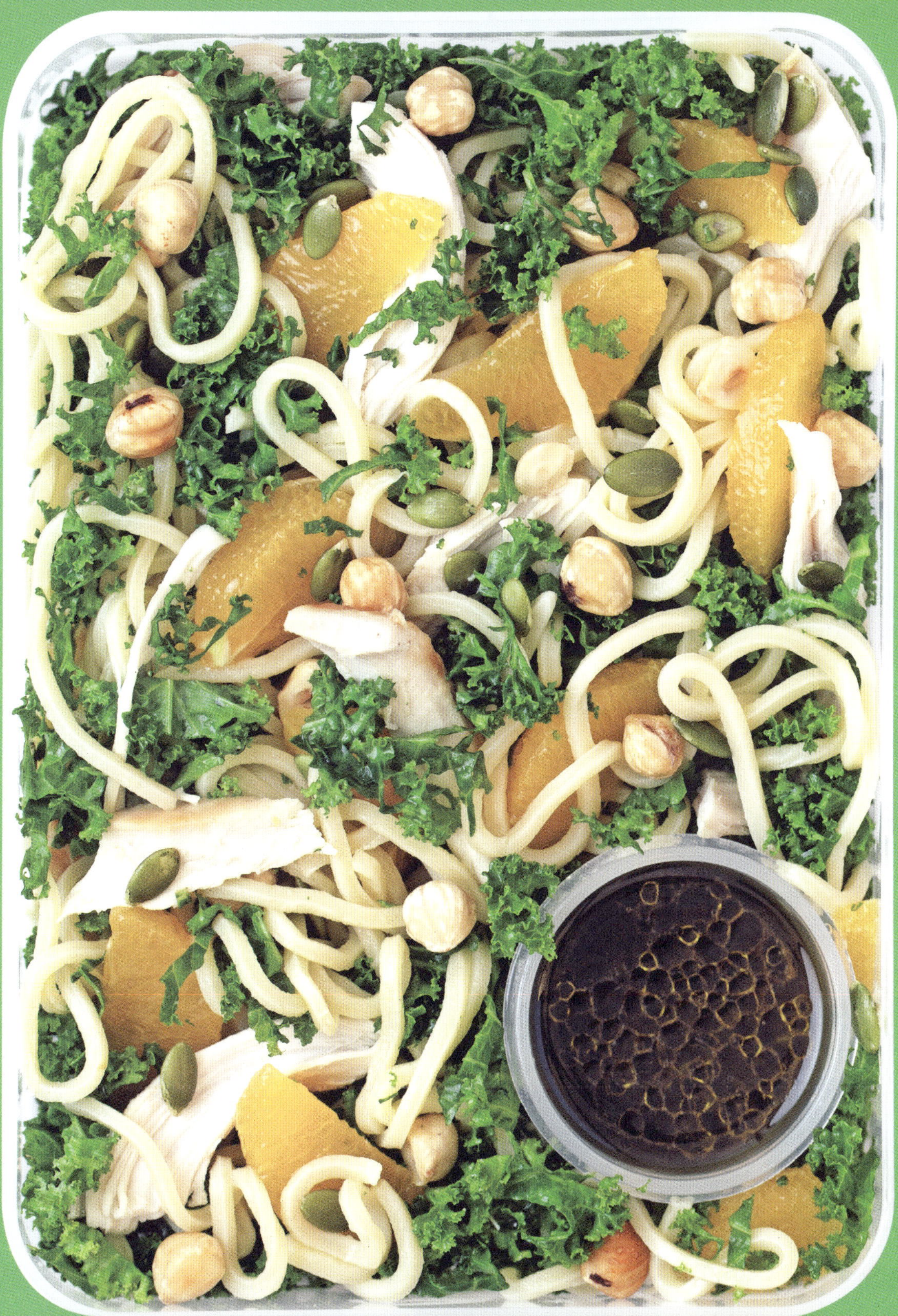

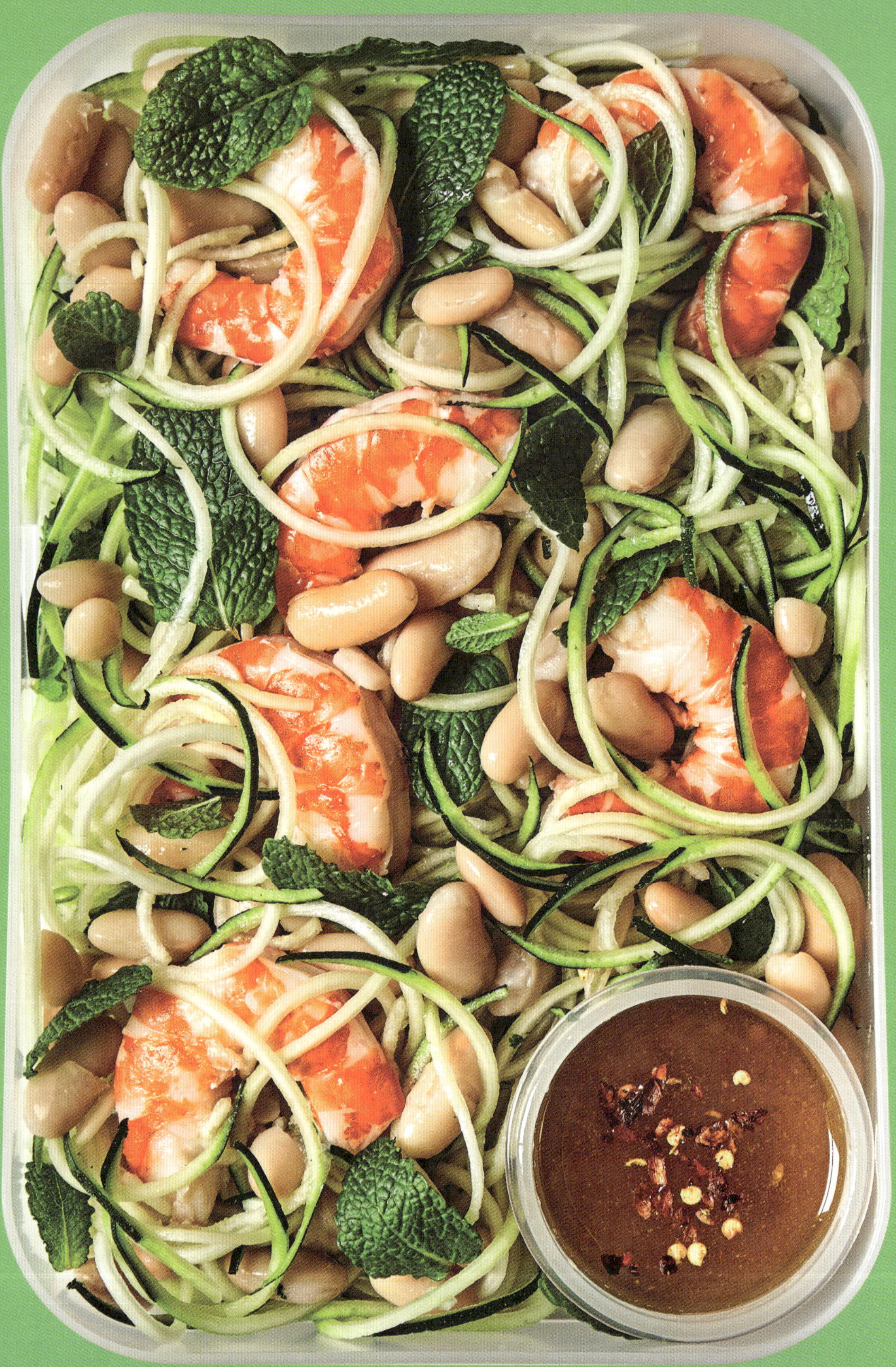

PROTEIN: 39 G NET CARBS: 23 G FAT: 30 G

Herby zoodles with prawns

Prawns provide substance here, while cannellini beans add another layer of protein power. Spiralised zucchini noodles keep the base light, and the preserved lemon dressing ties the fresh herbs together with a sharp finish.

- 1 zucchini (courgette), spiralised
- 120 g (4½ oz) cooked peeled prawns (shrimp), deveined
- 100 g (⅔ cup) tinned cannellini beans, drained and rinsed
- handful of mint leaves

PRESERVED LEMON DRESSING

- 2 tablespoons extra virgin olive oil
- 1½ tablespoons lemon juice
- ¼ preserved lemon skin, finely chopped
- pinch of chilli flakes

1. Place the salad ingredients in a bowl and toss lightly.
2. Combine the dressing ingredients in a small bowl, then season to taste with salt and pepper.
3. Pour the dressing over the salad just before serving and toss well to coat.

PROTEIN: 34 G NET CARBS: 10 G FAT: 12 G

Cajun salmon salad

Peppered hot-smoked salmon forms the centrepiece, with bell pepper, onion and greens offering freshness. The Cajun spice in the yoghurt-based dressing balances richness with heat, showing how seasoning blends can transform a protein-led dish. Cajun seasoning generally contains paprika, garlic powder, onion powder, cayenne pepper and salt. You can buy it from most supermarkets or a specialty grocer.

- 100 g (3½ oz) hot-smoked pepper-crusted salmon, flaked
- 100 g (⅔ cup) diced bell pepper (capsicum) - a mix of red and yellow, if possible
- 60 g (1½ cups) mixed salad greens
- 2 tablespoons diced red onion

CAJUN DRESSING

- 2 tablespoons high-protein Greek-style yoghurt
- 2 teaspoons lemon juice
- ½ teaspoon Cajun seasoning
- ¼ teaspoon minced garlic

1. Place the salad ingredients in a bowl and toss lightly.
2. Combine the dressing ingredients in a small bowl.
3. Pour the dressing over the salad just before serving and toss well to coat.

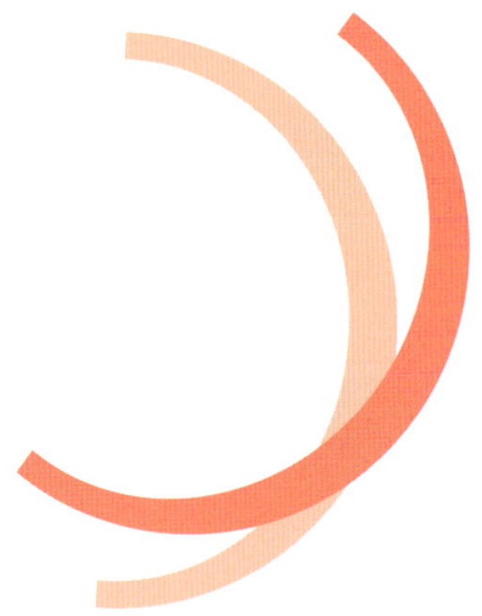

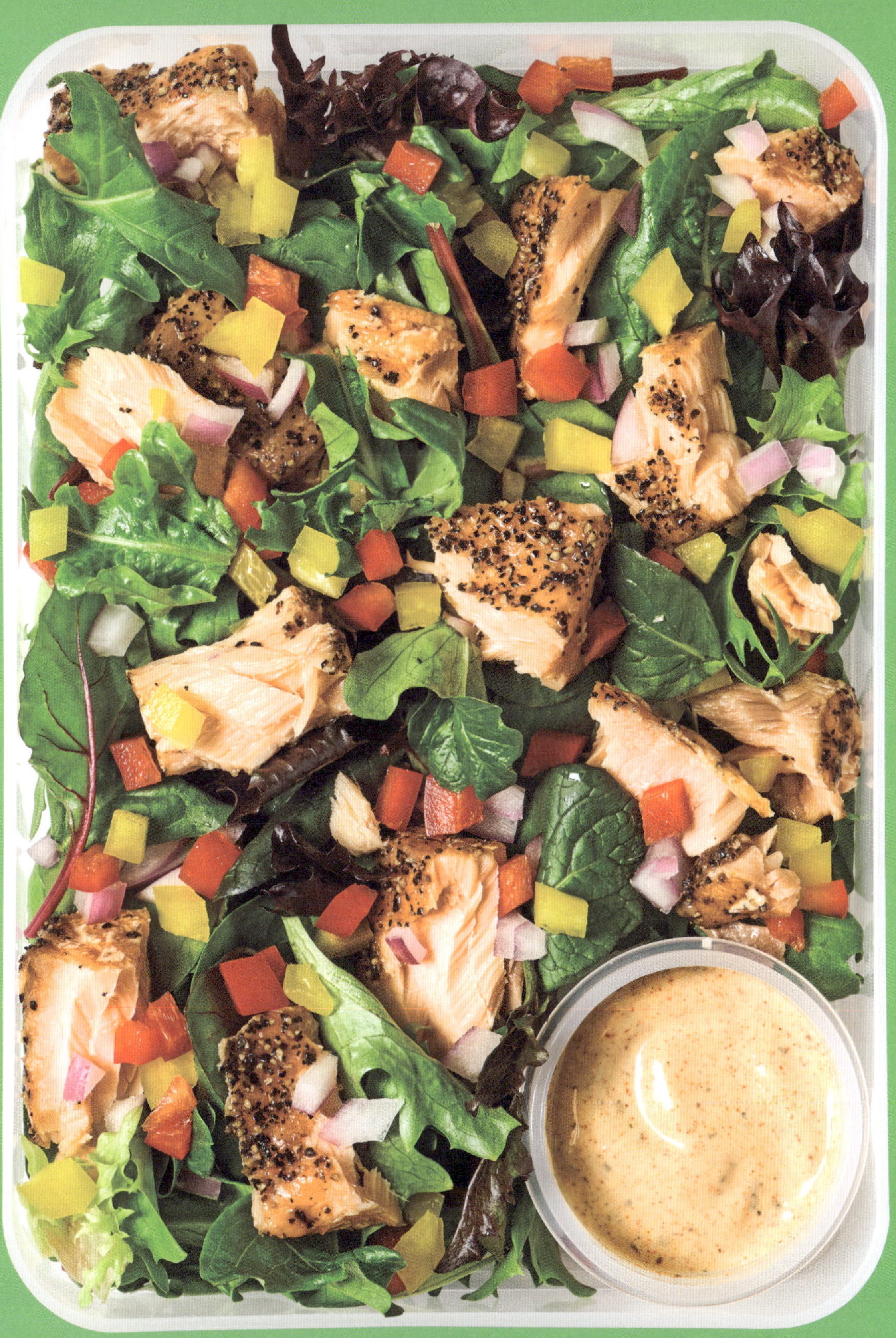

PROTEIN: 45 G NET CARBS: 10 G FAT: 42 G

Sesame cabbage chicken slaw

Shredded chicken anchors this salad, while Brazil nuts and sesame seeds add crunch and density. A miso-based dressing adds layers of umami, giving this otherwise light slaw plenty of backbone.

- 120 g (4½ oz) shredded cooked chicken
- 75 g (1 cup) finely shredded red cabbage
- small handful of coriander (cilantro) leaves
- 2 tablespoons chopped Brazil nuts
- 2 teaspoons toasted sesame seeds

SESAME-MISO DRESSING

- 1½ tablespoons toasted sesame oil
- 1 tablespoon rice vinegar
- 1½ teaspoons white (shiro) miso paste
- 1 teaspoon tamari sauce
- 1 teaspoon water
- ½ teaspoon minced ginger

1. Place the salad ingredients in a bowl and toss lightly.
2. Combine the dressing ingredients in a small bowl.
3. Pour the dressing over the salad just before serving and toss well to coat.

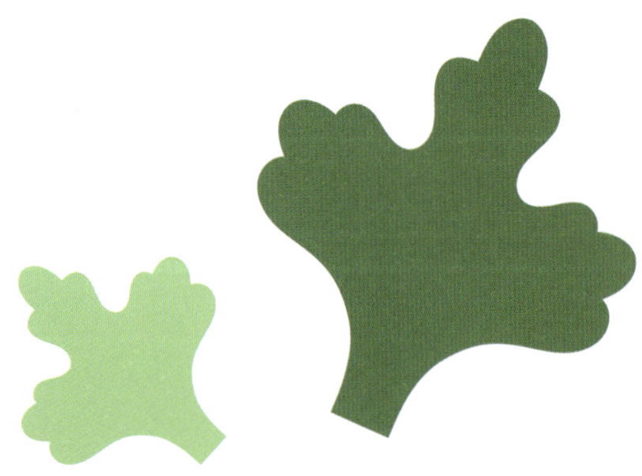

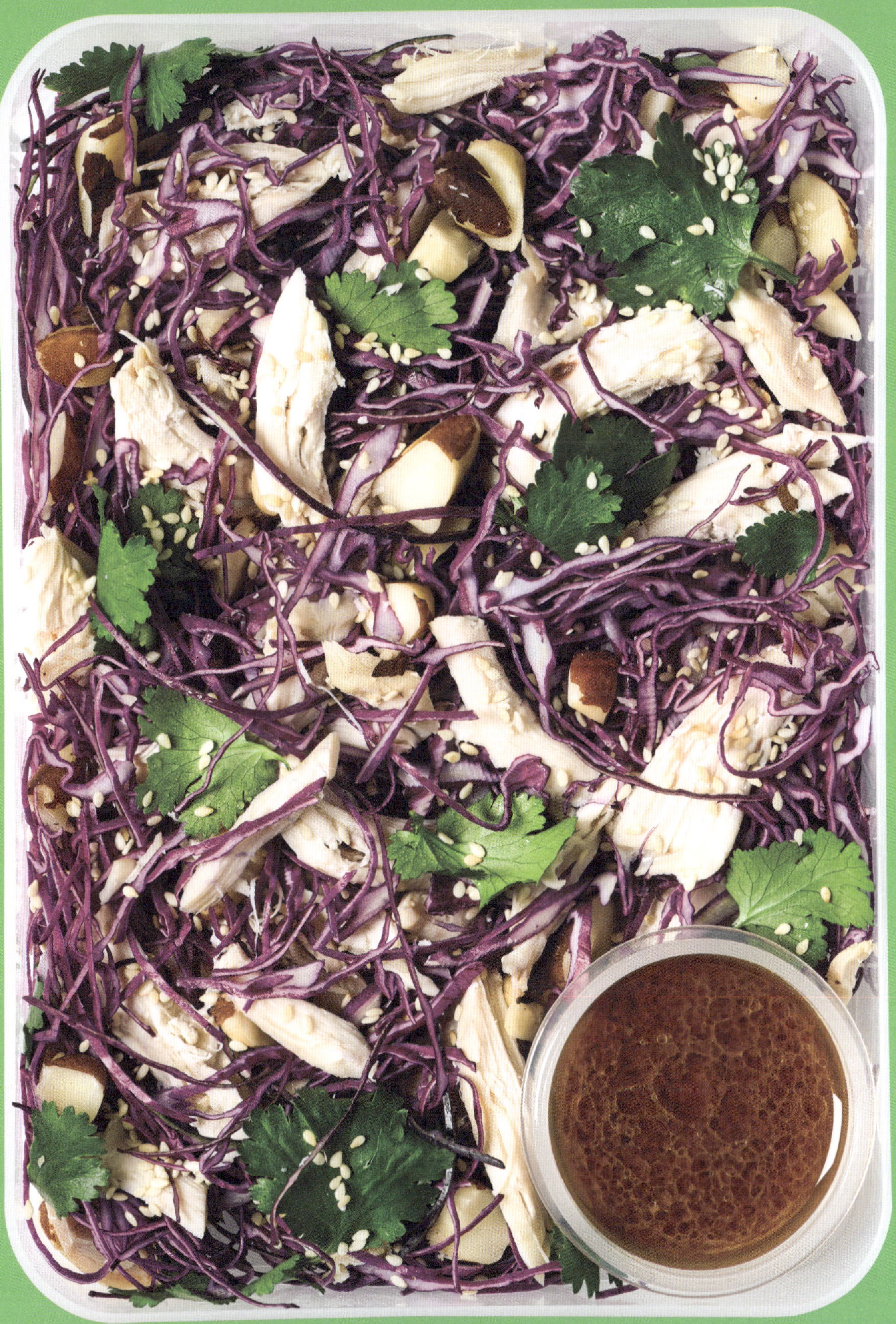

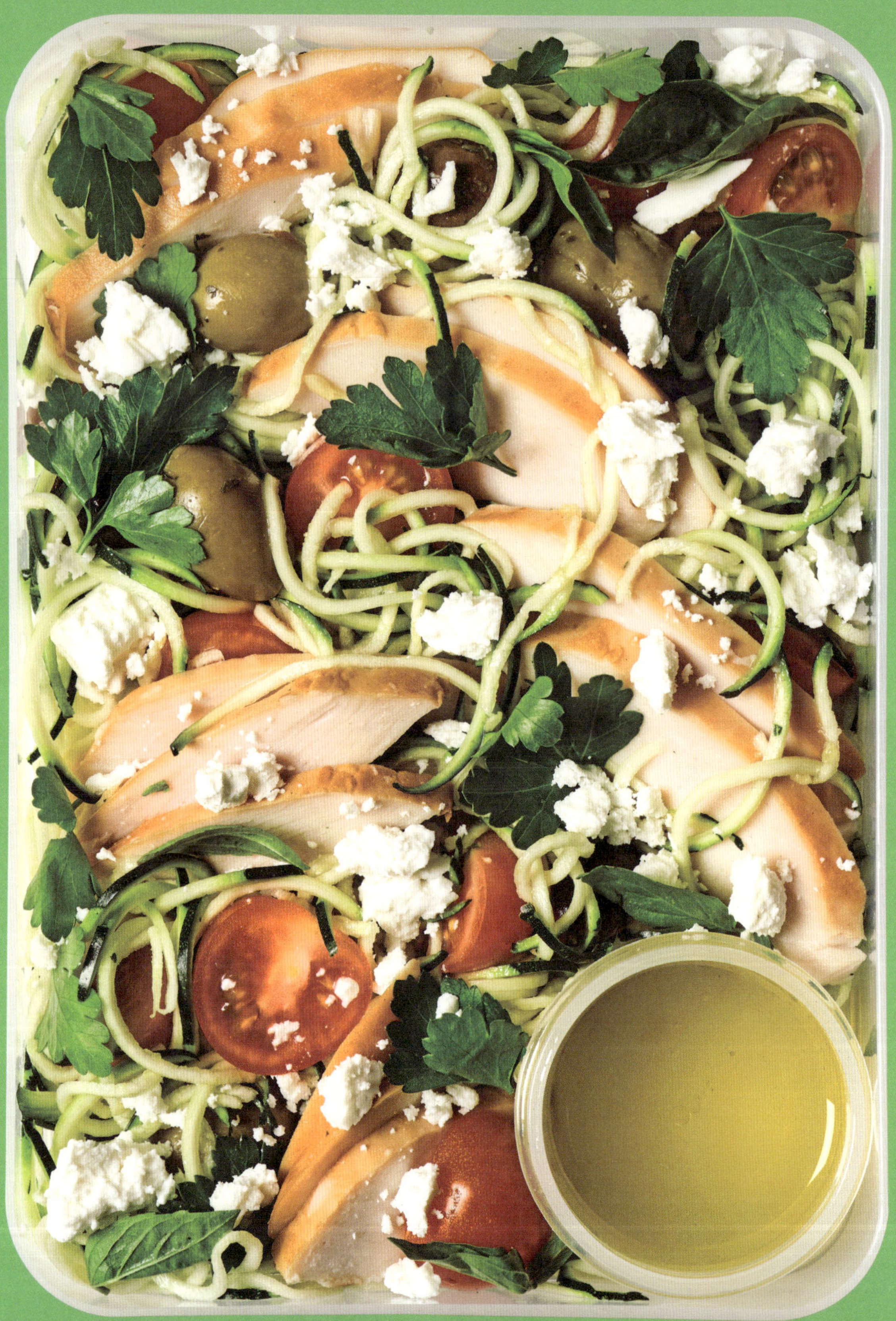

PROTEIN: 38 G NET CARBS: 12 G FAT: 43 G

Smoked chicken with herbs & zoodles

Smoked chicken ensures this salad has staying power, balanced by zucchini noodles and herbs. Feta and olives add a salty tang, while cherry tomatoes brighten the mix.

- 1 zucchini (courgette), spiralised
- 120 g (4½ oz) smoked chicken breast, sliced
- 100 g (3½ oz) cherry tomatoes, halved
- 50 g (⅓ cup) crumbled feta
- 30 g (¼ cup) marinated green olives
- small handful of parsley leaves
- small handful of basil leaves

LEMON VINAIGRETTE

- 1½ tablespoons extra virgin olive oil
- 1 tablespoon lemon juice

1. Place the salad ingredients in a bowl and toss lightly.
2. Combine the vinaigrette ingredients in a small bowl, then season to taste with salt and pepper.
3. Pour the vinaigrette over the salad just before serving and toss well to coat.

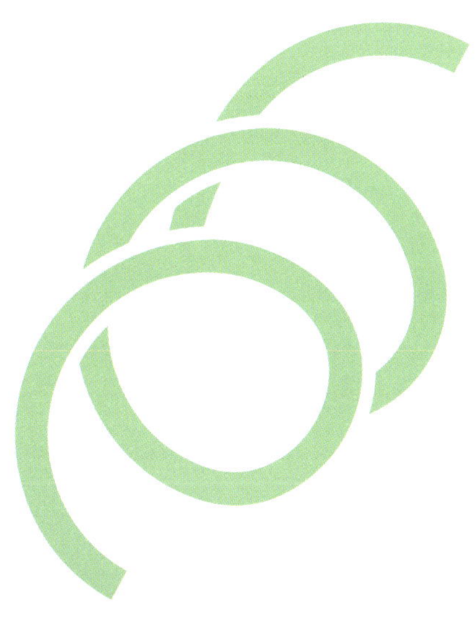

PROTEIN: 28 G NET CARBS: 9 G FAT: 17 G

Smoked salmon 'bagel' salad

All the satisfaction of a smoked salmon bagel without the bread. Salmon slices give richness, avocado adds creaminess, and the cottage cheese dressing rounds it out – proof that a few well-chosen components can carry a dish. 'Everything bagel' seasoning is available from most supermarkets – or make your own by mixing sesame seeds, poppy seeds, dried garlic and onion flakes with some sea salt.

- ½ avocado, diced
- 120 g (4½ oz) smoked salmon slices
- 60 g (2 cups) rocket (arugula) or watercress leaves
- ¼ red onion, finely sliced
- 2 teaspoons baby capers
- 1 teaspoon toasted sesame seeds
- lemon wedge, to serve

CREAMY DRESSING

- 2 tablespoons blended cottage cheese (2% fat)
- 1 tablespoon lemon juice
- 1 teaspoon 'everything bagel' seasoning mix

1. Place all the salad ingredients in a bowl, except the lemon wedge, and toss lightly.
2. Combine the dressing ingredients in a small bowl, then season to taste with pepper.
3. Pour the dressing over the salad just before serving and toss well to coat, then squeeze over the lemon.

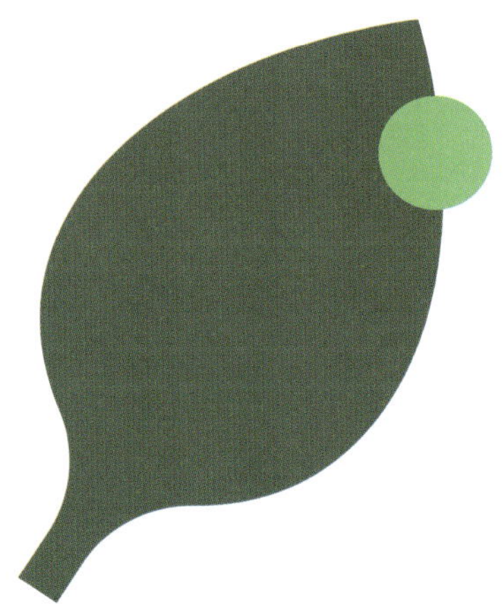

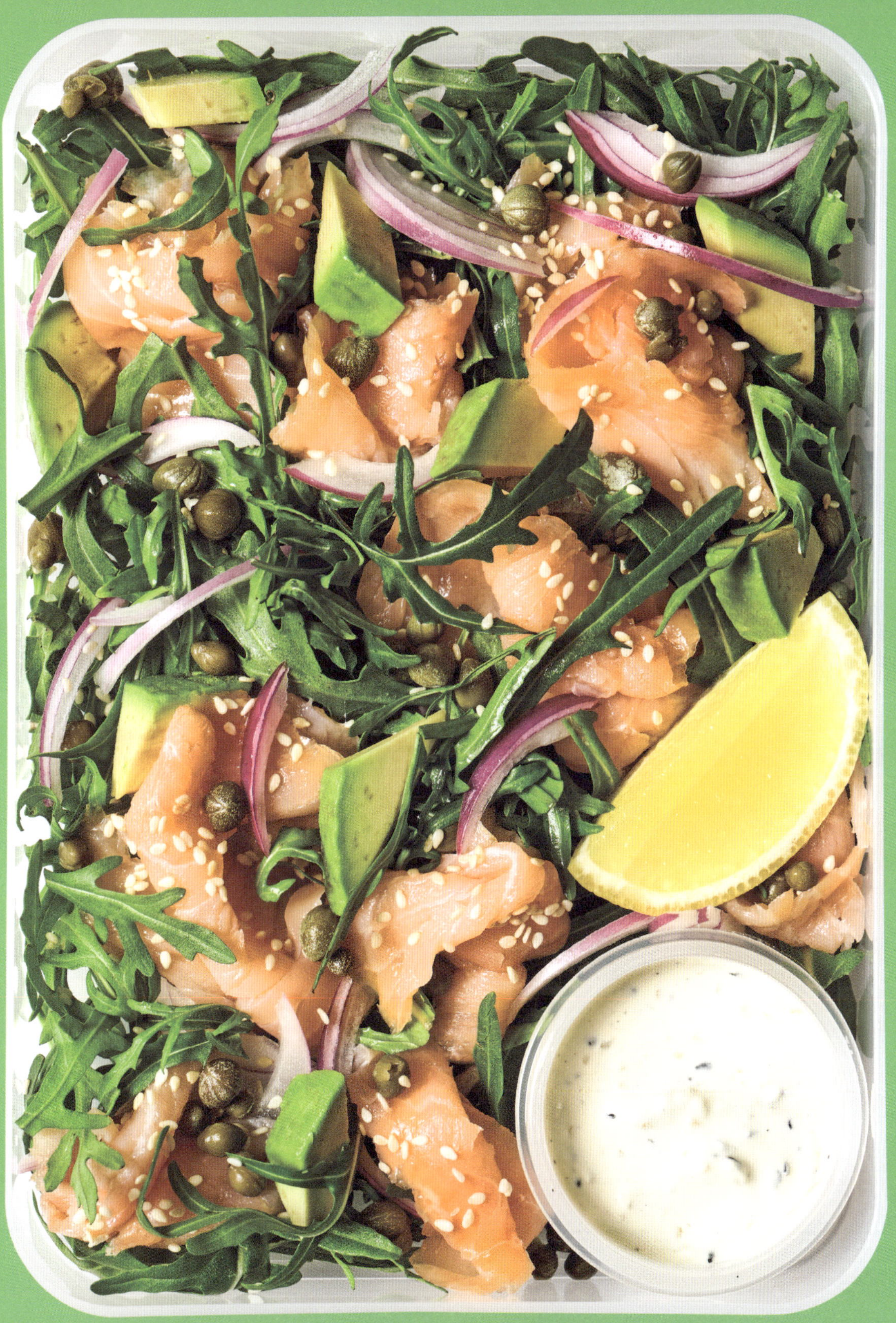

PROTEIN: 34 G   NET CARBS: 27 G   FAT: 18 G

Leafy chicken, mango & jalapeño salad

Chicken and mango create a classic sweet–savoury pairing. The jalapeño dressing provides heat and contrast, with lettuce and bell pepper adding crunch. Each element contributes, making the salad both refreshing and substantial.

100 g (⅔ cup) shredded cooked chicken

½ mango, diced

1 baby cos (romaine) lettuce, chopped

¼ red bell pepper (capsicum), diced

small handful of coriander (cilantro) leaves, roughly chopped

JALAPEÑO DRESSING

juice of ½ lime

3 pickled jalapeño slices, finely chopped

1 tablespoon extra virgin olive oil

1. Place the salad ingredients in a bowl and toss lightly, then season to taste with salt and pepper.
2. Combine the dressing ingredients in a small bowl.
3. Pour the dressing over the salad just before serving and toss well to coat.

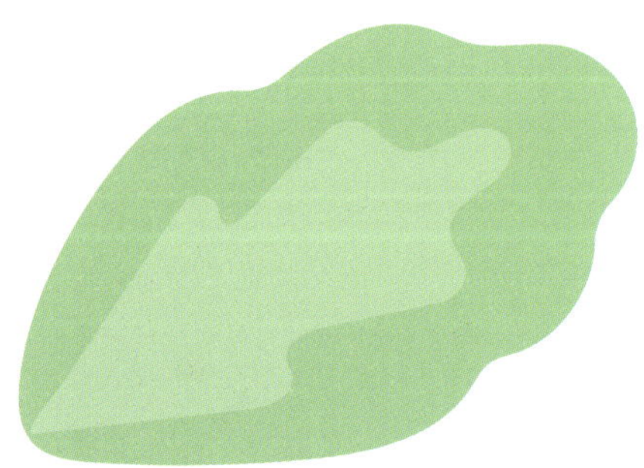

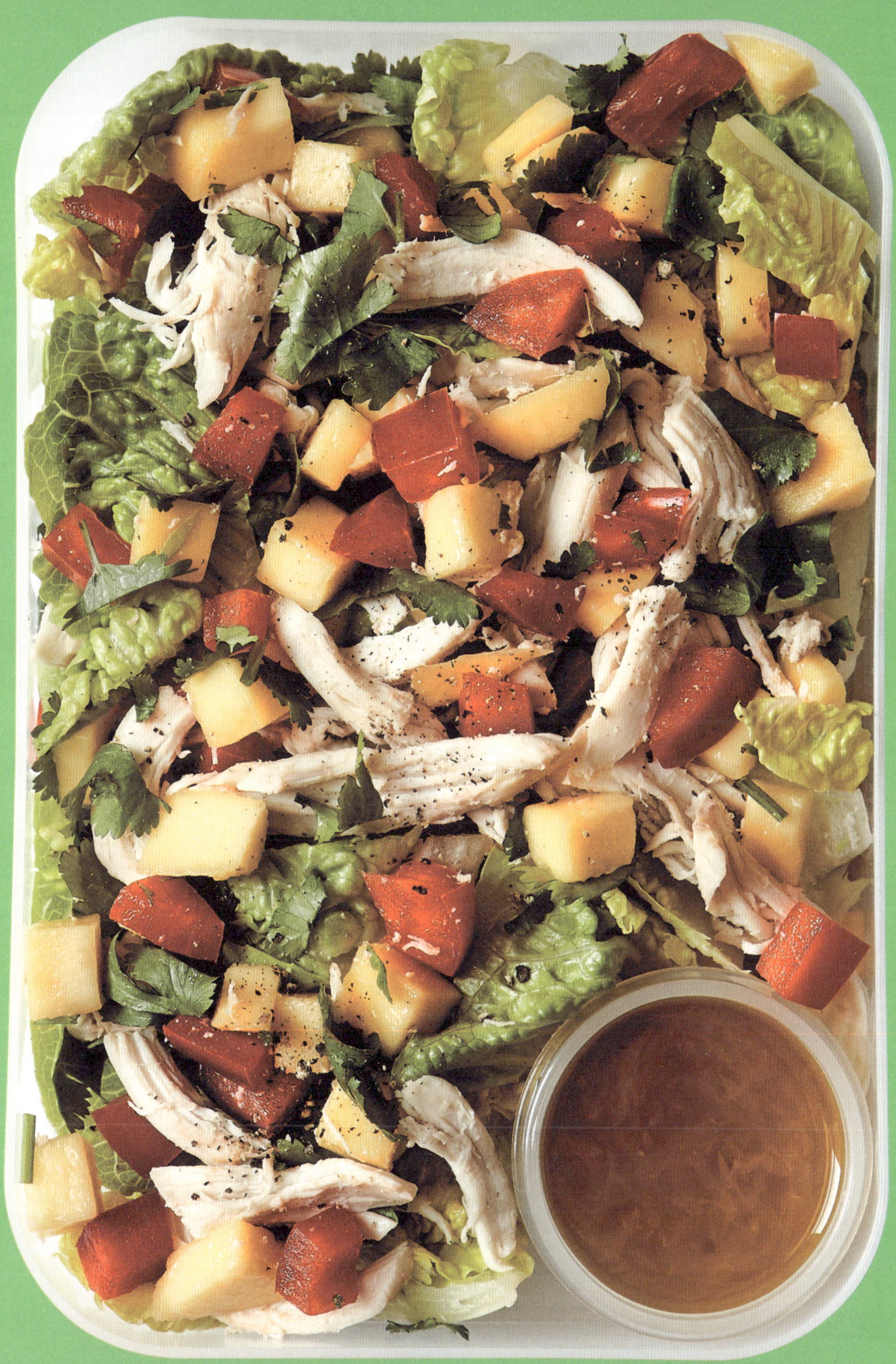

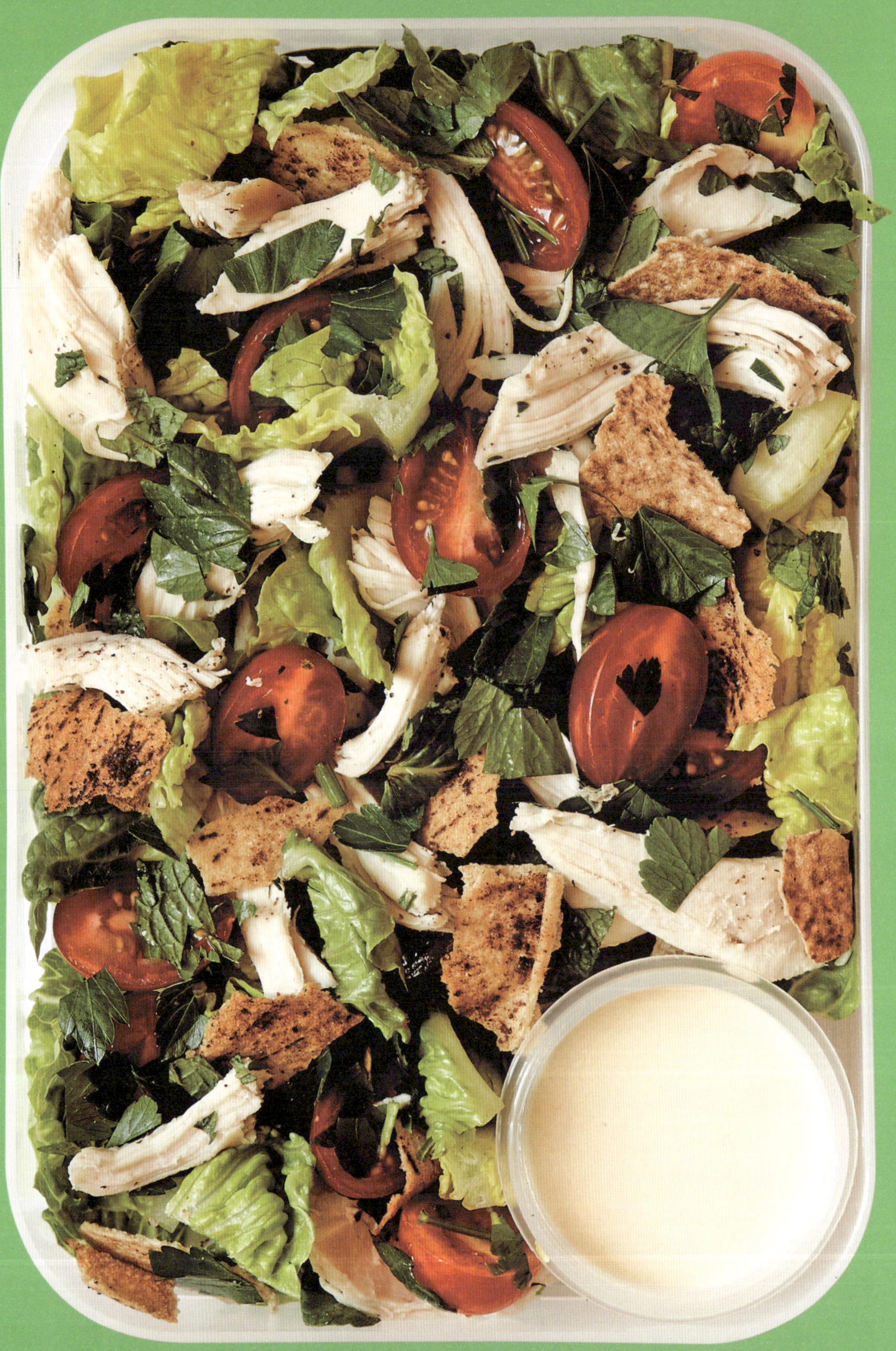

PROTEIN: 43 G NET CARBS: 43 G FAT: 14 G

Chicken fattoush with tahini-yoghurt dressing

Here, we've added shredded chicken to turn this Lebanese-style fattoush into a more filling meal. Toasted pita chips bring crunch, and the tahini–yoghurt dressing layers creaminess with nutty depth.

- 1 pita bread
- olive oil, for brushing
- sumac, for sprinkling
- 100 g (⅔ cup) shredded cooked chicken
- 1 baby cos (romaine) lettuce, chopped
- 100 g (3½ oz) grape (baby plum) tomatoes, halved
- small handful of mint leaves, chopped
- small handful of parsley leaves, chopped

TAHINI-YOGHURT DRESSING

- 1 tablespoon lemon juice
- 1 tablespoon tahini
- 1 tablespoon high-protein Greek-style yoghurt
- 1 teaspoon honey
- 2 teaspoons water

1. Lightly brush the pita bread with olive oil, sprinkle with sumac, then toast until golden. Set aside to cool, then break into pieces.
2. Place the remaining salad ingredients in a bowl and toss lightly, then season to taste with salt and pepper.
3. Combine the dressing ingredients in a small bowl.
4. Pour the dressing over the salad and toss through the pita bread just before serving.

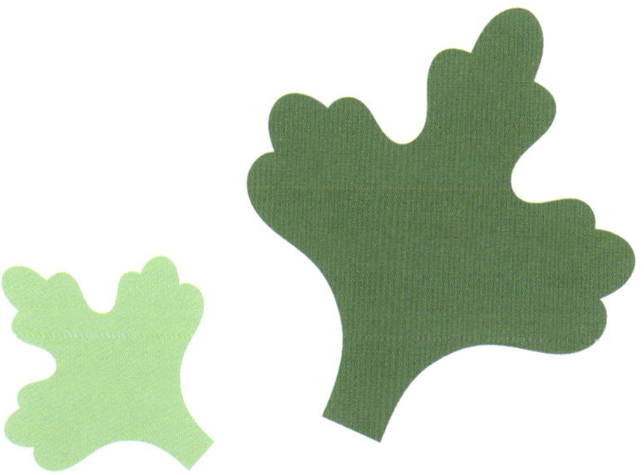

PROTEIN: 34 G NET CARBS: 36 G FAT: 16 G

Chicken, cabbage, pear & carrot zoodles

Shredded chicken is the core of this salad, while cabbage and carrot zoodles keep the dish fresh and crunchy. The pear adds sweetness, which is balanced by a sesame-ginger dressing. This is a prime example of how fruit and protein can work well together.

- 100 g (2/3 cup) shredded cooked chicken
- 2 white or purple carrots, spiralised
- 1 nashi pear, spiralised
- 75 g (1 cup) finely shredded red cabbage

GINGER VINAIGRETTE

- 1½ tablespoons rice vinegar
- 1½ tablespoons mirin
- 2 teaspoons toasted sesame oil
- 2 teaspoons toasted sesame seeds
- 1 teaspoon minced ginger

1. Place the salad ingredients in a bowl and toss lightly.
2. Combine the vinaigrette ingredients in a small bowl, then season to taste with salt and pepper.
3. Pour the vinaigrette over the salad just before serving and toss well to coat.

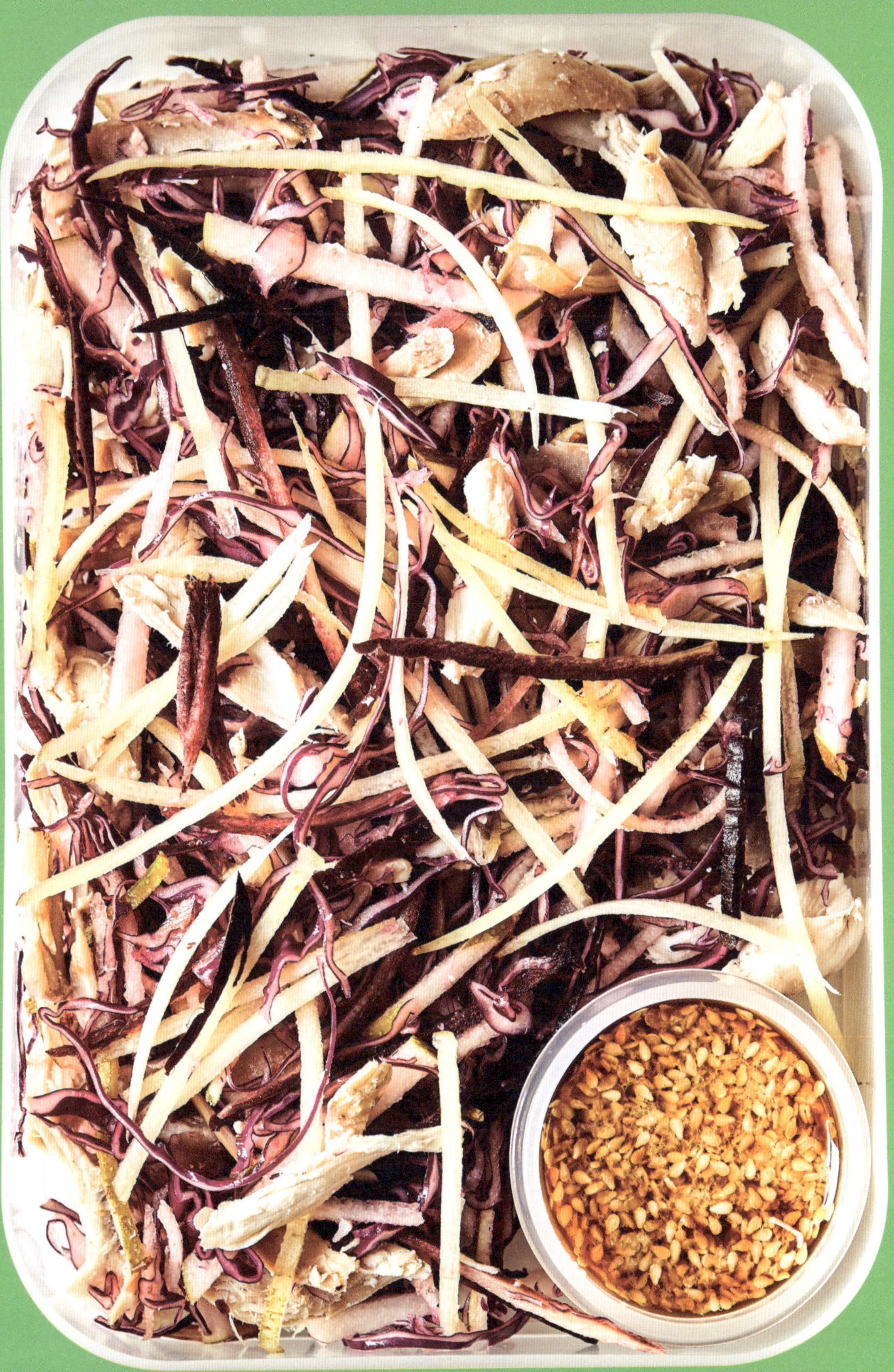

PROTEIN: 36 G NET CARBS: 36 G FAT: 25 G

Hot-smoked trout, quinoa & watercress salad

Hot-smoked trout adds both substance and flavour, while quinoa provides a grain-based counterpoint that's naturally sustaining. Watercress and cucumber bring freshness, with the horseradish dressing bringing a wonderfully sophisticated bite to this salad. If you can't find hot-smoked trout, salmon will do just as well.

- 75 g (2¾ oz) hot-smoked trout, flaked
- 150 g (1 cup) cooked and cooled quinoa
- 30 g (1 cup) watercress leaves
- ½ small short cucumber, diced
- juice of ½ lemon

CREAMY HORSERADISH DRESSING

- 2 teaspoons prepared horseradish
- juice of 1 lemon
- 2 teaspoons baby capers, chopped
- 1 tablespoon blended cottage cheese (2% fat)
- 1 tablespoon extra virgin olive oil

1. Place the salad ingredients in a bowl and toss lightly.
2. Combine the dressing ingredients in a small bowl, then season to taste with salt and pepper.
3. Pour the dressing over the salad just before serving and toss well to coat.

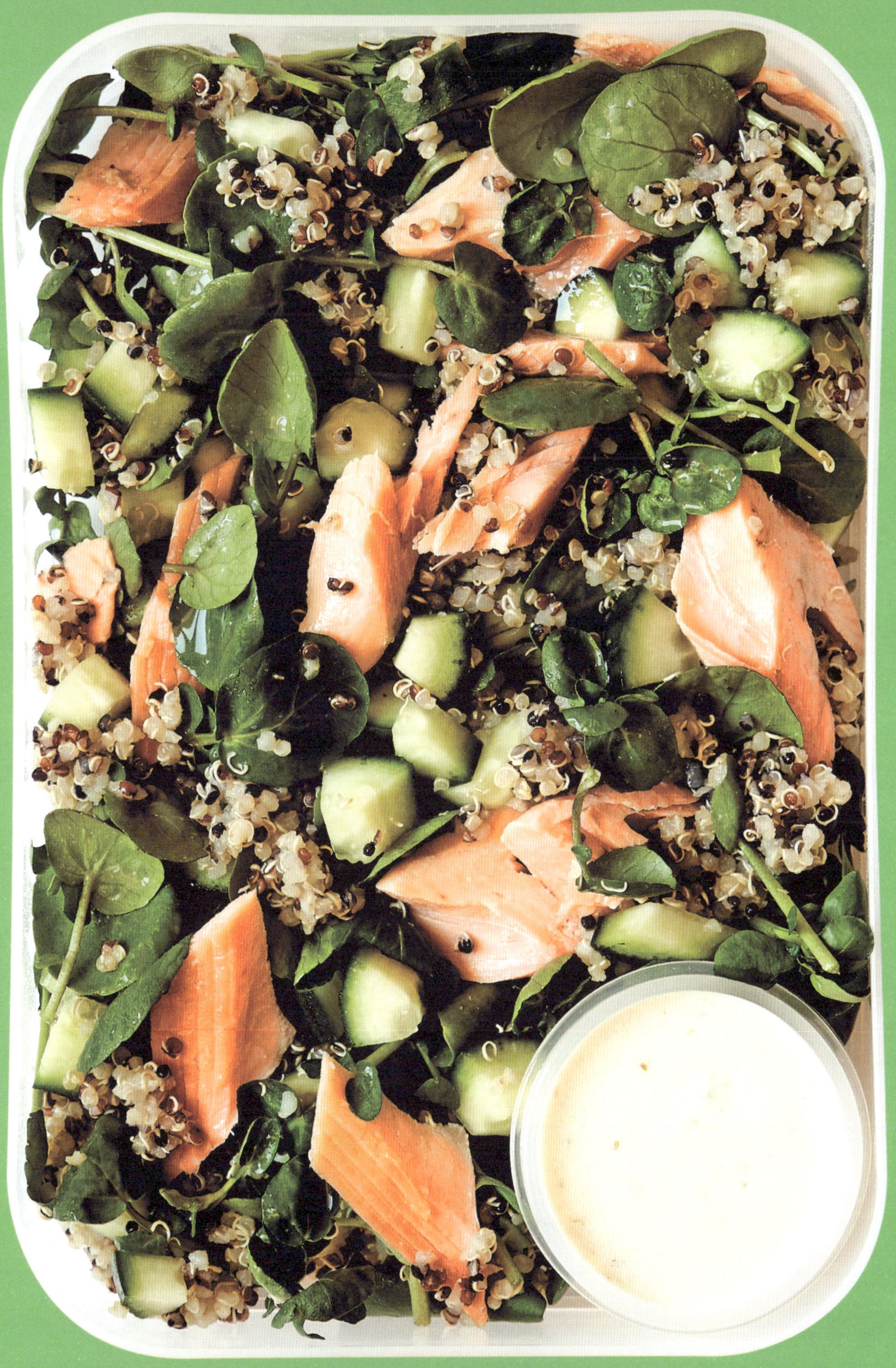

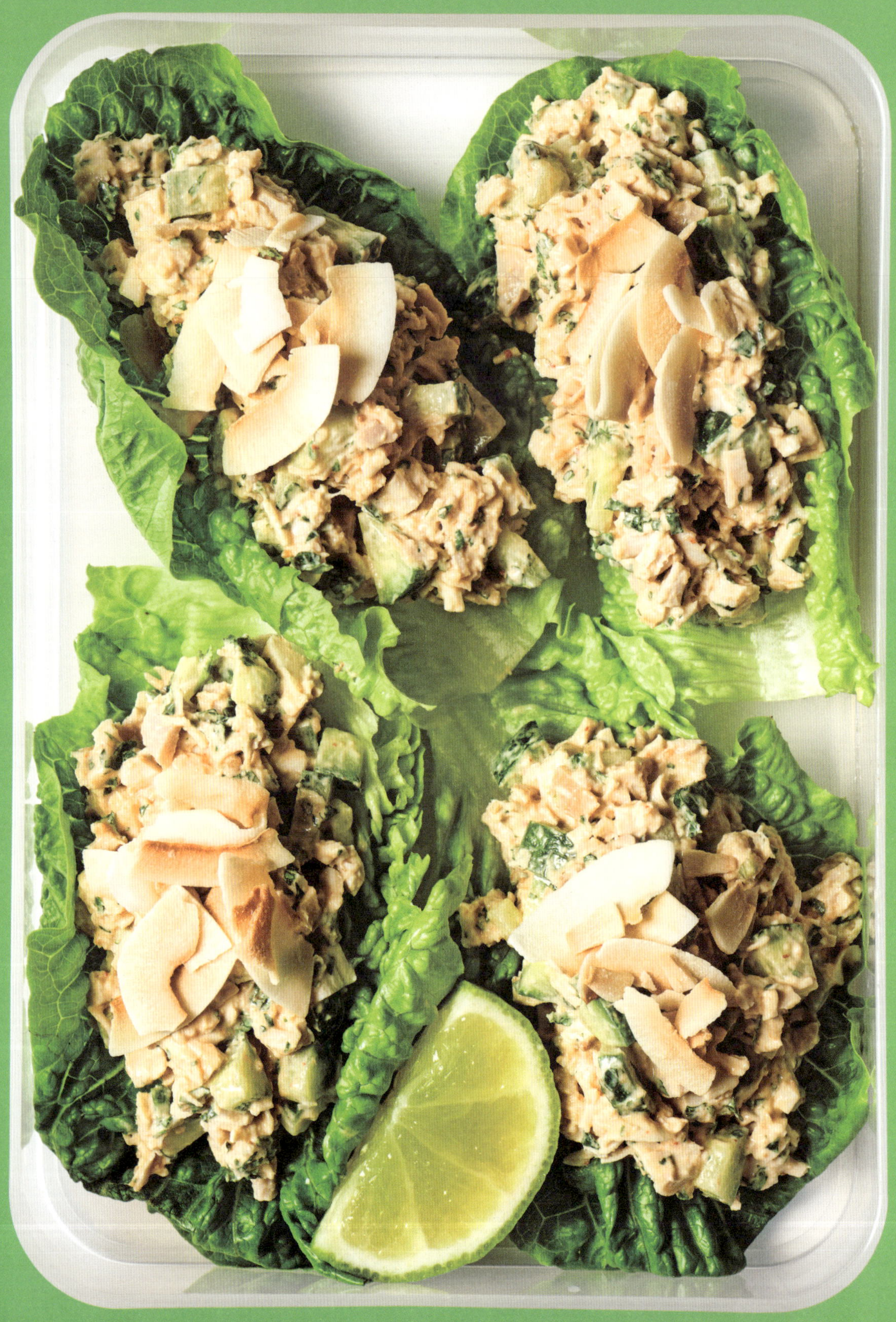

PROTEIN: 46 G   NET CARBS: 13 G   FAT: 21 G

Spiced chicken lettuce cups

Chicken makes these lettuce cups sturdy enough for a main meal. Coconut flakes provide crunch and richness, while herbs add freshness. These are light to eat but will keep you feeling satisfied well beyond the final bite.

- 120 g (4½ oz) shredded cooked chicken
- 90 g (½ cup) diced short cucumber
- handful of mixed Asian herbs, such as Thai basil, Vietnamese mint and coriander (cilantro) leaves
- 4 baby cos (romaine) lettuce leaves
- 2 tablespoons toasted flaked coconut
- lime wedge, to serve

CREAMY LIME-CHILLI DRESSING

- 2 tablespoons coconut yoghurt
- 1 tablespoon lime juice
- 1 tablespoon almond butter
- 1 teaspoon sriracha or hot sauce

1. In a bowl, whisk together all the dressing ingredients.
2. Add the chicken, cucumber and herbs to the dressing and toss to combine.
3. Spoon the chicken mixture into your lettuce leaves just before serving, then scatter over the toasted coconut flakes and finish with a squeeze of lime juice.

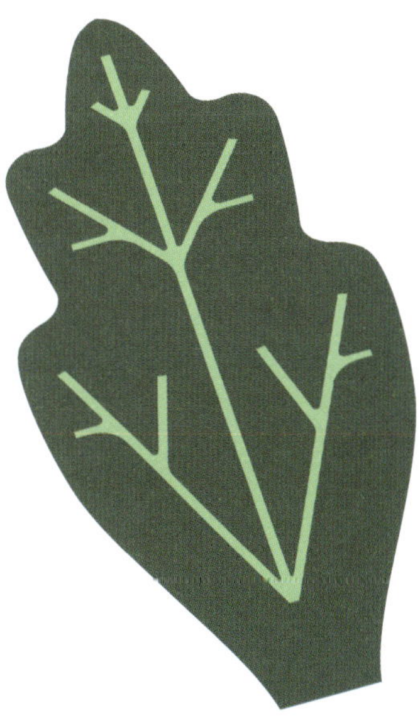

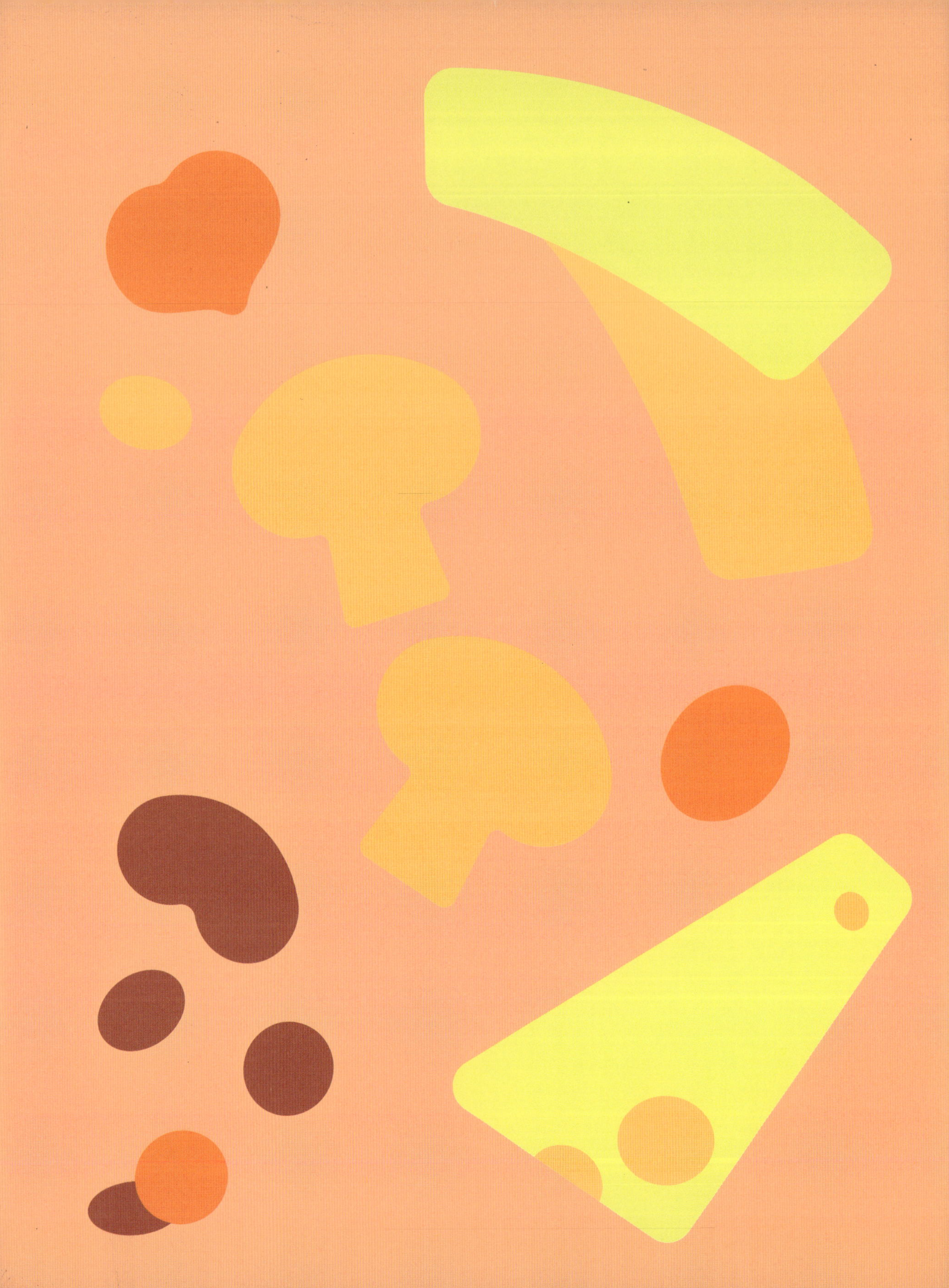

plant

power

PROTEIN: 26 G NET CARBS: 14 G FAT: 28 G

Tofu taco salad bowl

Plain tofu can be a little flavourless on its own, but mixing it with smoky chipotle sauce gives it plenty of flavour, with barely any effort on your part. If you have time, marinating the tofu for a few hours or overnight amps up the flavour even more.

- 150 g (5½ oz) firm tofu, drained and diced
- 1 tablespoon chipotle sauce
- ½ avocado, diced
- 55 g (1½ cups) shredded iceberg lettuce
- 5 cherry tomatoes, halved
- 2 radishes, sliced
- 2 tablespoons pumpkin seeds

LIME & SOUR CREAM DRESSING

- 2 tablespoons blended cottage cheese (2% fat)
- 1 tablespoon sour cream
- 1 tablespoon lime juice
- 2 teaspoons chopped coriander (cilantro) leaves
- pinch of onion powder

1. Toss the tofu in a bowl with the chipotle sauce, coating well. Combine with the remaining salad ingredients and toss lightly.
2. Combine the dressing ingredients in a small bowl, then season to taste with salt and pepper.
3. Pour the dressing over the salad just before serving and toss well to coat.

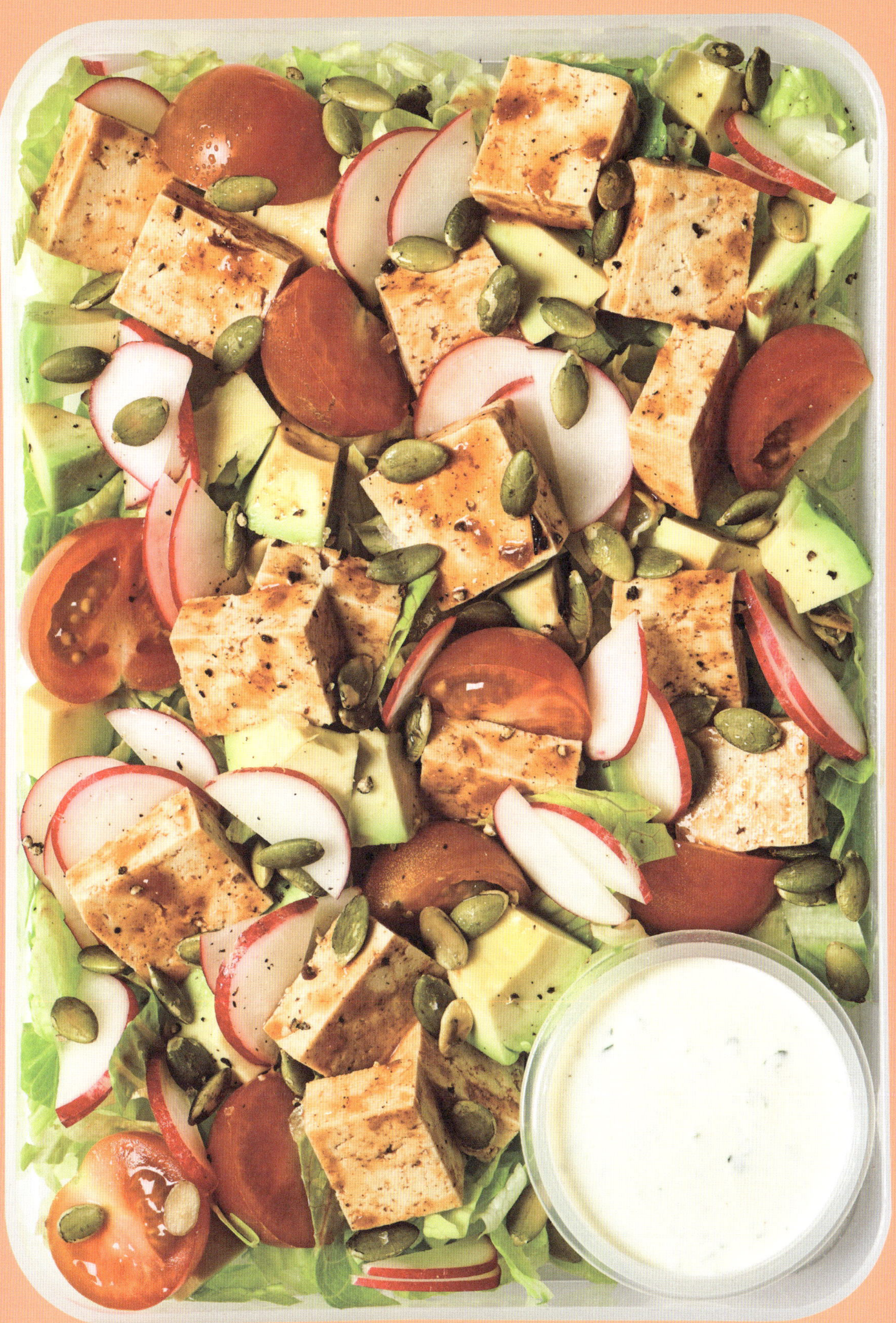

PROTEIN: 27 G NET CARBS: 84 G FAT: 14 G

Chipotle black bean nacho salad

Black beans do the heavy lifting here – a pantry-friendly way to make a salad feel like a meal. Corn, bell pepper and yoghurt bring freshness and creaminess, while tortilla chips add crunch for scooping.

- 200 g (7 oz) tinned black beans, drained and rinsed
- 100 g (3½ oz) tinned sweet corn kernels, drained and rinsed
- ½ green bell pepper (capsicum), diced
- 2 spring onions (scallions), finely sliced
- ½ teaspoon salt
- juice of ½ lime
- handful of coriander (cilantro) leaves, chopped
- 50 g (1¾ oz) tortilla chips

CHIPOTLE DRESSING

- ¼ teaspoon minced garlic
- 2 teaspoons chipotle in adobo hot sauce
- juice of ½ lime
- 2 tablespoons high-protein Greek-style yoghurt

1. Place the salad ingredients in a bowl, except the tortilla chips, and toss lightly.
2. Combine the dressing ingredients in a small bowl, then season to taste with salt and pepper.
3. Pour the dressing over the salad just before serving and toss well to coat.
4. Use the tortilla chips to scoop up the bean mixture.

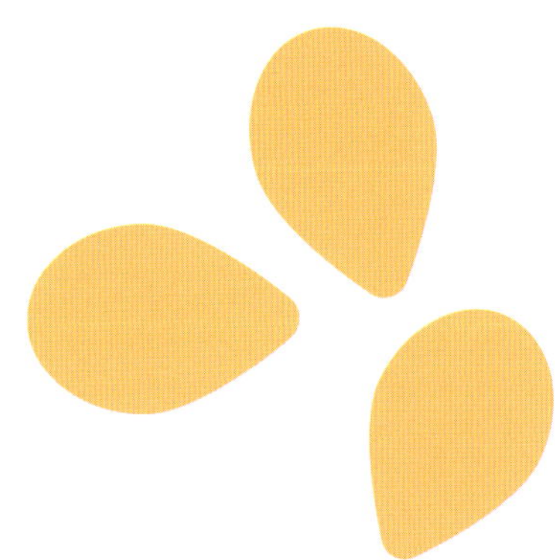

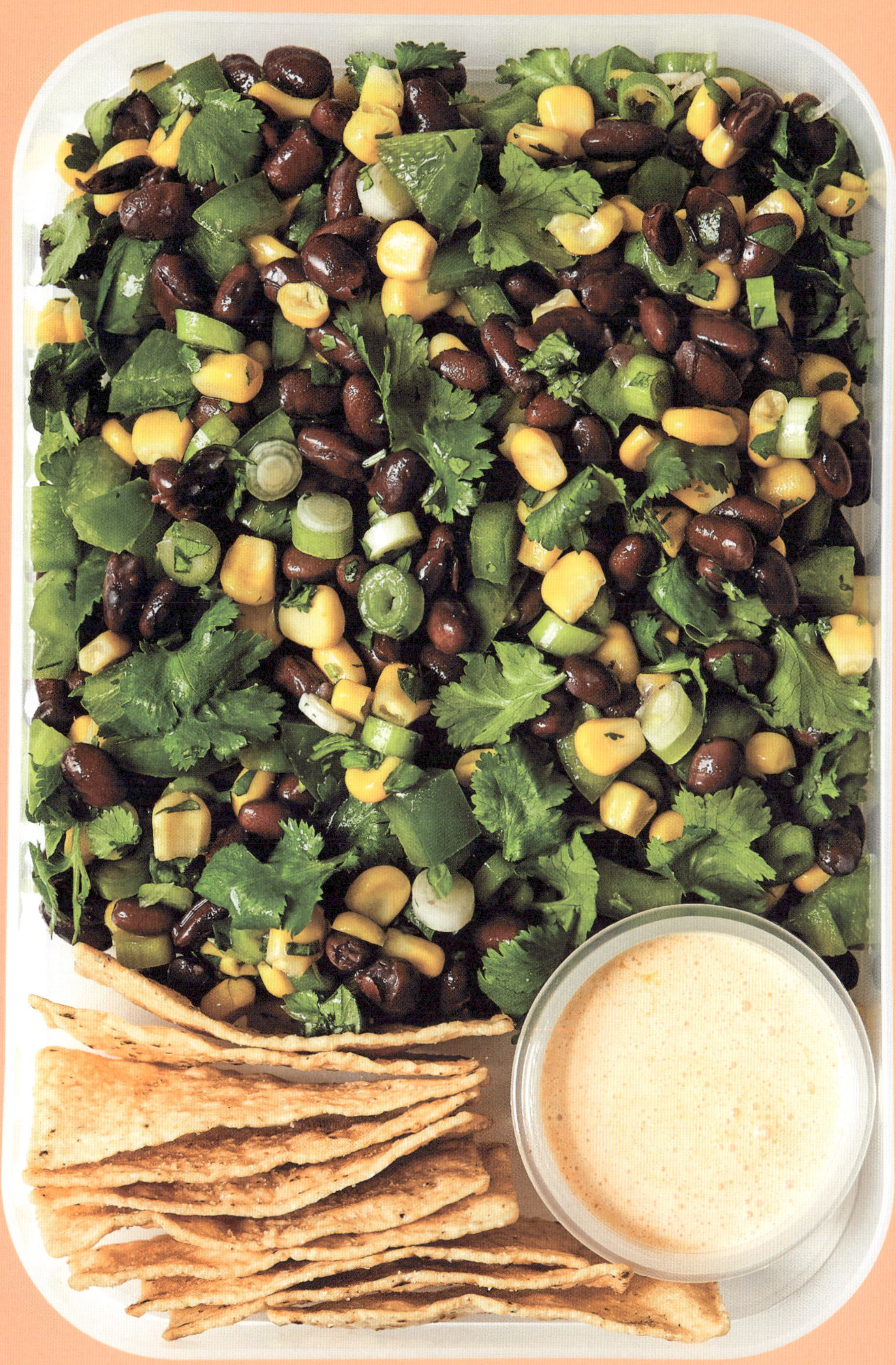

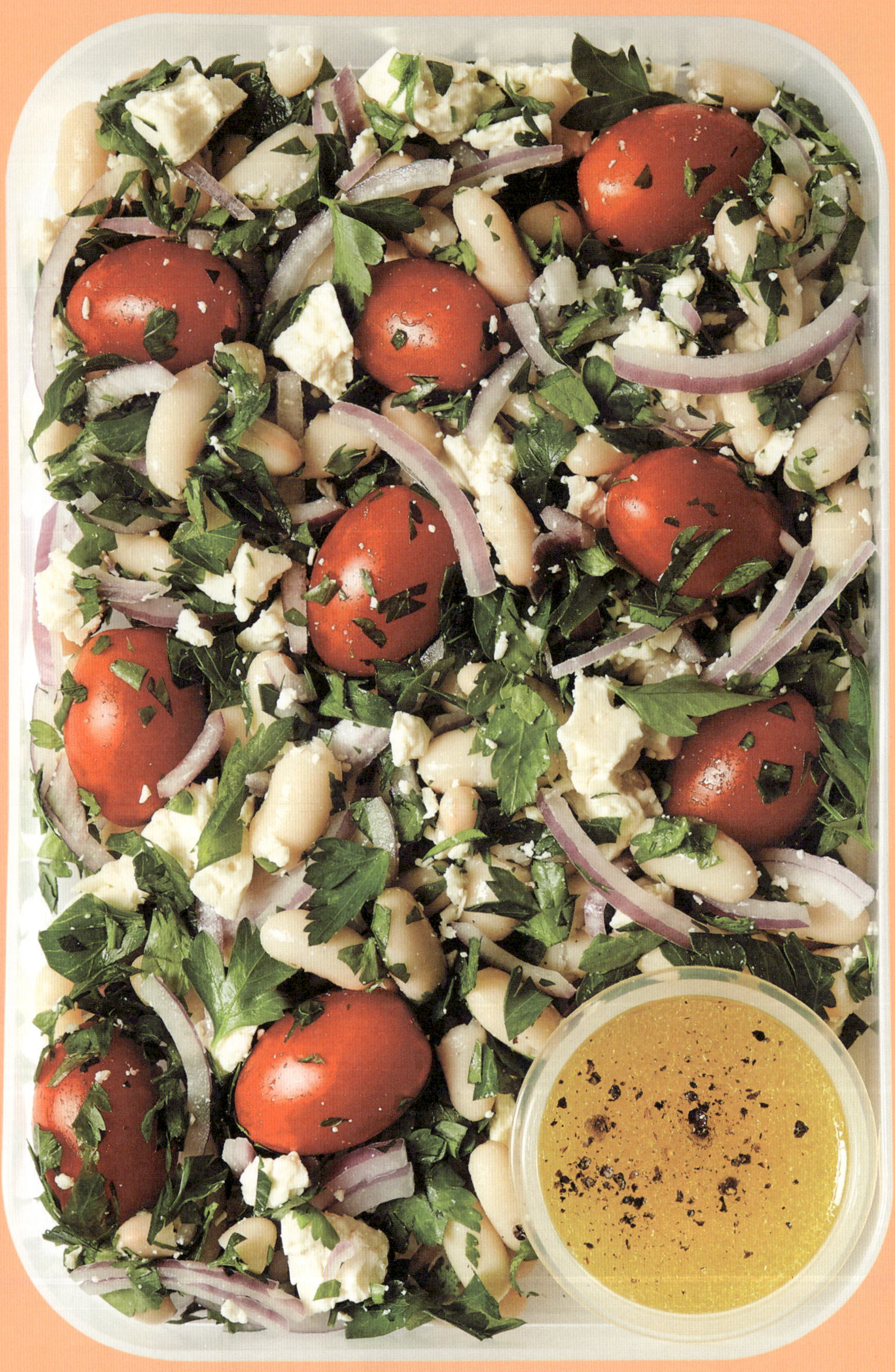

PROTEIN: 25 G NET CARBS: 32 G FAT: 31 G

Cannellini bean & feta salad

Cannellini beans offer a soft, creamy base that's naturally sustaining. Feta and fresh parsley sharpen the flavours, showing how a tin of beans plus a salty cheese can anchor a quick lunch. You can use butter (lima) beans or even chickpeas (garbanzo beans) instead of the cannellini beans if you prefer.

- 170 g (6 oz) tinned cannellini beans, drained and rinsed
- ¼ red onion, finely sliced
- 100 g (3½ oz) grape (baby plum) tomatoes
- 50 g (⅓ cup) crumbled feta
- small handful of parsley, roughly chopped

LEMON & GARLIC DRESSING

- ½ teaspoon minced garlic
- juice of ½ lemon
- 2 teaspoons apple cider vinegar
- 1½ tablespoons extra virgin olive oil

1. Place the salad ingredients in a bowl and toss lightly, then season to taste with salt and pepper.
2. Combine the dressing ingredients in a small bowl and season with pepper.
3. Pour the dressing over the salad just before serving and toss well to coat.

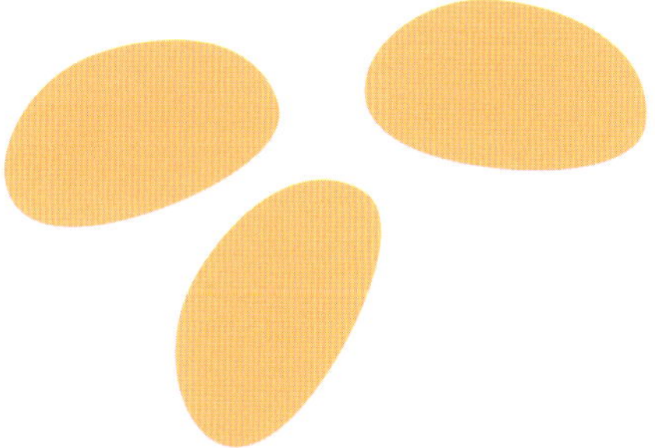

PROTEIN: 25 G NET CARBS: 45 G FAT: 34 G

Lentil, beetroot & feta salad

Earthy lentils pair beautifully with sweet beetroot and tangy feta. Using pre-cooked beetroot keeps prep simple – just add greens and a balsamic vinaigrette for balance. Pre-cooked beetroot is available in vacuum-sealed packs from the supermarket. Look for varieties with no added sugar or preservatives.

- 4 cooked baked beetroot (beets), quartered
- 1 short cucumber, halved lengthways and sliced
- 150 g (5½ oz) tinned brown lentils, drained and rinsed
- 30 g (1 oz) feta, crumbled
- 30 g (⅔ cup) baby spinach leaves
- handful of mint leaves

BALSAMIC DRESSING

- 1 tablespoon balsamic vinegar
- 1 teaspoon dijon mustard
- 2 tablespoons extra virgin olive oil

1. Place the salad ingredients in a bowl and toss lightly.
2. Combine the dressing ingredients in a small bowl, then season to taste with salt and pepper.
3. Pour the dressing over the salad just before serving and toss well to coat.

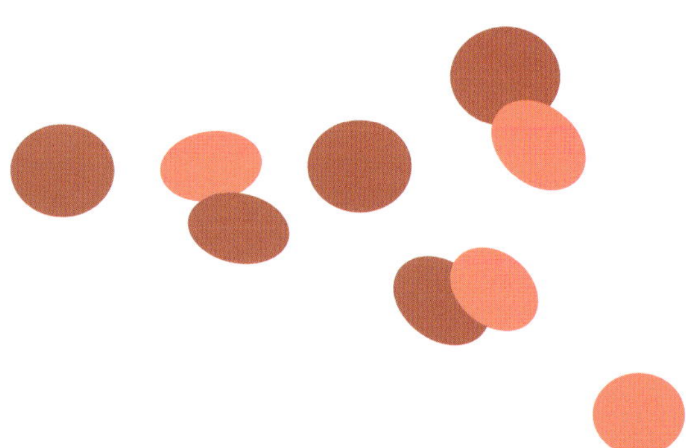

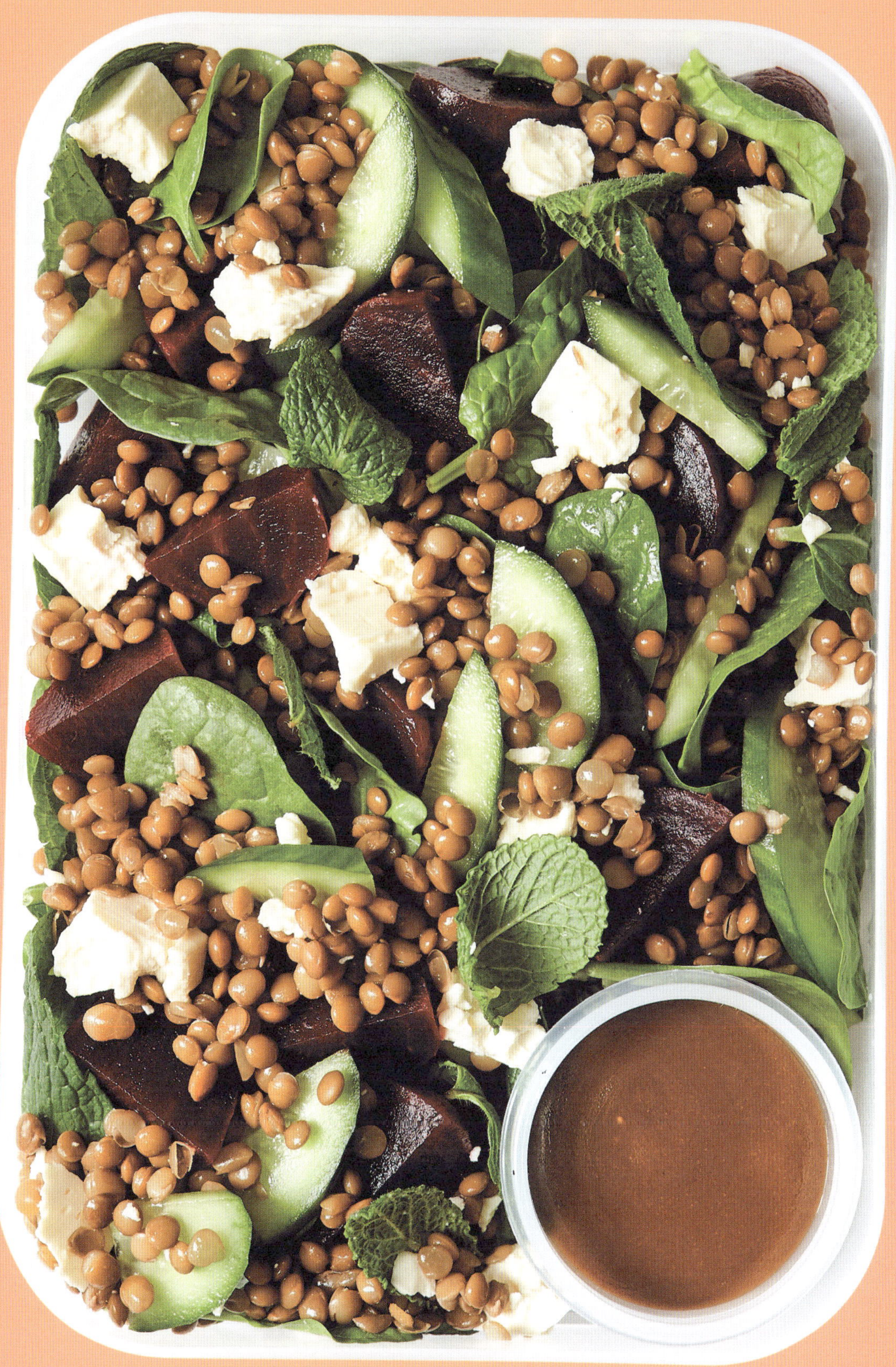

PROTEIN: 25 G NET CARBS: 38 G FAT: 44 G

Chickpea chopped salad

Chickpeas make this a deliciously hearty meal, but this recipe works brilliantly with any legume, so feel free to substitute cannellini or borlotti (cranberry) beans, or even lentils! Whatever you have on hand in your pantry will work in this simple salad.

- 150 g (5½ oz) tinned chickpeas (garbanzo beans), drained and rinsed
- 1 small short cucumber, diced
- ¼ green bell pepper (capsicum), diced
- ¼ red onion, finely sliced
- 80 g (2¾ oz) grape (baby plum) tomatoes
- 60 g (2 oz) feta, crumbled
- handful of parsley, finely chopped

OREGANO & PAPRIKA DRESSING

- juice of ½ lemon
- pinch of dried oregano
- pinch of smoked paprika
- 2 tablespoons extra virgin olive oil

1. Place the salad ingredients in a bowl and toss lightly.
2. Combine the dressing ingredients in a small bowl, then season to taste with salt and pepper.
3. Pour the dressing over the salad just before serving and toss well to coat.

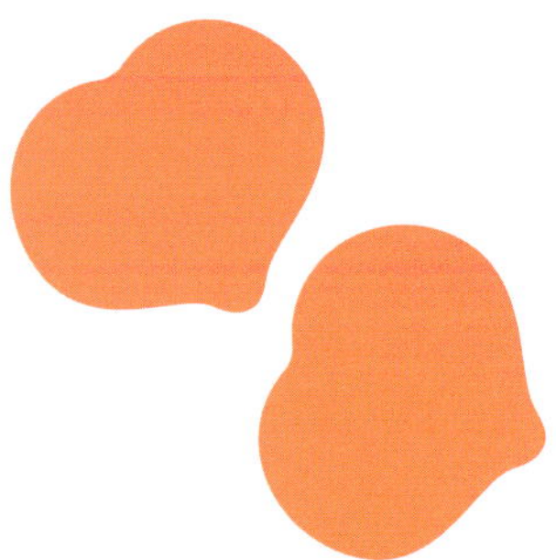

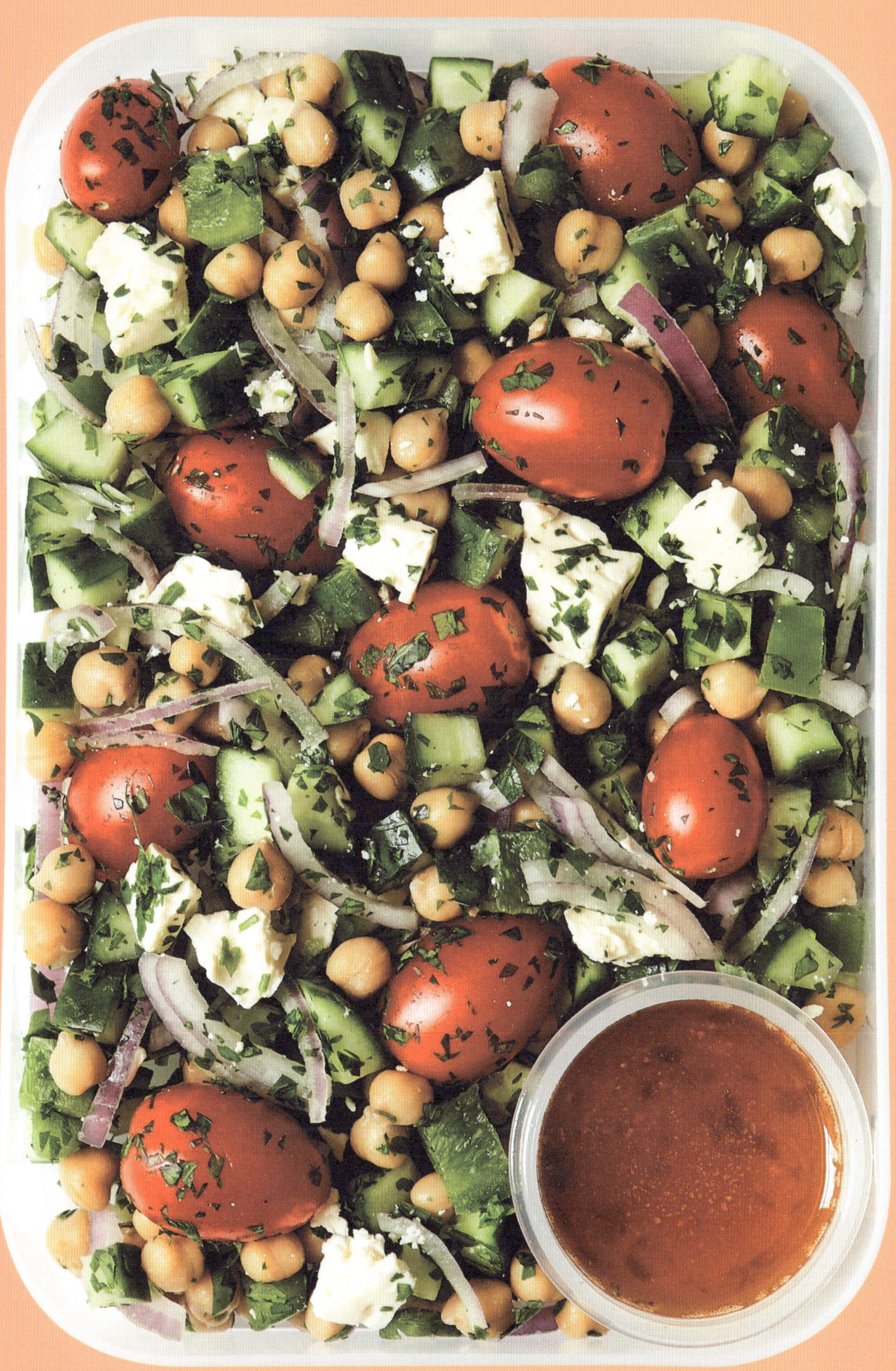

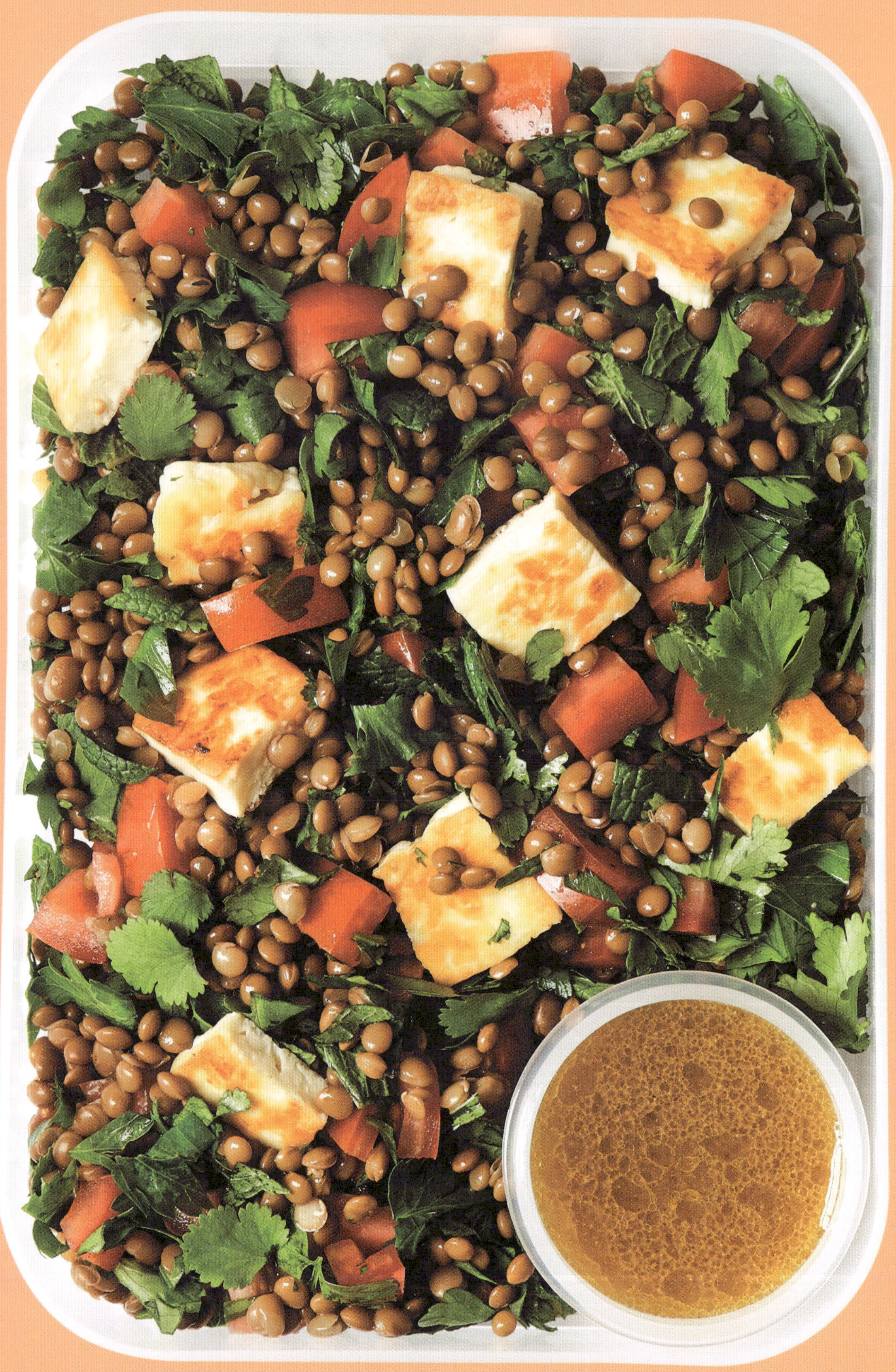

PROTEIN: 26 G NET CARBS: 28 G FAT: 42 G

Lentil, haloumi & herb salad

Seared haloumi adds a savoury chew that works well with lentils and lots of herbs. Short on time? Scoops of cottage cheese makes a no-cook high-protein alternative that still feels substantial. If you prefer a bit more flavour, you could crumble over fresh goat's cheese or feta instead.

- 50 g (1¾ oz) haloumi, sliced
- 1 teaspoon olive oil
- 150 g (⅔ cup) tinned brown lentils, drained and rinsed
- 1 tomato, diced
- handful each of mint, parsley and coriander (cilantro) leaves, chopped

LEMON & CUMIN DRESSING

- juice of ½ lemon
- 1 teaspoon ground cumin
- 2 tablespoons extra virgin olive oil

1. Fry the haloumi in the olive oil for 1–2 minutes on each side until golden, then cut into cubes.
2. Place the salad ingredients in a bowl and toss lightly.
3. Combine the dressing ingredients in a small bowl, then season to taste with salt and pepper.
4. Pour the dressing over the salad just before serving and toss well to coat.

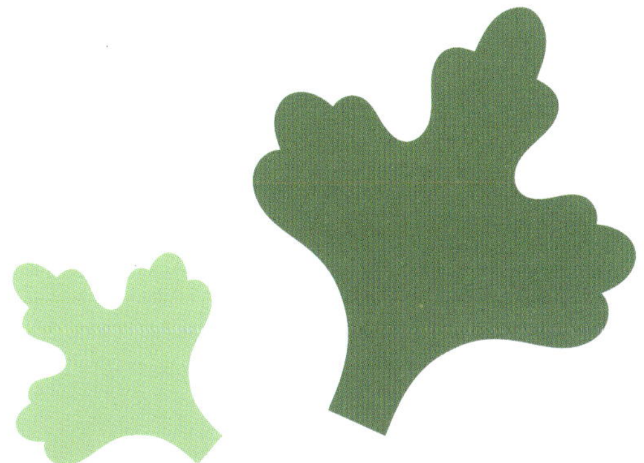

PROTEIN: 26 G NET CARBS: 34 G FAT: 43 G

Lentil, zucchini & mint salad

Lentils give body to delicate zucchini ribbons. A handful of seeds – sunflower or pumpkin seeds – adds texture and extra staying power, while mint keeps things fresh. You can try goat's cheese in this recipe instead of the feta. You can also mix up the herbs and use whatever you have in your fridge.

- 1 zucchini (courgette), cut into ribbons using a vegetable peeler
- juice of ½ lemon
- pinch of salt
- 150 g (5½ oz) tinned brown lentils, drained and rinsed
- large handful of mint leaves, larger leaves chopped
- small handful of parsley, chopped
- 30 g (1 oz) feta, crumbled
- 2 tablespoons seeds, such as sunflower seeds and pumpkin seeds

LEMON DRESSING

- zest and juice of ½ lemon
- 1 teaspoon white wine vinegar
- 2 tablespoons extra virgin olive oil

1. Combine the zucchini, lemon juice and salt in a bowl. Use your hands to massage the lemon juice into the zucchini. Add the remaining salad ingredients and toss lightly.
2. Combine the dressing ingredients in a small bowl, then season to taste with salt and pepper.
3. Pour the dressing over the salad just before serving and toss well to coat.

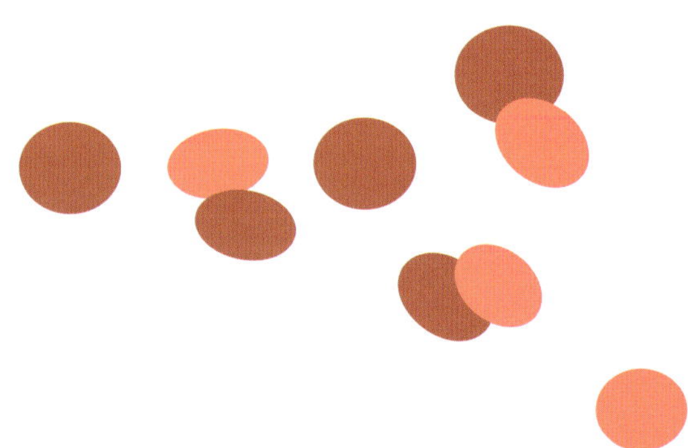

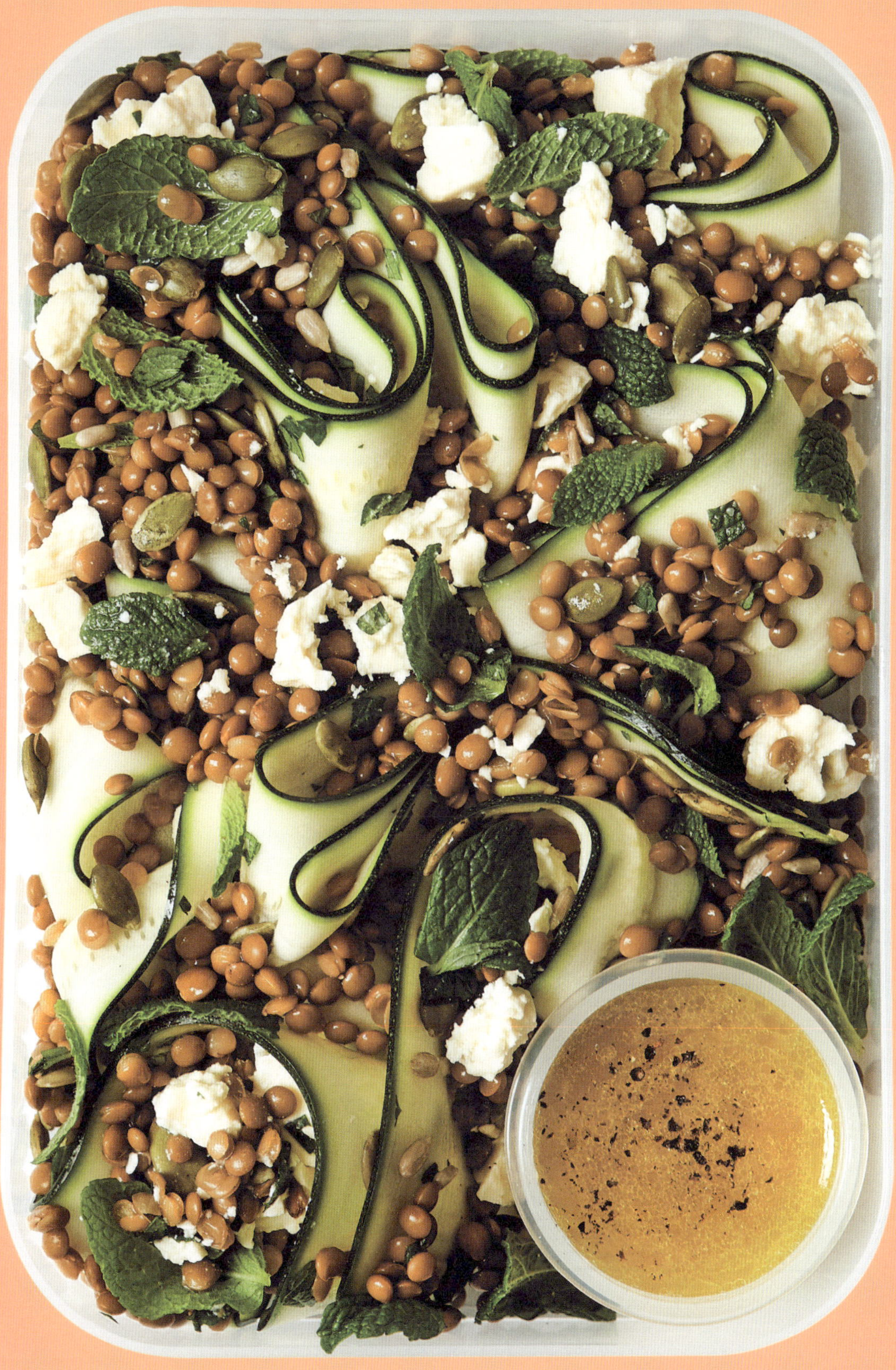

PROTEIN: 29 G NET CARBS: 12 G FAT: 61 G

Grilled haloumi & broccolini salad

Haloumi is a salty cheese that has a high melting point, which makes it perfect for grilling or frying. It's also full of protein and a good source of fat, making it a great way to bulk out a meal. Feel free to replace it with feta for a quicker no-cook option.

- 100 g (3½ oz) haloumi, sliced
- 1 tablespoon olive oil
- 100 g (3½ oz) broccolini florets, blanched and cooled
- 30 g (1 cup) rocket (arugula) leaves
- 2 tablespoons pomegranate seeds
- 1 tablespoon dukkah

CREAMY LEMON & SHALLOT VINAIGRETTE

- 1 tablespoon lemon juice
- 1 tablespoon extra virgin olive oil
- 1 tablespoon dijonnaise
- 2 teaspoons chopped shallot

1. Fry the haloumi in the olive oil for 1–2 minutes on each side, until golden.
2. Place the remaining salad ingredients together in a bowl, toss lightly and top with the haloumi.
3. Combine the vinaigrette ingredients in a small bowl and season to taste with salt and pepper.
4. Pour the vinaigrette over the salad just before serving and toss well to coat.

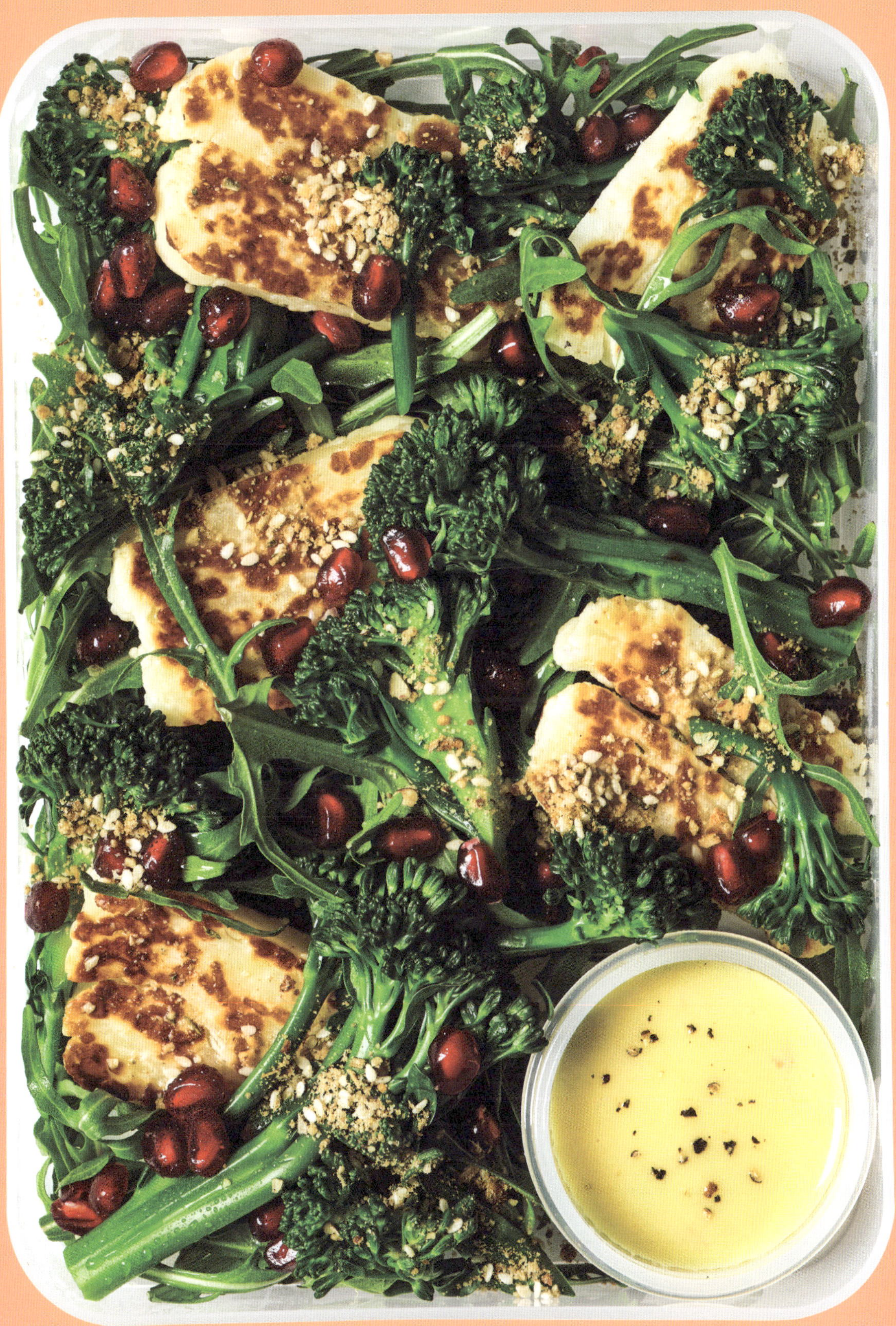

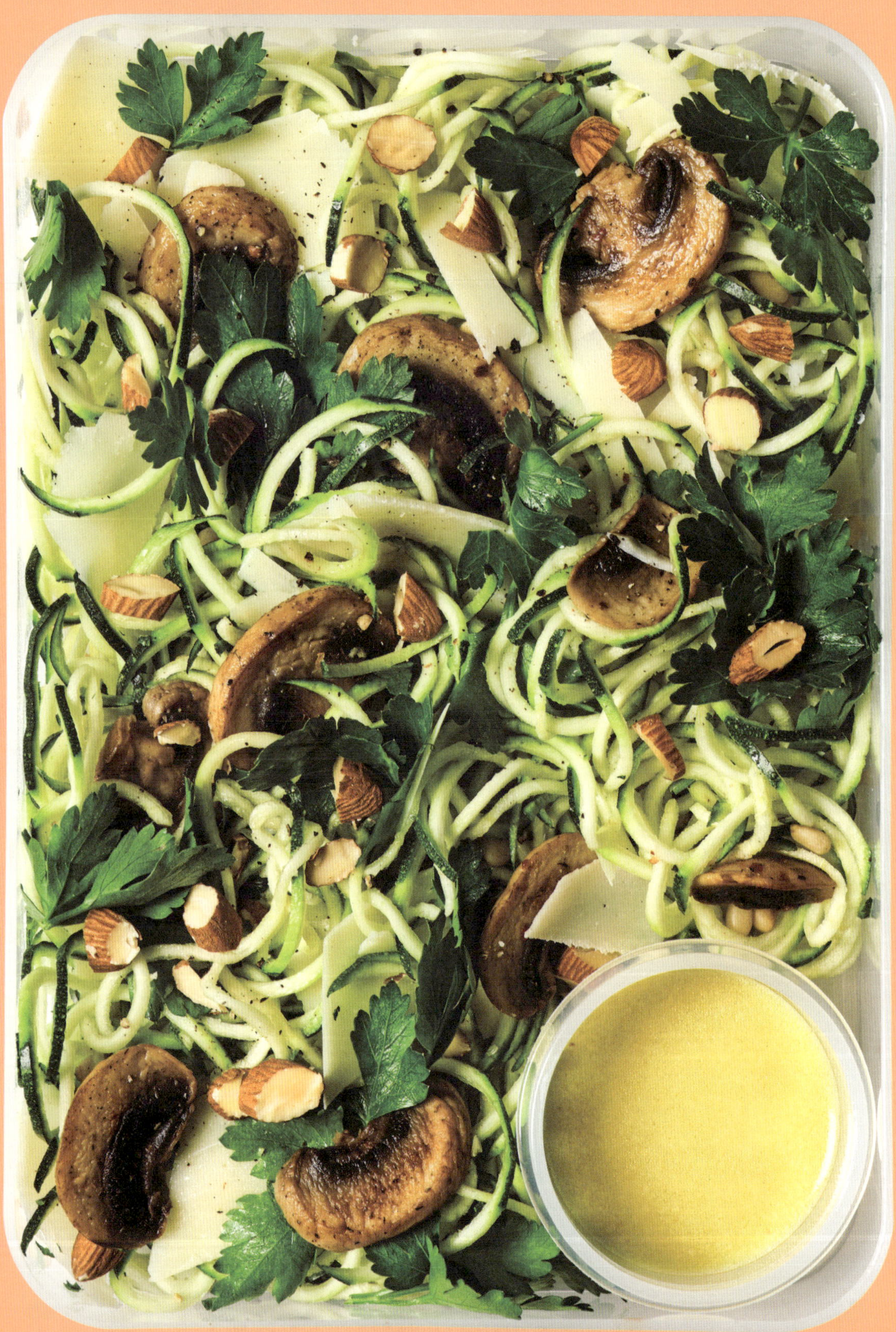

PROTEIN: 30 G NET CARBS: 10 G FAT: 51 G

Zucchini salad with parmesan & mushrooms

Zoodles are a light base, so the parmesan and mushrooms step in to provide richness and bite. Finish with toasted nuts for texture – a small handful goes a long way.

- 1 tablespoon salted butter
- 40 g (1½ oz) button mushrooms, sliced
- pinch of chilli flakes
- 1 zucchini (courgette), spiralised
- 60 g (2 oz) shaved parmesan
- small handful of parsley leaves
- 1 tablespoon toasted pine nuts
- 1 tablespoon toasted chopped almonds

LEMON-MUSTARD VINAIGRETTE

- 1 tablespoon extra virgin olive oil
- 1 tablespoon lemon juice
- 1 teaspoon dijon mustard
- ¼ teaspoon minced garlic

1. Melt the butter in a frying pan and sauté the mushrooms over high heat for about 3 minutes, until golden. Season with chilli flakes, salt and pepper.
2. Place the remaining salad ingredients in a bowl, toss lightly and top with the mushrooms.
3. Combine the vinaigrette ingredients in a small bowl and season to taste with salt and pepper.
4. Pour the vinaigrette over the salad just before serving and toss well to coat.

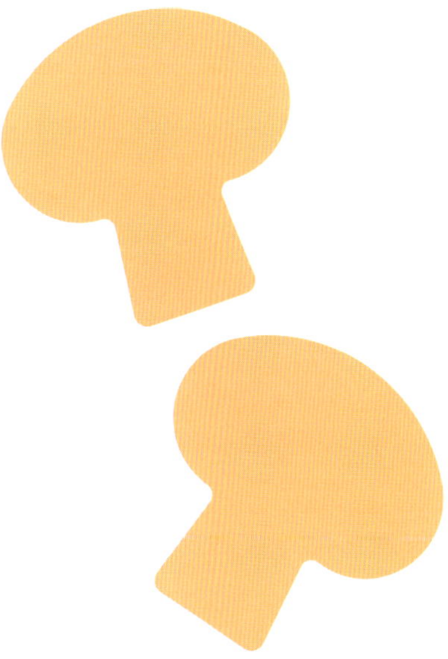

PROTEIN: 33 G NET CARBS: 68 G FAT: 49 G

Goat's cheese, lentil & baby beetroot soba noodles

Pear, goat's cheese and walnuts are a classic French-style combination, often served in a salad along with lettuce. Adding lentils, noodles and beetroot, as we do here, yields a truly hearty meal.

- 180 g (6½ oz) cooked soba noodles, prepared as per packet instructions
- 110 g (4 oz) tinned lentils, drained and rinsed
- 1 baby beetroot (beet), peeled and finely sliced
- ½ nashi pear, finely sliced
- 50 g (1¾ oz) goat's cheese, crumbled
- 25 g (¼ cup) toasted walnuts, chopped

SHALLOT & LEMON VINAIGRETTE

- 5 teaspoons extra virgin olive oil
- 1 tablespoon lemon juice
- 2 teaspoons minced red Asian shallot
- ½ teaspoon dijon mustard

1. Place the salad ingredients in a bowl and toss lightly.
2. Combine the vinaigrette ingredients in a small bowl, then season to taste with salt and pepper.
3. Pour the vinaigrette over the salad just before serving and toss well to coat.

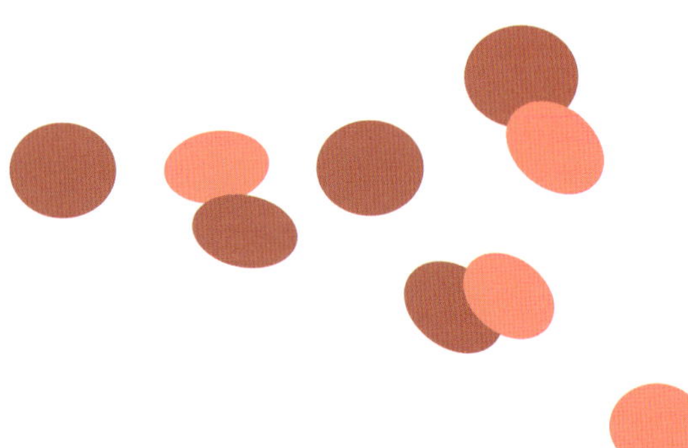

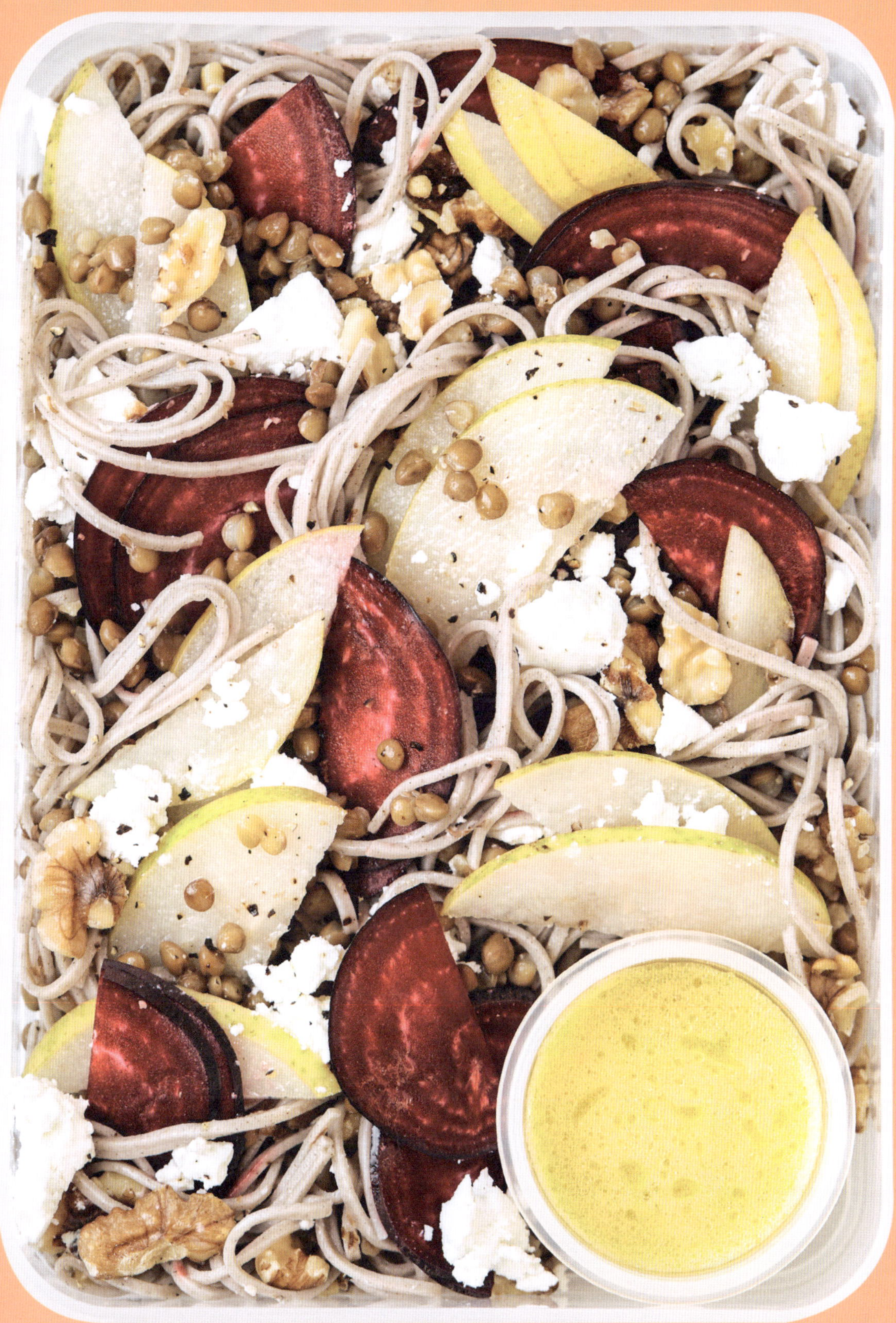

PROTEIN: 27 G   NET CARBS: 17 G   FAT: 26 G

Smoked tofu 'spring roll' salad

Smoked tofu brings depth without extra effort – all you have to do is dice it and toss it through your salad. Paired with shirataki noodles and plenty of herbs, this is a no-fuss way to make a plant-led salad more satisfying.

- 85 g (3 oz) smoked tofu, drained and diced
- 70 g (2½ oz) shirataki noodles, prepared as per packet instructions
- 1 short cucumber, spiralised
- ¼ red bell pepper (capsicum), sliced
- 40 g (¼ cup) grated carrot
- 1 spring onion (scallion), sliced
- small handful of mint leaves
- small handful of coriander (cilantro) leaves

ALMOND BUTTER DRESSING

- 2 tablespoons almond butter
- 2 teaspoons tamari sauce or coconut aminos
- 2 teaspoons lime juice
- ½ teaspoon minced ginger

1. Place the salad ingredients in a bowl and toss lightly.
2. In a small bowl, whisk the dressing ingredients until smooth.
3. Pour the dressing over the salad just before serving and toss well to coat.

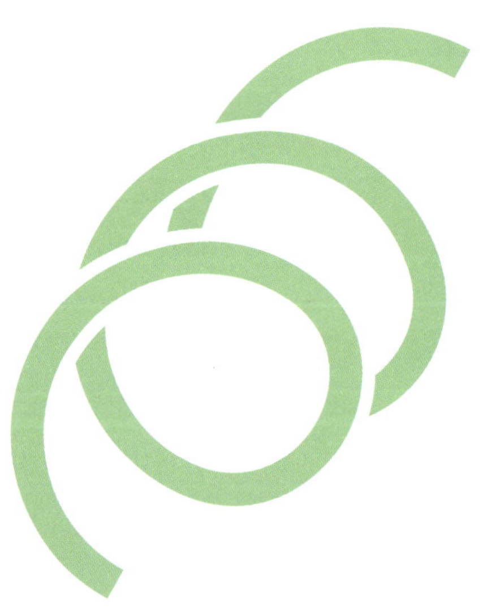

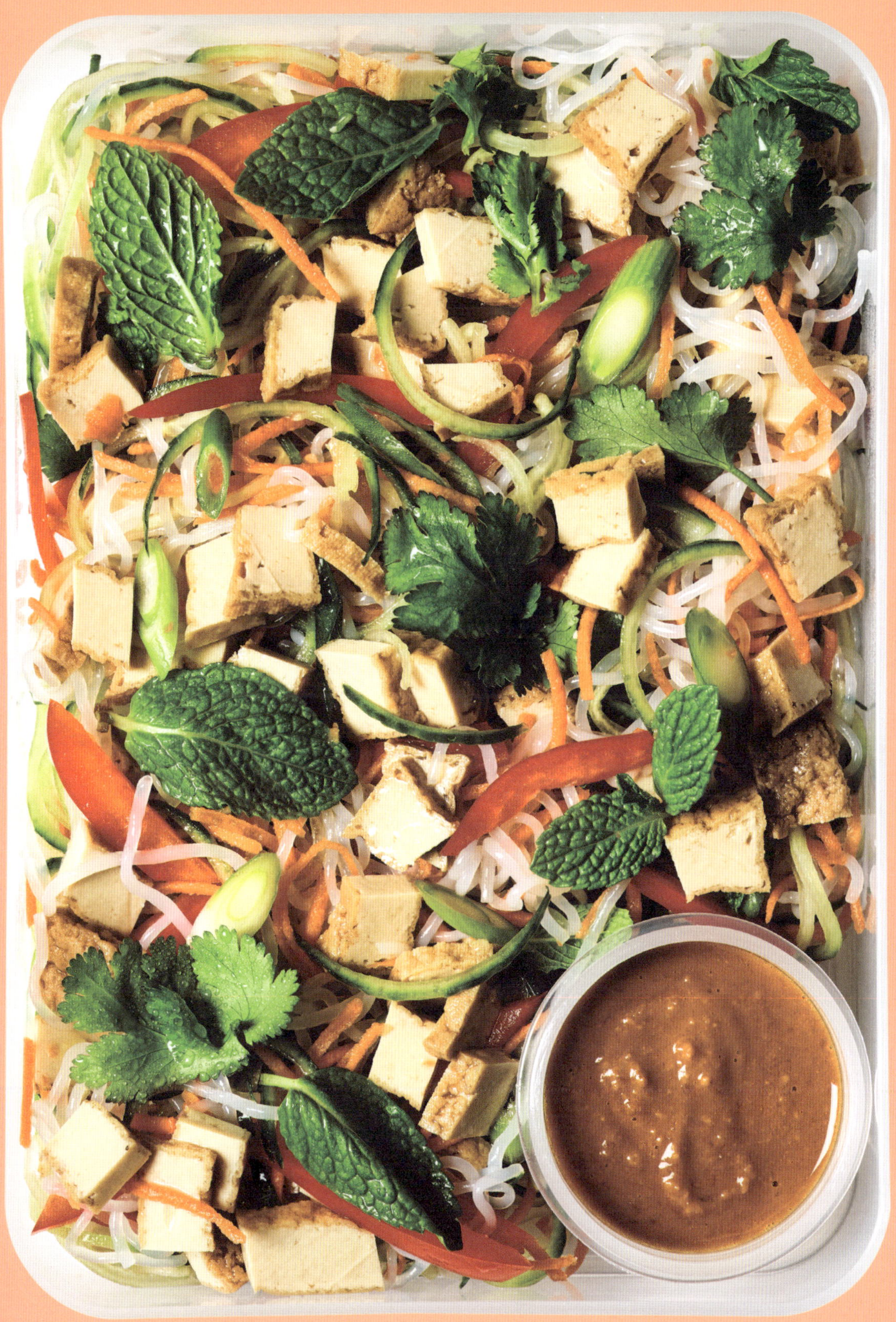

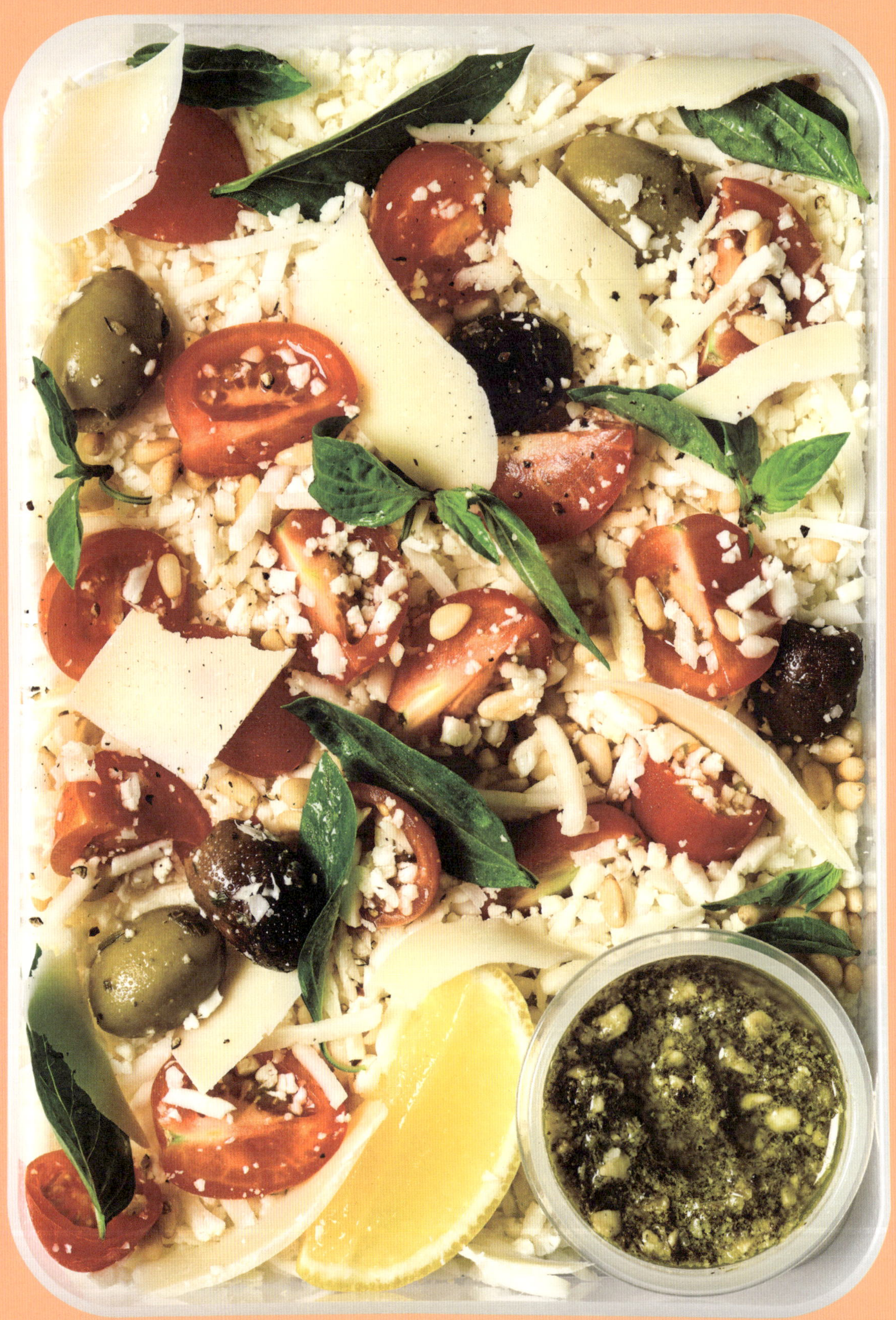

PROTEIN: 26 G NET CARBS: 11 G FAT: 50 G

Italian cauliflower rice salad

Cauliflower rice keeps things light, while parmesan and olives lend a savoury punch. Stirring pesto through the 'rice' is an easy trick to add body without cooking. Cauliflower rice is available ready-made from some supermarkets and greengrocers, or you can easily prepare it yourself. Either grate fresh cauliflower with a box grater or pulse it in a food processor.

- 150 g (1½ cups) cauliflower rice
- 100 g (3½ oz) cherry tomatoes, halved or quartered
- 30 g (¼ cup) marinated pitted olives, halved
- 45 g (1½ oz) shaved parmesan
- 2 tablespoons toasted pine nuts
- small handful of basil leaves
- lemon wedge, to serve

LEMON PESTO DRESSING

- 3 tablespoons store-bought basil pesto
- 1 tablespoon lemon juice

1. Place all the salad ingredients in a bowl, except the lemon wedge, and toss lightly.
2. Combine the dressing ingredients in a small bowl, then season to taste with salt and pepper.
3. Pour the dressing over the salad just before serving and toss well to coat, then squeeze over the lemon.

PROTEIN: 26 G NET CARBS: 46 G FAT: 37 G

Lentil, ricotta & beetroot salad

Lentils form the base, while ricotta adds a gentle creaminess that binds everything together. Use golden or red beetroot – whichever you can find – and finish with a white balsamic dressing.

170 g (6 oz) tinned lentils, drained and rinsed

120 g (4½ oz) raw yellow beetroot (beet), very finely sliced

70 g (2½ oz) ricotta, crumbled

30 g (1 cup) torn radicchio leaves

WHITE BALSAMIC DRESSING

2 tablespoons extra virgin olive oil

1½ tablespoons white balsamic vinegar

1 teaspoon dijon mustard

1 teaspoon honey

1. Place the salad ingredients in a bowl and toss lightly.
2. Combine the dressing ingredients in a small bowl, then season to taste with salt and pepper.
3. Pour the dressing over the salad just before serving and toss well to coat.

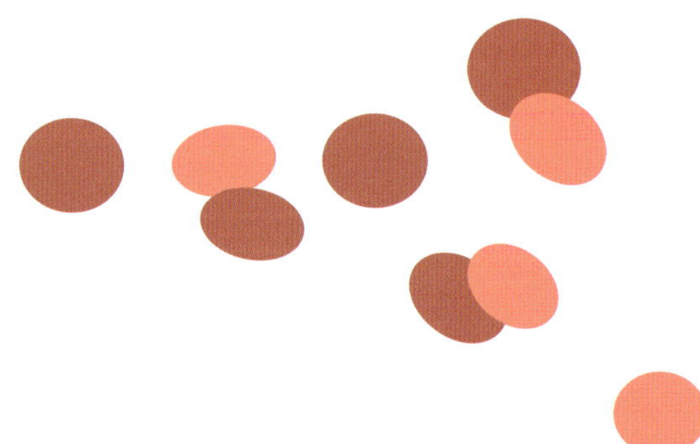

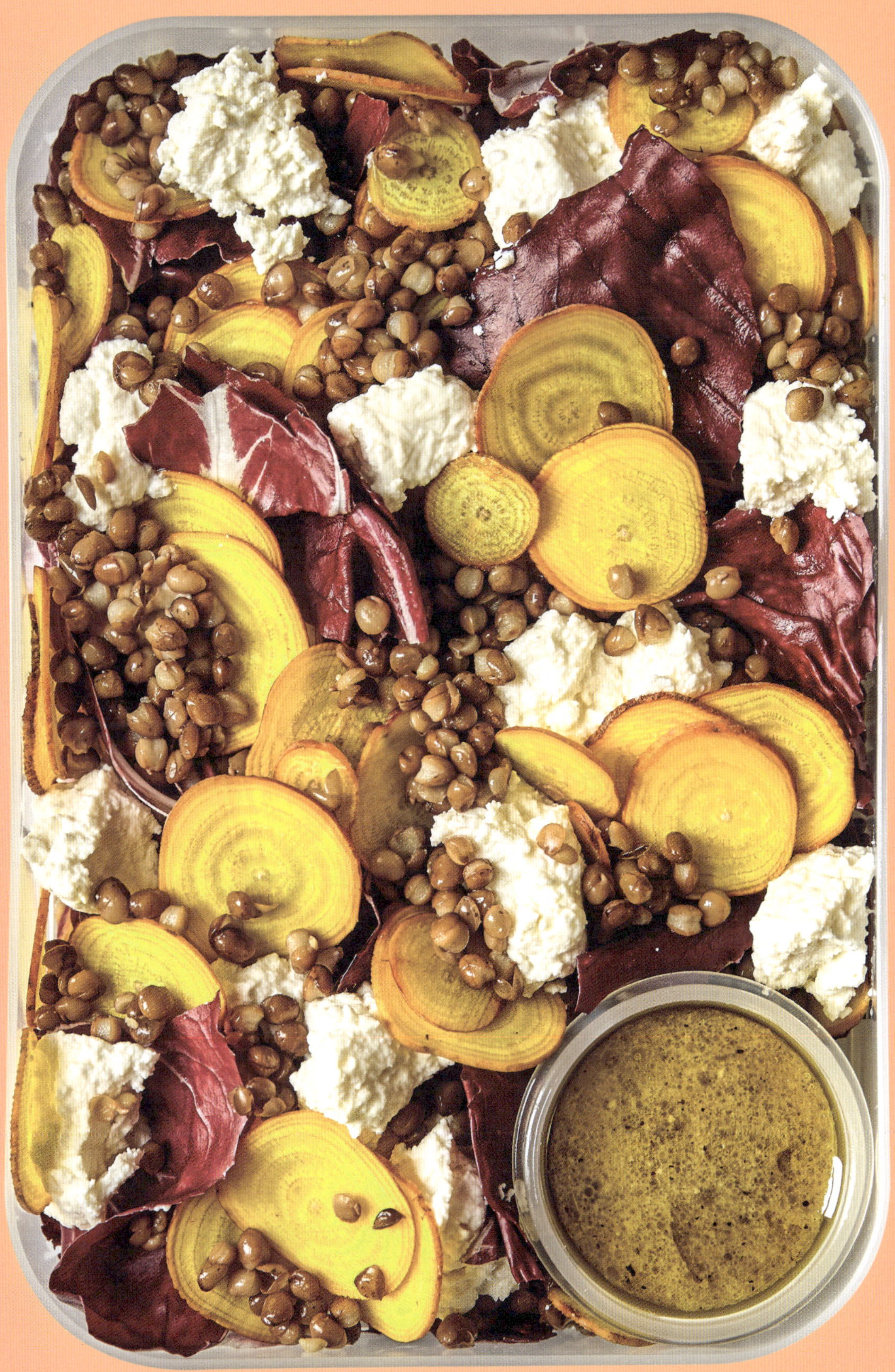

PROTEIN: 25 G NET CARBS: 5 G FAT: 58 G

Veggie chopped salad

A simple mix of chopped vegetables becomes a meal with the addition of egg and blue cheese. If you prefer milder flavours, swap the blue for feta or add avocado to make this salad dairy-free.

1 hard-boiled egg, chopped

1 celery stalk, chopped

3 radishes, chopped

55 g (1½ cups) chopped cos (romaine) lettuce

75 g (2¾ oz) blue cheese, crumbled

1 tablespoon chopped toasted almonds

SHALLOT & MUSTARD VINAIGRETTE

2 tablespoons extra virgin olive oil

1 tablespoon red wine vinegar

2 teaspoons minced shallot

½ teaspoon dijon mustard

1. Place the salad ingredients in a bowl and toss lightly.
2. Combine the vinaigrette ingredients in a small bowl, then season to taste with salt and pepper.
3. Pour the vinaigrette over the salad just before serving and toss well to coat.

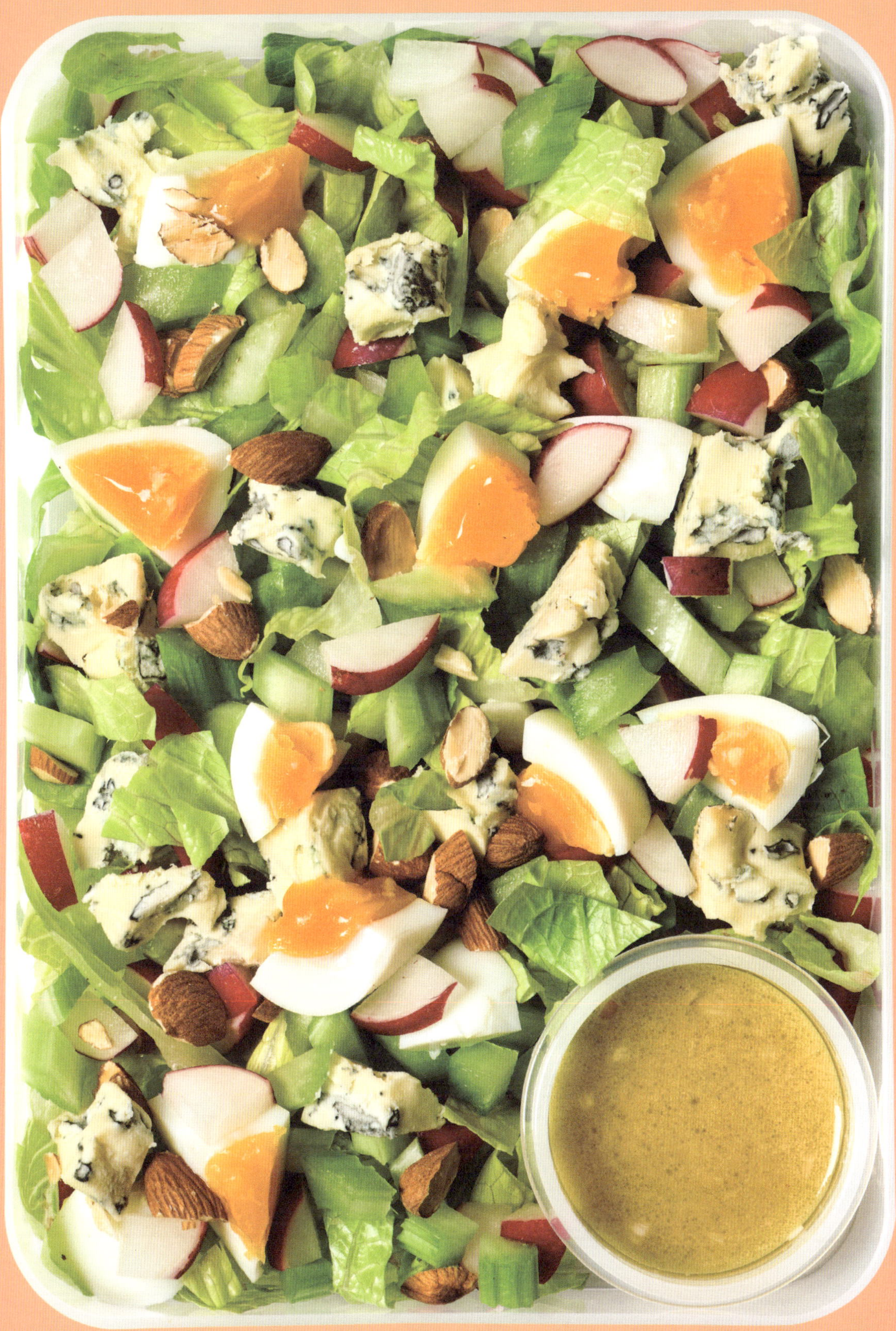

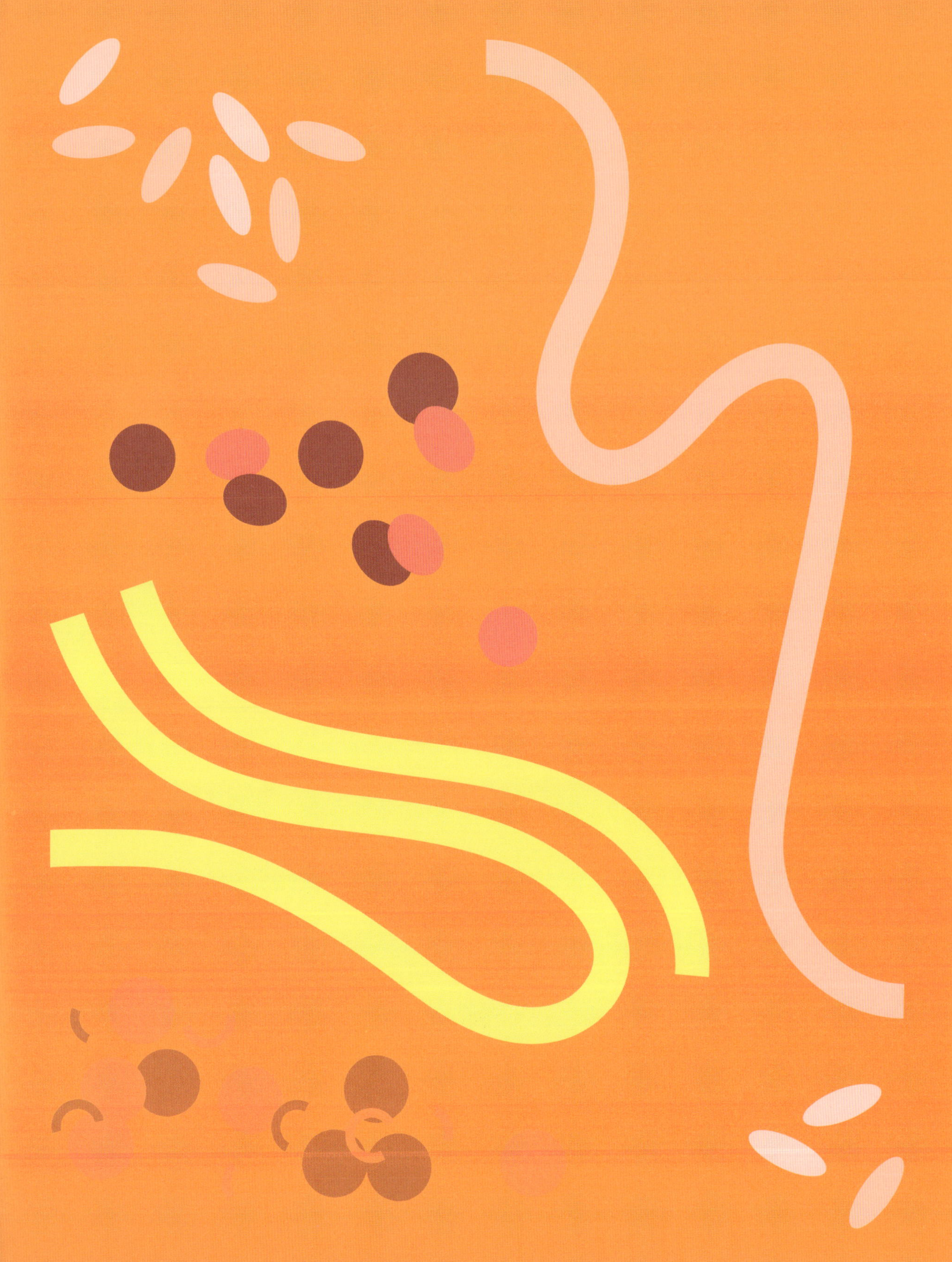

grains &

good carbs

PROTEIN: 43 G NET CARBS: 33 G FAT: 54 G

Chicken & quinoa salad with salsa verde dressing

Quinoa is a complete plant protein, and pairing it with chicken makes this salad especially sustaining. Salsa verde adds brightness and brings a lively flavour to this simple and satiating salad.

- 100 g (⅔ cup) shredded cooked chicken
- 150 g (1 cup) cooked and cooled quinoa
- 1 spring onion (scallion), sliced
- 1 celery stalk, sliced
- ¼ green chilli, finely sliced
- 2 radishes, cut into wedges
- 30 g (1 oz) toasted pine nuts

SALSA VERDE DRESSING

- small handful each of basil, mint and parsley, very finely chopped
- ½ teaspoon minced garlic
- 1 tablespoon white wine vinegar
- 2 tablespoons extra virgin olive oil

1. Place the salad ingredients in a bowl and toss lightly.
2. Combine the dressing ingredients in a small bowl, then season to taste with salt and pepper.
3. Pour the dressing over the salad just before serving and toss well to coat.

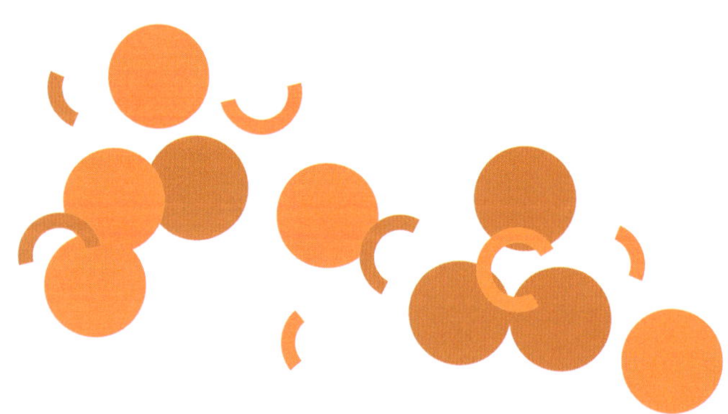

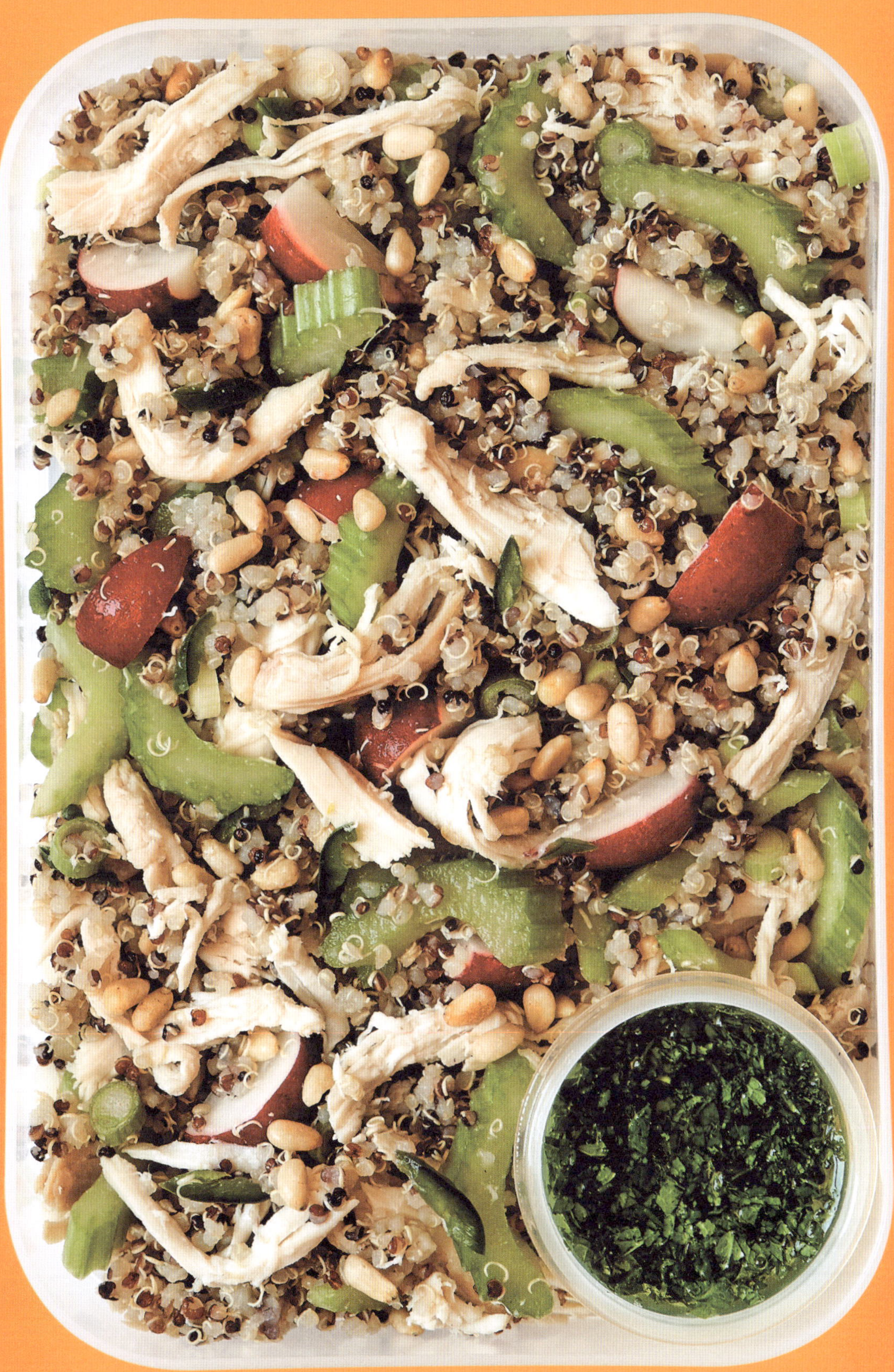

PROTEIN: 49 G NET CARBS: 123 G FAT: 29 G

Salmon poke bowl with black rice

Black rice is rich and nutty, and the salmon provides a clean-tasting protein hit. Avocado and edamame beans balance the bowl with creaminess and crunch.

- 150 g (5½ oz) cooked and cooled black rice
- 100 g (3½ oz) raw sashimi-grade salmon, diced
- ½ avocado, diced
- 75 g (½ cup) podded edamame beans (soybeans), blanched

SWEET CHILLI-SOY DRESSING

- 1½ tablespoons soy sauce or tamari
- 1½ tablespoons sweet chilli sauce
- 2 teaspoons rice vinegar
- 1 teaspoon toasted sesame oil
- 1 spring onion (scallion), finely sliced

1. Place the salad ingredients in a bowl and toss lightly.
2. Combine the dressing ingredients in a small bowl.
3. Pour the dressing over the salad just before serving and toss well to coat.

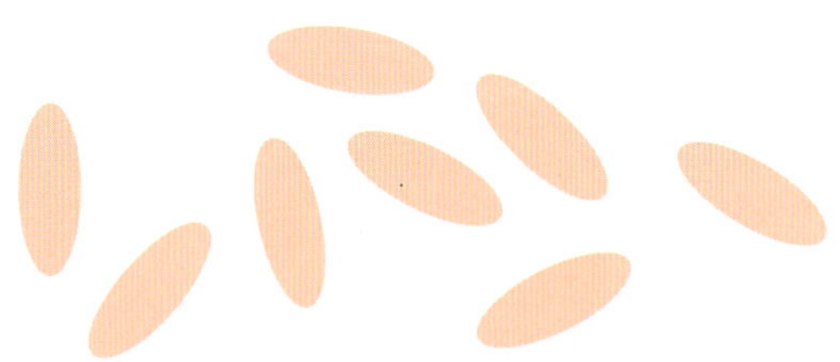

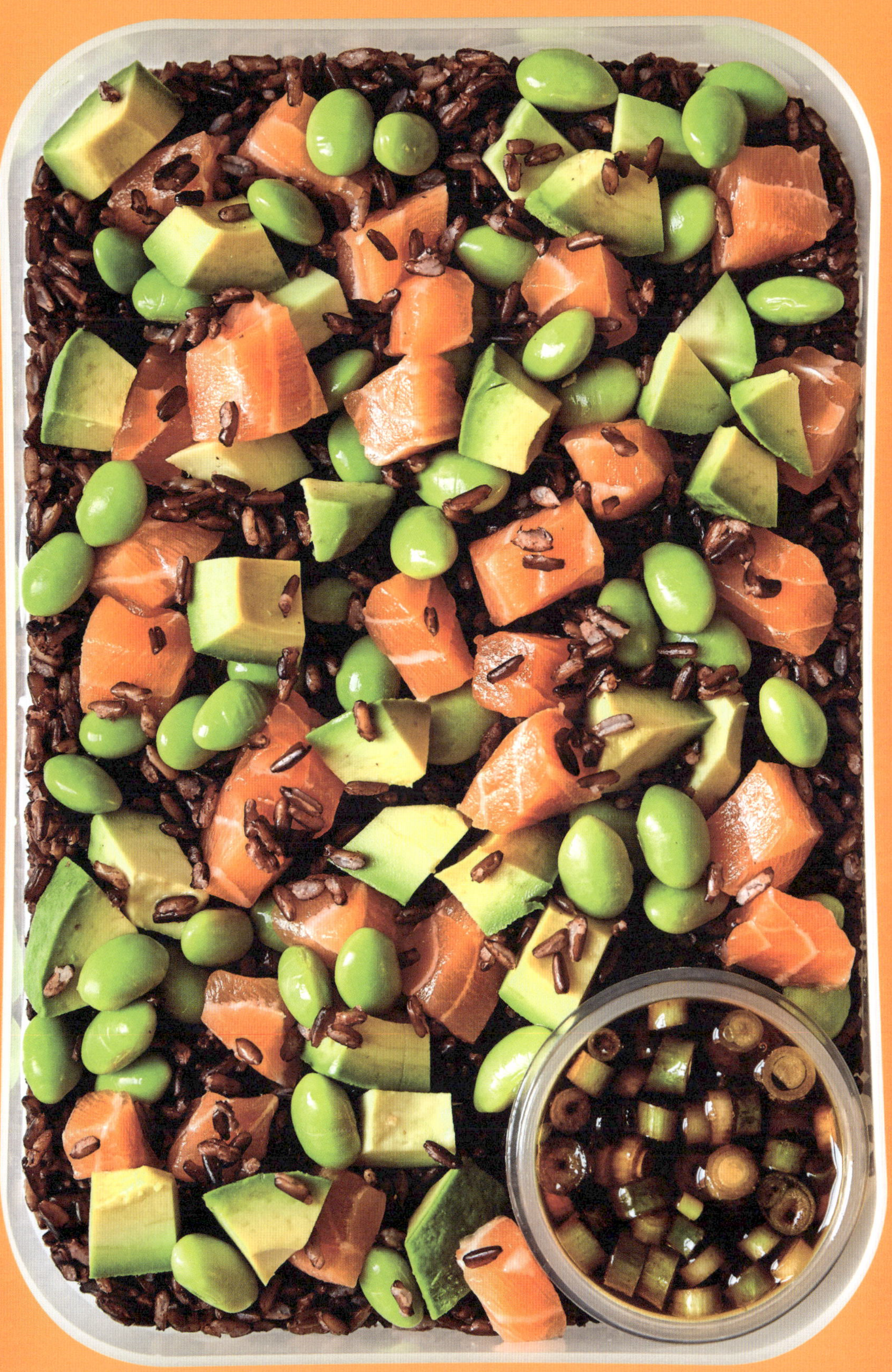

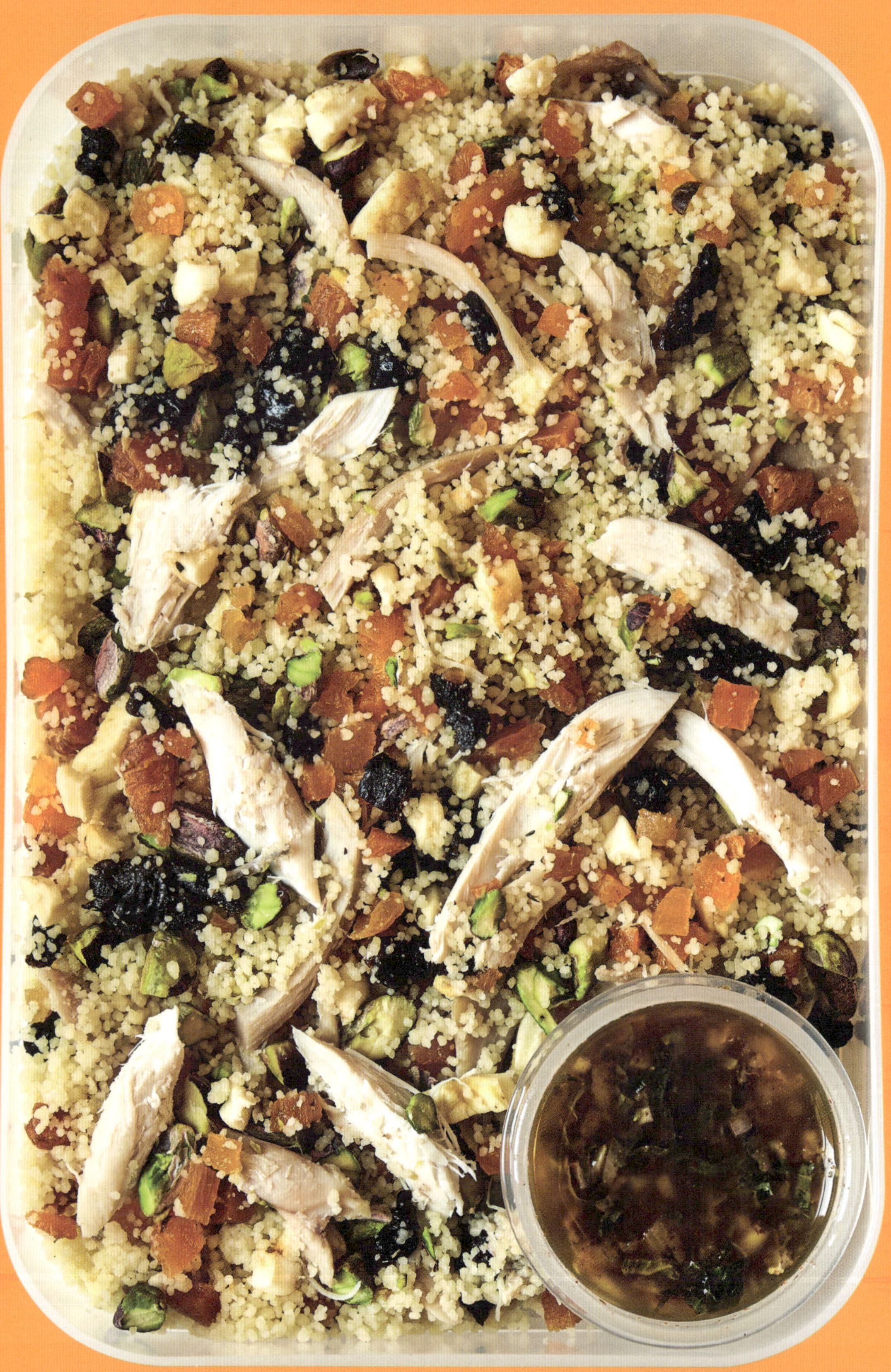

PROTEIN: 41 G NET CARBS: 90 G FAT: 38 G

Chicken & couscous salad with pistachio

The lean chicken and nutty pistachios in this recipe provide plenty of protein, all wrapped up with fruity pops and a bright lemony flavour.

- 150 g (1 cup) cooked and cooled couscous
- 100 g (⅔ cup) shredded cooked chicken
- 70 g (2½ oz) diced mixed dried fruits, such as apricot, cherries and figs
- 2 tablespoons chopped pistachios

LEMON & SUMAC DRESSING

- 2 tablespoons extra virgin olive oil
- zest and juice of ½ lemon
- 1 tablespoon finely diced shallot
- 2 teaspoons chopped mint leaves
- ½ teaspoon ground sumac

1. Place the salad ingredients in a bowl and toss lightly.
2. Combine the dressing ingredients in a small bowl, then season to taste with salt and pepper.
3. Pour the dressing over the salad just before serving and toss well to coat.

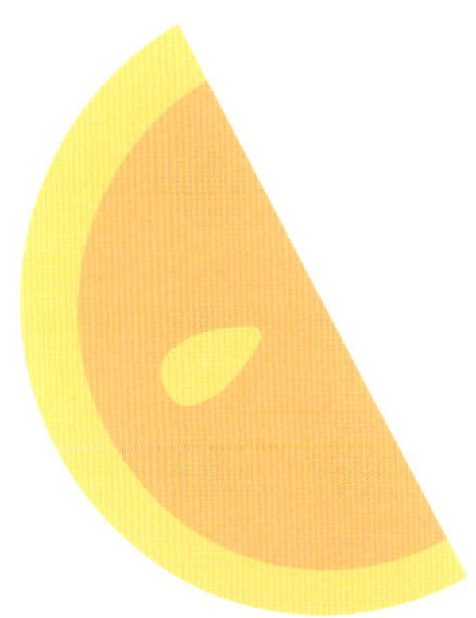

PROTEIN: 44 G NET CARBS: 30 G FAT: 60 G

Chicken & peach burghul salad with maple dressing

Burghul provides a tender base, while juicy peaches and grilled chicken keep this bowl both fresh and filling. A maple–mustard dressing ties all the elements together.

- 45 g (¼ cup) burghul
- 60 ml (¼ cup) just-boiled chicken stock or water
- 1 ripe peach, sliced into wedges
- 1 teaspoon lime juice
- 100 g (⅔ cup) shredded cooked chicken
- 30 g (1 oz) feta, crumbled
- small handful of basil leaves
- 30 g (¼ cup) chopped toasted pecans

MAPLE-MUSTARD DRESSING

- 1½ teaspoons pure maple syrup
- 1 tablespoon apple cider vinegar
- 1 teaspoon dijon mustard
- 2 tablespoons extra virgin olive oil

1. Place the burghul in a jar or heatproof container with a tight-fitting lid. Pour in the stock or water and cover with the lid.
2. Place the peach in a bowl and gently toss in the lime juice. Add the remaining salad ingredients, except the pecans, and toss lightly.
3. Combine the dressing ingredients in a small bowl, then season to taste with salt and pepper.
4. Before serving, fluff the burghul with a fork and add to the salad along with the pecans and the dressing. Toss well to coat.

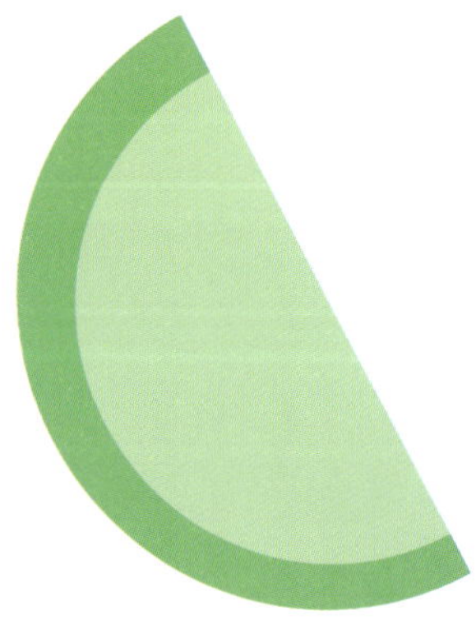

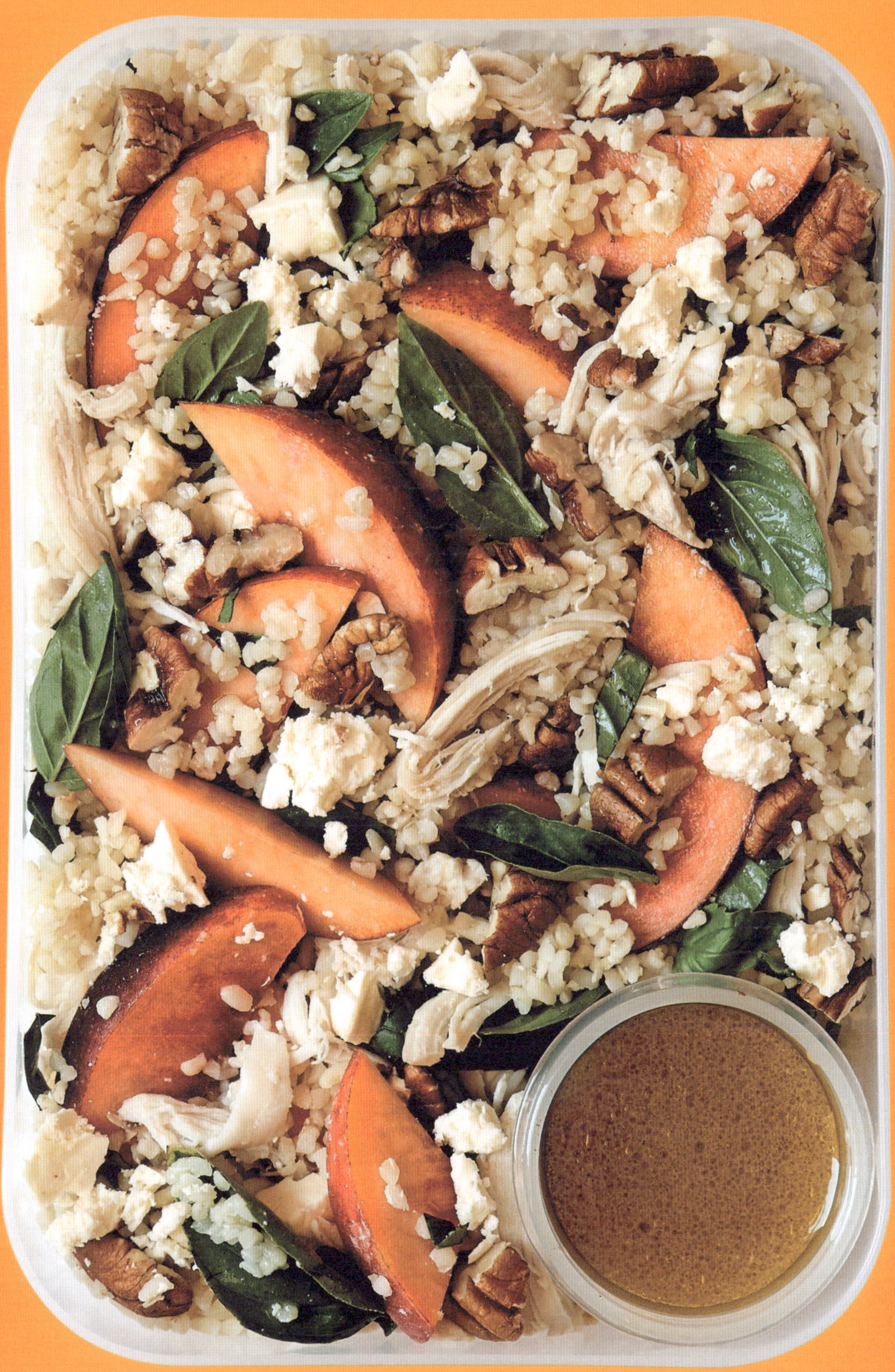

PROTEIN: 51 G NET CARBS: 53 G FAT: 53 G

Chicken & couscous salad with pomegranate & feta

Tiny couscous grains soak up the flavours of chicken, feta and herbs. This recipe calls for frozen pomegranate seeds for the sake of convenience, but you can definitely use fresh seeds if you have them. To save some prep time, remove the seeds from the pomegranate and store in the fridge in an airtight container for up to 3 days.

- 150 g (1 cup) cooked and cooled couscous
- 100 g (2/3 cup) shredded cooked chicken
- 90 g (3 oz) frozen pomegranate seeds
- 30 g (1/4 cup) slivered almonds
- 30 g (1 oz) feta, crumbled
- small handful of mint leaves, chopped
- small handful of parsley leaves, chopped

POMEGRANATE DRESSING

- 1 tablespoon red wine vinegar
- 1 teaspoon pomegranate molasses
- 2 tablespoons extra virgin olive oil

1. Place the salad ingredients in a bowl and toss lightly.
2. Combine the dressing ingredients in a small bowl, then season to taste with salt and pepper.
3. Pour the dressing over the salad just before serving and toss well to coat.

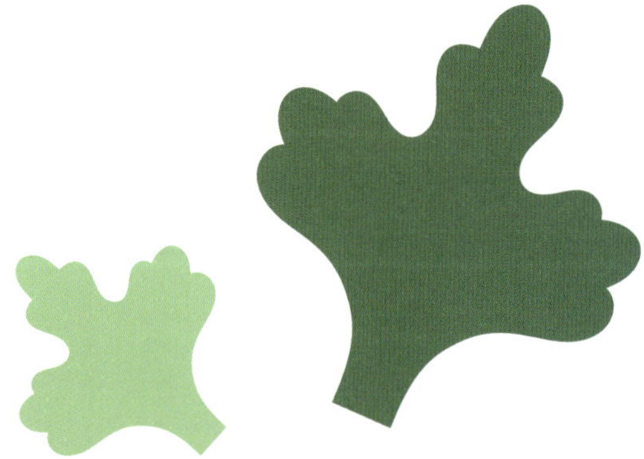

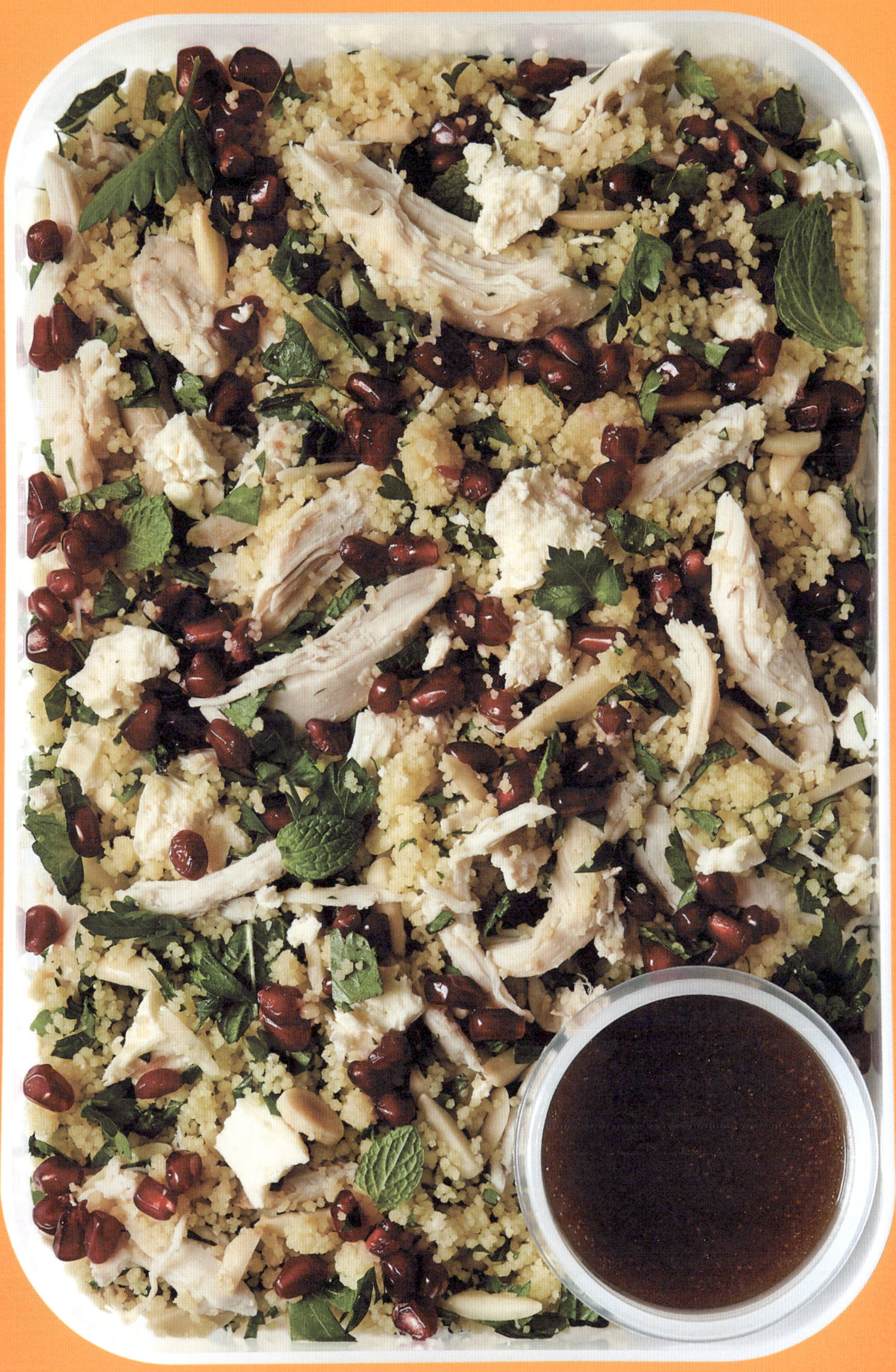

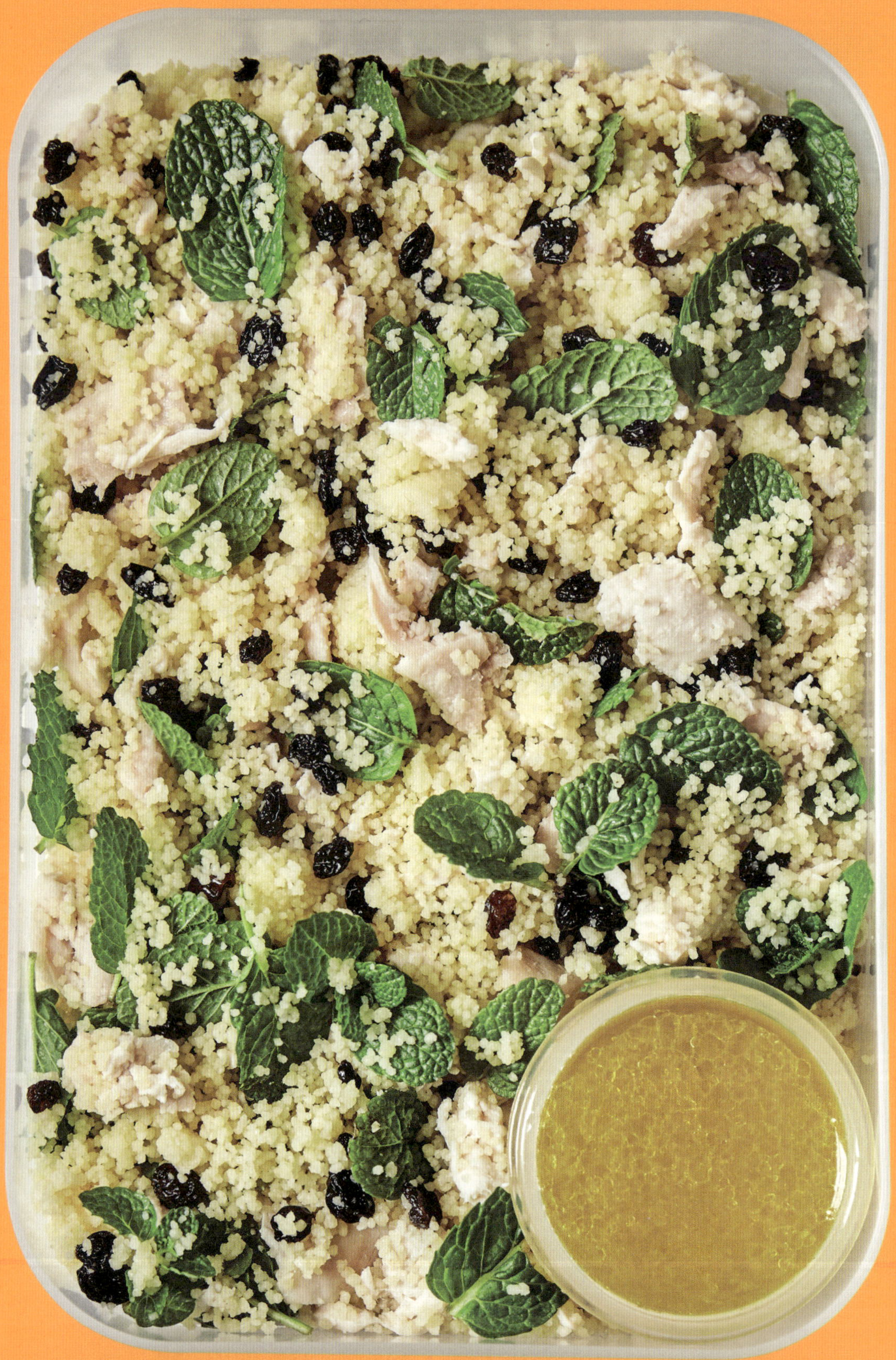

PROTEIN: 39 G NET CARBS: 55 G FAT: 31 G

Chicken, mint & couscous salad

A simple combination of chicken and couscous is lifted with plenty of mint and lemon. It's proof that a small portion of meat plus a grain can form a balanced meal.

150 g (1 cup) cooked and cooled couscous

100 g (⅔ cup) shredded cooked chicken

large handful of roughly torn mint leaves

3 tablespoons currants

LEMON DRESSING

2 tablespoons extra virgin olive oil

juice of ½ lemon

1. Place the salad ingredients in a bowl and toss lightly.
2. Combine the dressing ingredients in a small bowl, then season to taste with salt and pepper.
3. Pour the dressing over the salad just before serving and toss well to coat.

PROTEIN: 53 G NET CARBS: 76 G FAT: 51 G

Gochujang, corn & chicken soba noodle salad

Soba noodles offer slow-release energy, and chicken adds even more protein power. The tangy chilli oil dressing ties together the noodles, corn and greens into a punchy dish.

- 1 tablespoon salted butter
- 1–1½ teaspoons chilli crisp oil
- 1 teaspoon gochujang paste
- 100 g (⅔ cup) tinned sweet corn kernels, drained and rinsed
- 180 g (6½ oz) cooked soba noodles, prepared as per packet instructions
- 100 g (⅔ cup) shredded cooked chicken
- 40 g (1½ oz) feta, crumbled
- 2 tablespoons crispy fried shallots
- handful of coriander (cilantro) leaves

SESAME & LIME DRESSING

- 4 teaspoons lime juice
- 2 teaspoons toasted sesame oil
- ½ teaspoon chilli oil
- ½ teaspoon sesame seeds

1. Place a frying pan over medium heat. Add the butter, chilli crisp oil, gochujang paste and corn and sauté for about 3 minutes. Season to taste with salt and pepper.
2. Add the drained noodles to a bowl. Toss the chilli corn through, along with the remaining salad ingredients.
3. Combine the dressing ingredients in a small bowl.
4. Pour the dressing over the salad just before serving and toss well to coat.

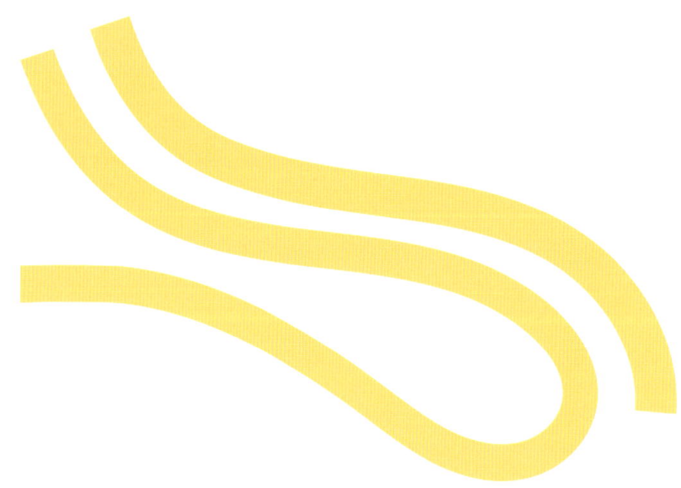

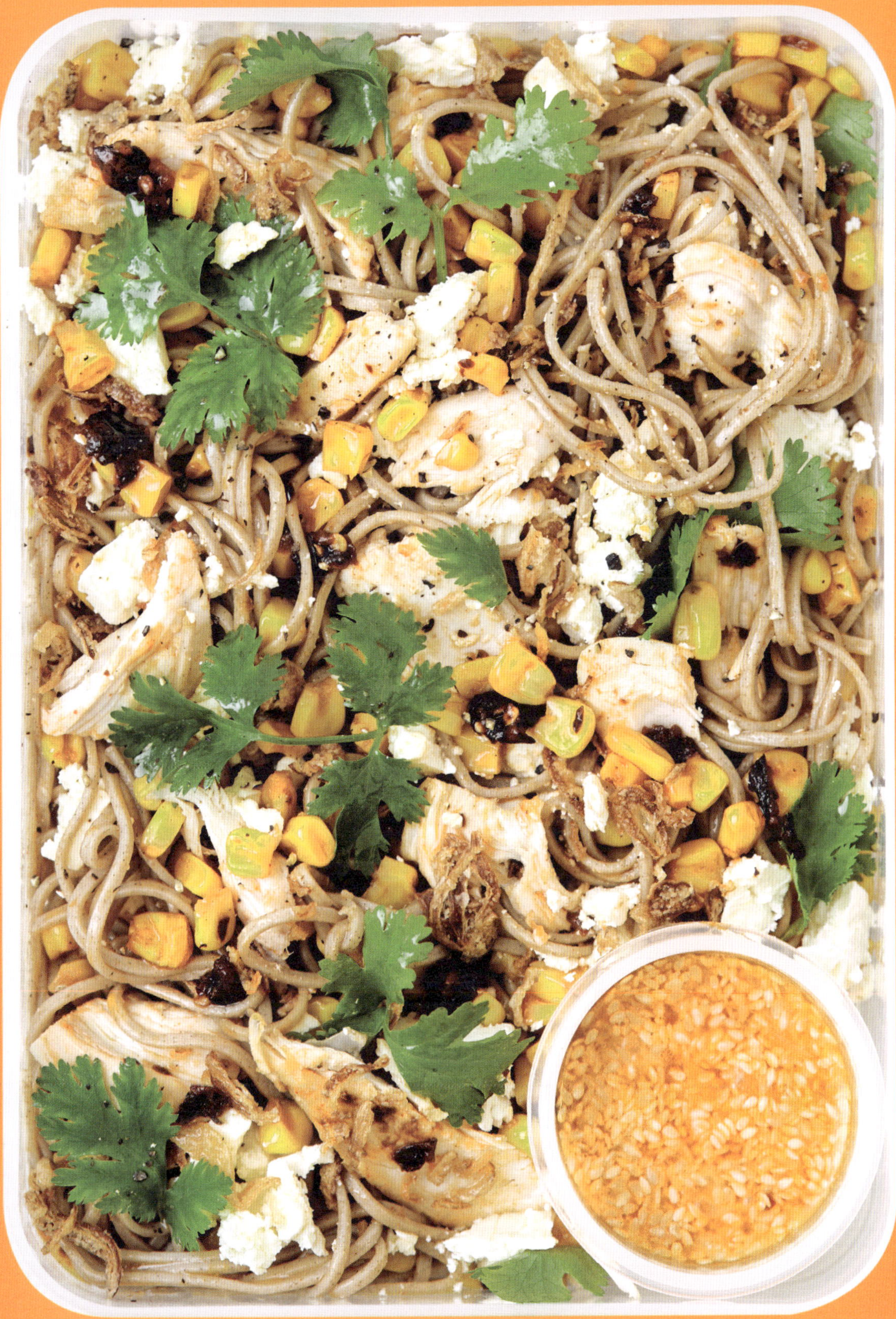

PROTEIN: 44 G NET CARBS: 41 G FAT: 21 G

Chicken soba noodle salad with sesame dressing

Soba noodles and shredded chicken are a classic pairing – both light yet filling. The dressing on this salad is a lighter take on the wildly popular sesame-infused Japanese condiment known as goma, usually made with mayonnaise. You can, of course, add some kewpie mayo – just thin it out with a little water and add a little less sugar, as kewpie is quite sweet.

- 180 g (6½ oz) cooked soba noodles, prepared as per packet instructions
- sesame oil, for drizzling
- 100 g (⅔ cup) shredded cooked chicken
- 1 spring onion (scallion), finely sliced
- 50 g (1¾ oz) snow peas (mangetout), sliced
- 60 g (2 oz) shredded carrot

SESAME DRESSING

- 1 tablespoon toasted sesame seeds
- 1 tablespoon rice vinegar
- 1 tablespoon light soy sauce
- ¾ teaspoon caster (superfine) sugar
- 2 teaspoons sesame oil

1. Toss the soba noodles with a little sesame oil. Add the remaining salad ingredients and toss lightly.
2. Combine the dressing ingredients in a small bowl.
3. Pour the dressing over the salad just before serving and toss well to coat.

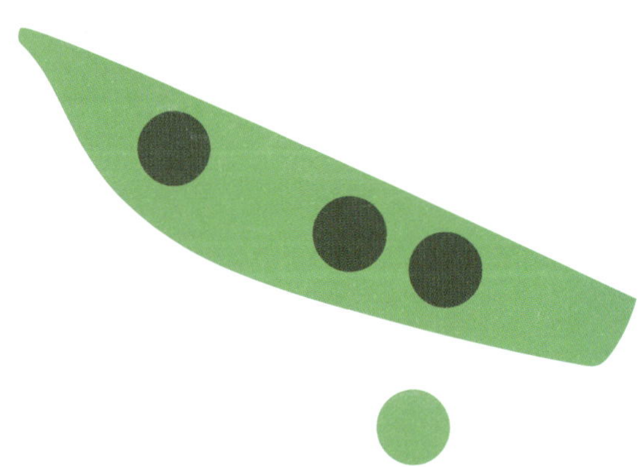

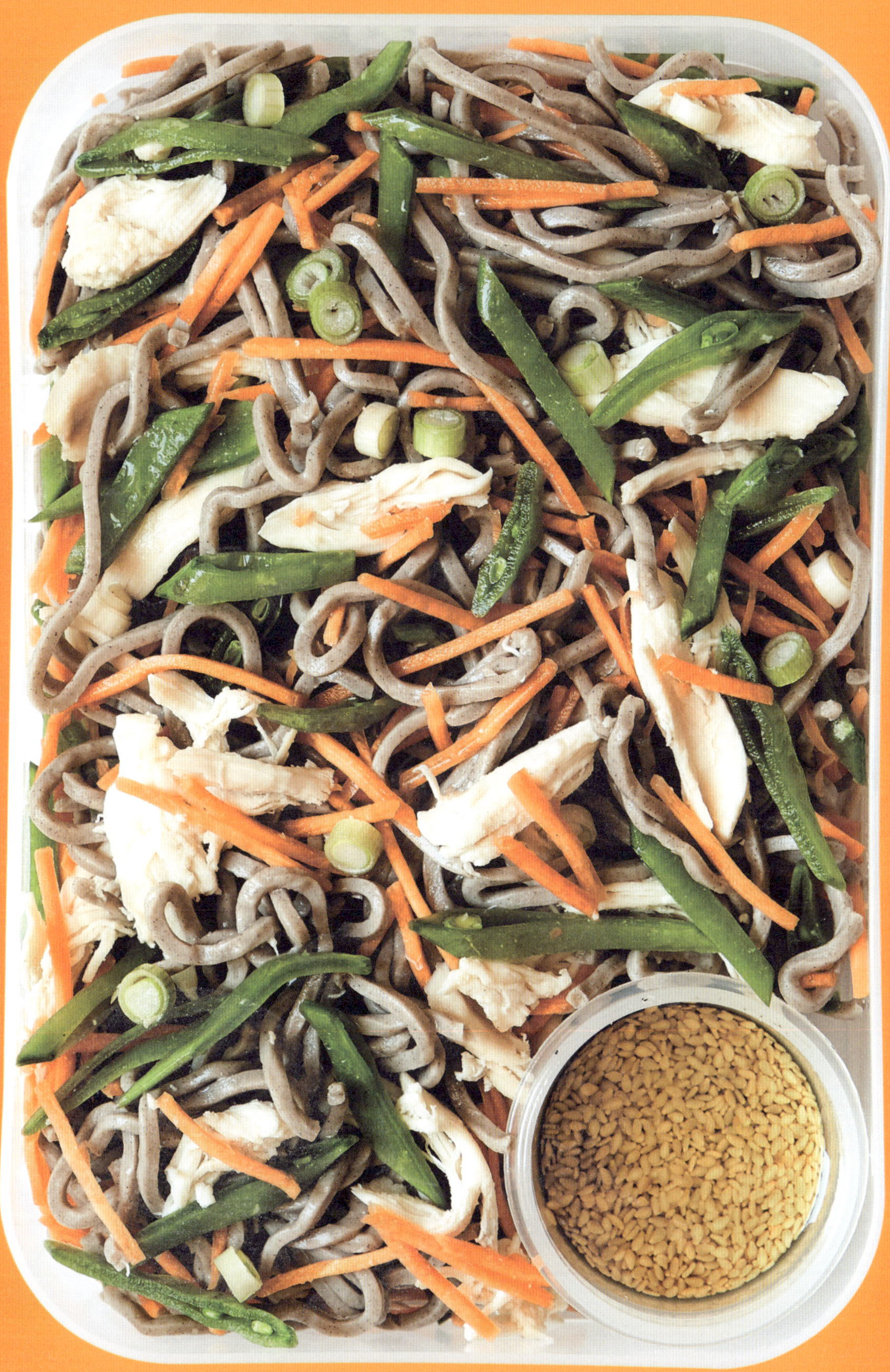

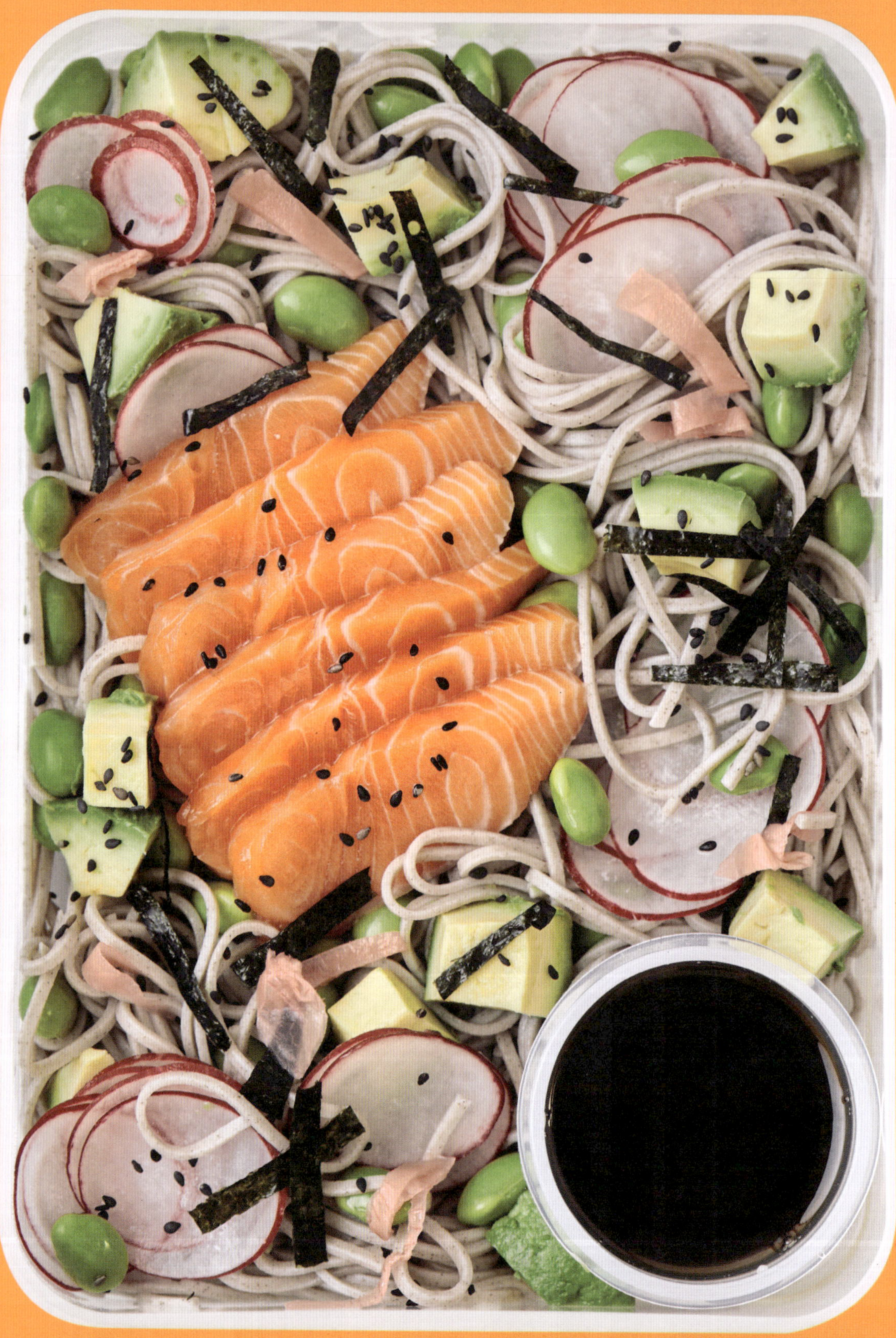

PROTEIN: 36 G NET CARBS: 38 G FAT: 44 G

Salmon sashimi soba salad

With a nod to Japanese cuisine, this soba noodle salad combines silky salmon, creamy avocado, moreish edamame beans and crunchy radishes. Edamame beans can be found in the frozen vegetable section of larger supermarkets.

- 180 g (6½ oz) cooked soba noodles, prepared as per packet instructions
- toasted sesame oil, for drizzling
- 50 g (⅓ cup) podded edamame beans (soybeans), blanched
- ½ avocado, diced
- 2 radishes, finely sliced
- 2 teaspoons toasted black sesame seeds
- 2 teaspoons sliced pickled ginger
- 80 g (2¾ oz) raw sashimi-grade salmon, sliced
- ¼ toasted nori sheet, finely sliced

PONZU SESAME DRESSING

- 3½ teaspoons ponzu sauce
- 1 teaspoon rice vinegar
- 1 teaspoon extra virgin olive oil
- 1 teaspoon toasted sesame oil

1. Toss the noodles in a bowl with a little sesame oil. Add the remaining salad ingredients, except the sashimi and nori, and toss lightly. Arrange the sashimi slices on top.
2. Combine the dressing ingredients in a small bowl.
3. Drizzle the dressing and sprinkle the nori over the salad just before serving.

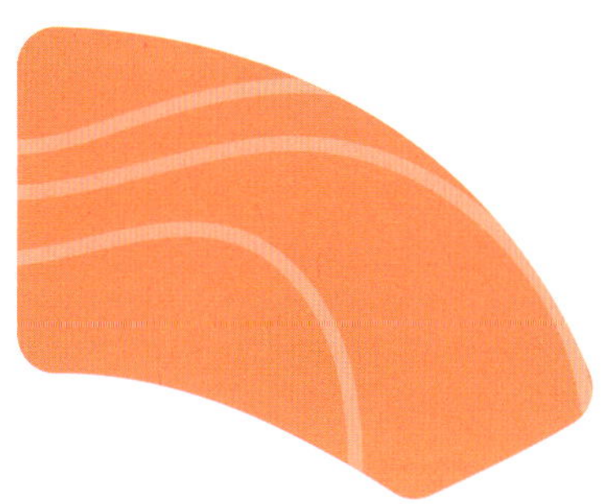

PROTEIN: 52 G NET CARBS: 82 G FAT: 58 G

Broccolini, chicken & honey-chilli soba noodles

Honey and chilli balance out the earthy soba noodles, while the fried shallots and tamari almonds add some real crunch. With chicken and broccolini, it's a simple stir-through salad that's hearty enough for dinner. You can swap the broccolini for shaved cabbage, if you like.

- 180 g (6½ oz) cooked soba noodles, prepared as per packet instructions
- 3 broccolini stems, blanched and sliced
- 100 g (⅔ cup) shredded cooked chicken
- small handful of coriander (cilantro) leaves
- 40 g (¼ cup) spiced tamari almonds, chopped
- 2 tablespoons crispy fried shallots

HONEY, CHILLI & GINGER DRESSING

- 2 tablespoons chilli crisp oil
- 1 teaspoon rice vinegar
- 1 teaspoon honey
- 1 teaspoon kecap manis (sweet soy sauce)
- ½ teaspoon minced ginger

1. Place the salad ingredients in a bowl and toss lightly.
2. Combine the dressing ingredients in a small bowl.
3. Pour the dressing over the salad just before serving and toss well to coat.

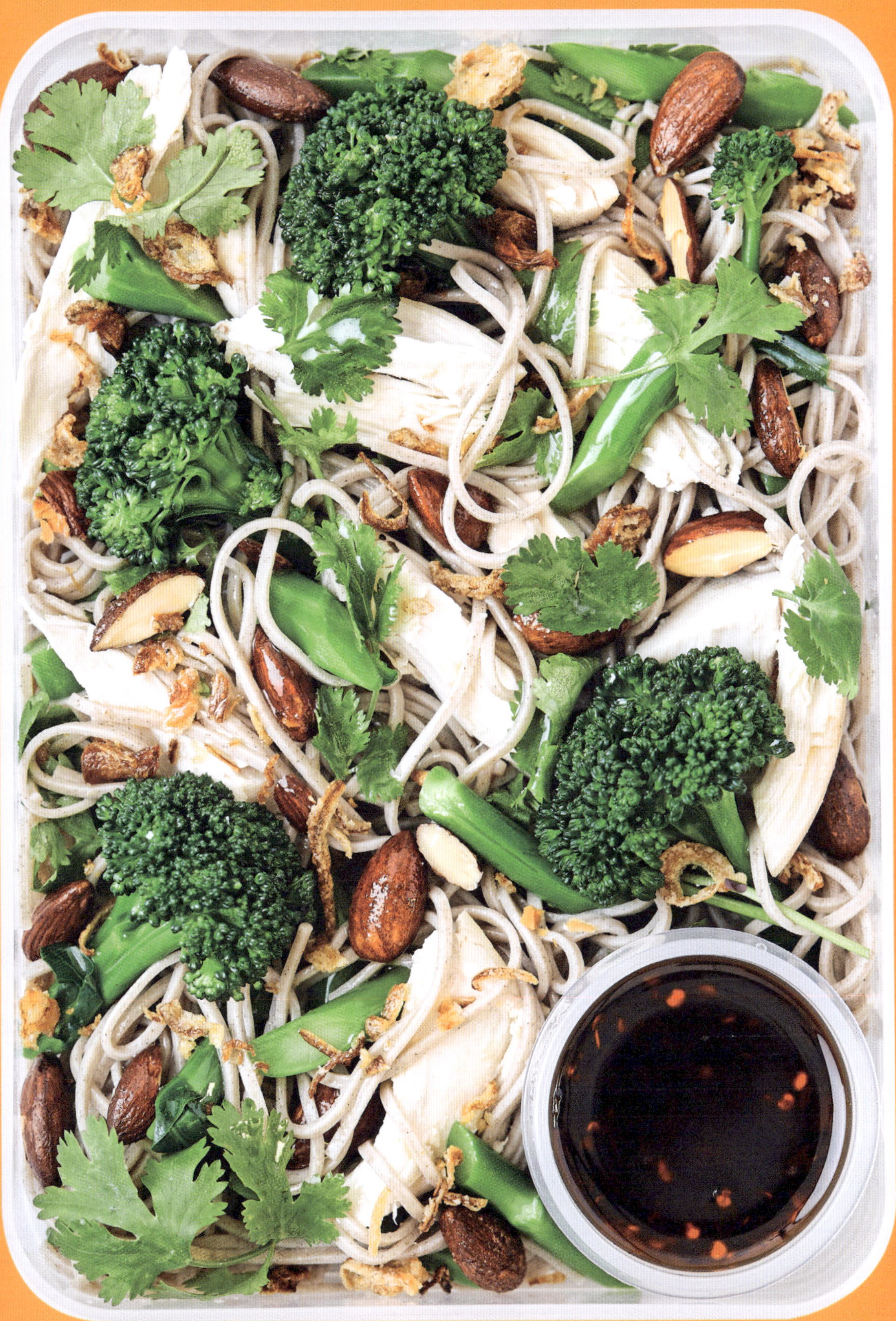

PROTEIN: 49 G NET CARBS: 40 G FAT: 19 G

Chicken soba salad with artichoke, spinach & green olives

Chicken and soba noodles set the base, while artichoke, spinach and olives add Mediterranean flavour. It's a travel-inspired twist that still comes together quickly. The lemony dressing adds a perfect creaminess.

- 180 g (6½ oz) cooked soba noodles, prepared as per packet instructions
- 100 g (⅔ cup) shredded cooked chicken
- 2-3 marinated artichoke hearts, quartered
- 30 g (⅔ cup) baby spinach leaves
- 30 g (¼ cup) pitted Sicilian green olives
- small handful of parsley leaves
- 2 tablespoons finely grated parmesan

CREAMY LEMON & CAPER DRESSING

- 2 tablespoons blended cottage cheese (2% fat)
- 1½ tablespoons lemon juice
- 1 teaspoon baby capers, chopped

1. Place the salad ingredients in a bowl and toss lightly.
2. Combine the dressing ingredients in a small bowl, then season to taste with pepper.
3. Pour the dressing over the salad just before serving and toss well to coat.

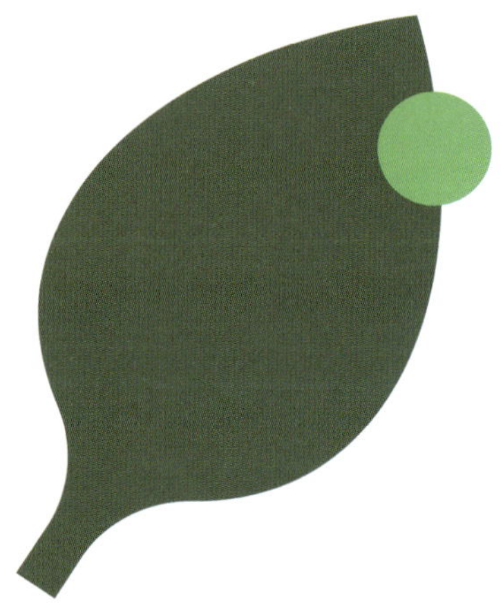

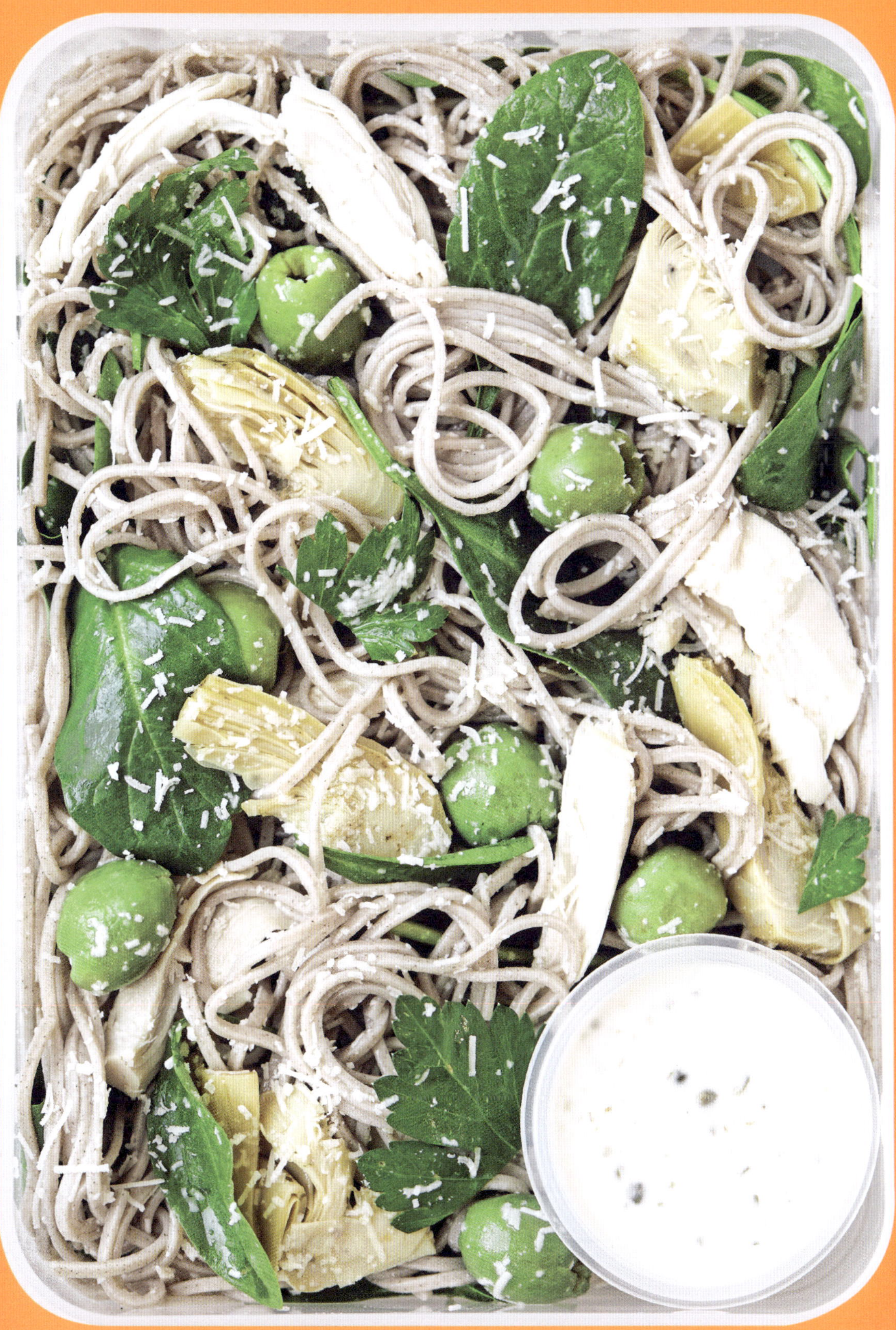

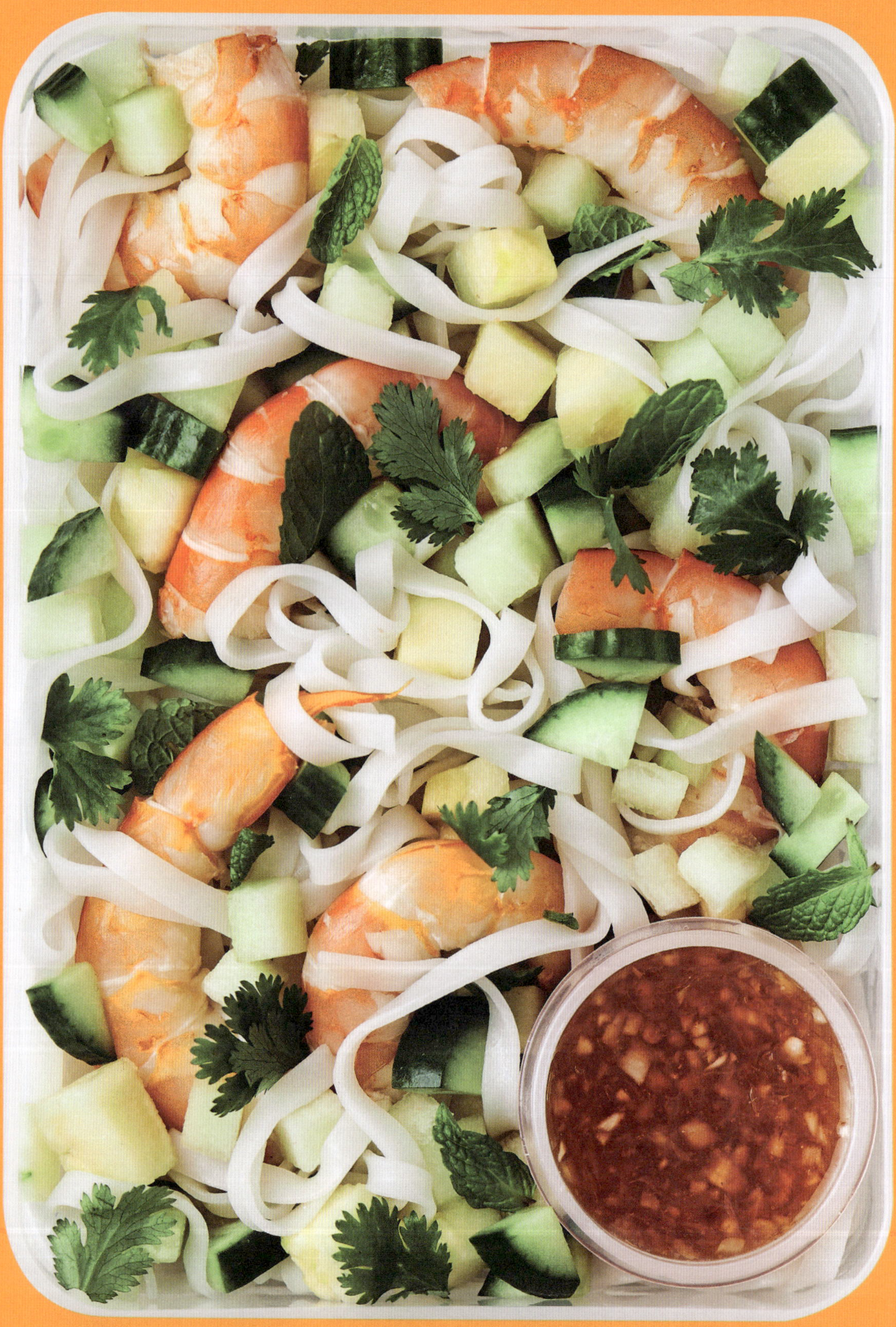

PROTEIN: 33 G NET CARBS: 52 G FAT: 1 G

Prawn, pineapple & melon noodle salad

Prawns are light yet satisfying, and fruit keeps this salad refreshing. It's a sweet–savoury combination that works beautifully on hot days. If you like things a little spicier, toss in a finely chopped red chilli.

80 g (2¾ oz) dried flat rice stick or pad Thai noodles, prepared as per packet instructions

120 g (4½ oz) cooked prawns (shrimp), peeled and deveined

65 g (⅓ cup) finely diced pineapple

60 g (⅓ cup) diced honeydew melon

60 g (⅓ cup) diced short cucumber

small handful of mint leaves

small handful of coriander (cilantro) leaves

SHALLOT & GINGER DRESSING

2 tablespoons sweet chilli sauce

1 tablespoon lime juice

2 teaspoons finely chopped red Asian shallot

½ teaspoon minced ginger

1. Place the salad ingredients in a bowl and toss lightly.
2. Combine the dressing ingredients in a small bowl.
3. Pour the dressing over the salad just before serving and toss well to coat.

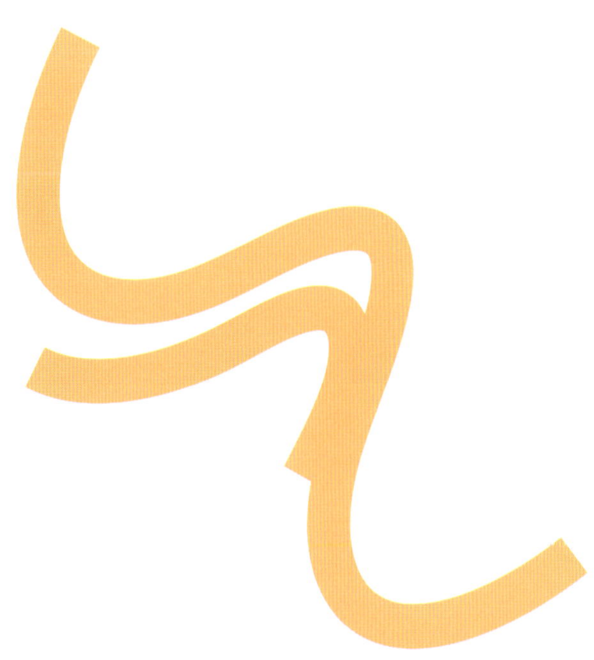

PROTEIN: 38 G NET CARBS: 49 G FAT: 29 G

Chicken & rice salad with ginger-soy dressing

If you prefer a nuttier flavour – and a little more fibre – in your salad, opt for brown rice here. Micro herbs can be found in most good-quality greengrocers.

- 150 g (5½ oz) cooked and cooled rice
- 100 g (⅔ cup) shredded cooked chicken
- 50 g (1¾ oz) snow peas (mangetout), sliced
- large handful of mixed micro herbs

GINGER-SOY DRESSING

- 1½ tablespoons macadamia oil or other mild-flavoured oil
- 1 tablespoon rice vinegar
- 1 tablespoon tamari or soy sauce
- 2 teaspoons minced ginger
- 1 teaspoon toasted sesame oil

1. Place the salad ingredients in a bowl and toss lightly.
2. Combine the dressing ingredients in a small bowl, then season to taste with salt and pepper.
3. Pour the dressing over the salad just before serving and toss well to coat.

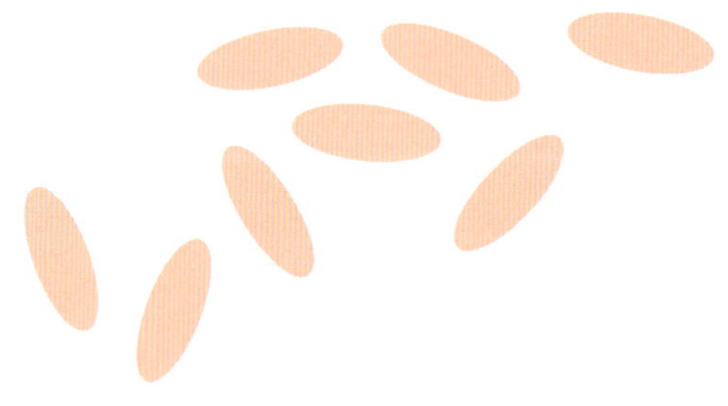

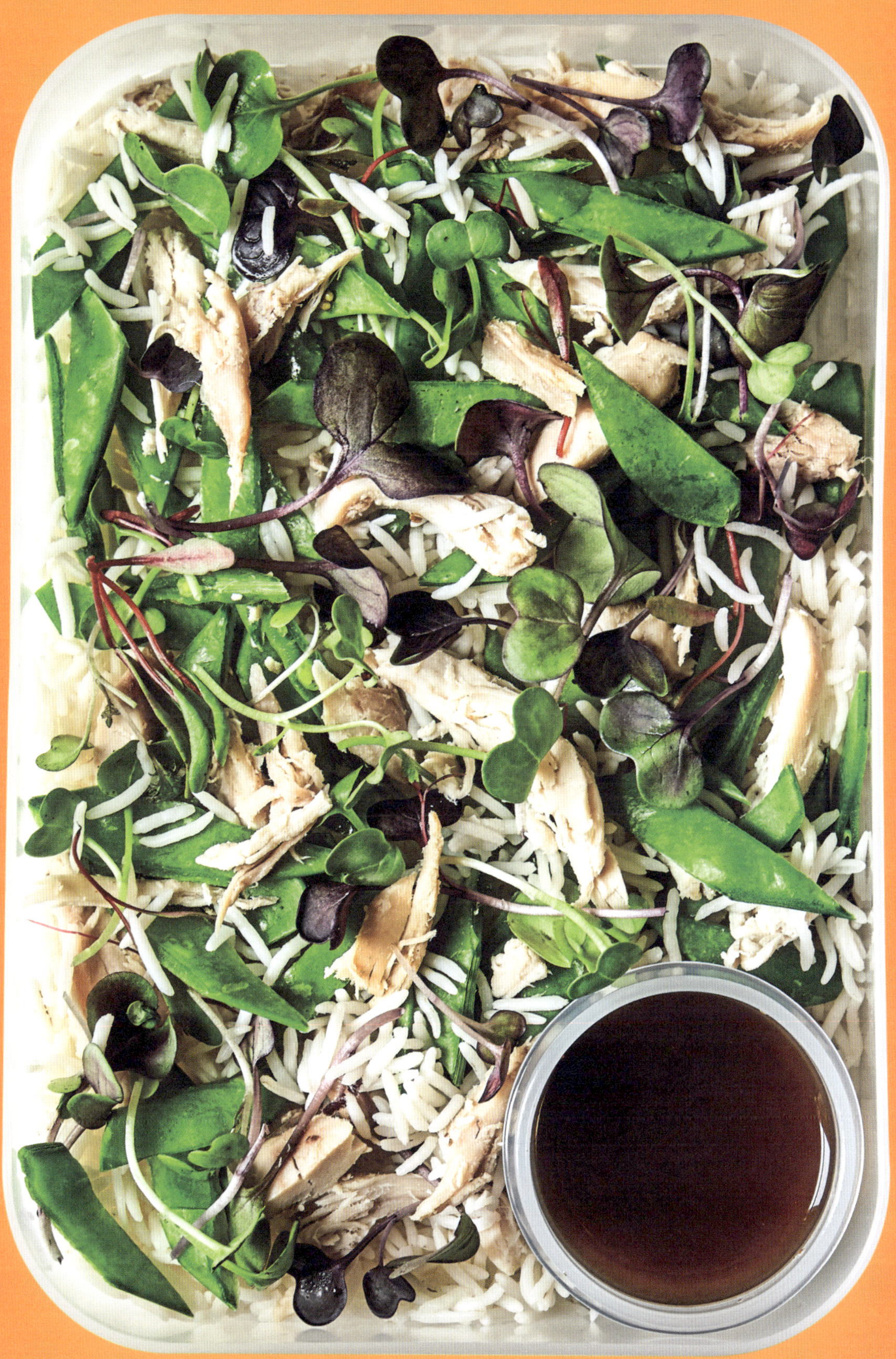

PROTEIN: 53 G   NET CARBS: 68 G   FAT: 37 G

Creamy turmeric noodles with chicken, herbs & lime

Shredded chicken and fresh herbs stop the dish from feeling heavy, while lime adds tang. The turmeric in the dressing adds a lovely yellow hue to this tasty salad. If you're not a fan of coriander, simply omit it from the dish or replace it with parsley – and if you can't get hold of Vietnamese mint, use regular mint instead.

180 g (6½ oz) hokkien noodles, prepared as per packet instructions

100 g (⅔ cup) shredded cooked chicken

1 small spring onion (scallion), finely sliced

small handful of coriander (cilantro) leaves

small handful of Vietnamese mint leaves

25 g (¼ cup) toasted flaked almonds

lime wedges, to serve

TURMERIC DRESSING

2 tablespoons tahini

2 tablespoons water

1 tablespoon lime juice

1–1½ teaspoons agave syrup, honey or maple syrup

1 teaspoon rice vinegar

¼ teaspoon ground turmeric

1. Place the dressing ingredients in a bowl and whisk to combine. Add the noodles and toss well to coat. Add the remaining ingredients, except the lime wedges, and toss again.
2. Squeeze the lime over just before serving.

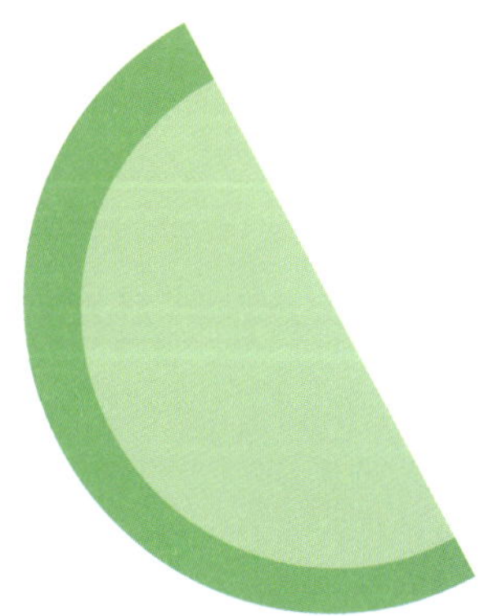

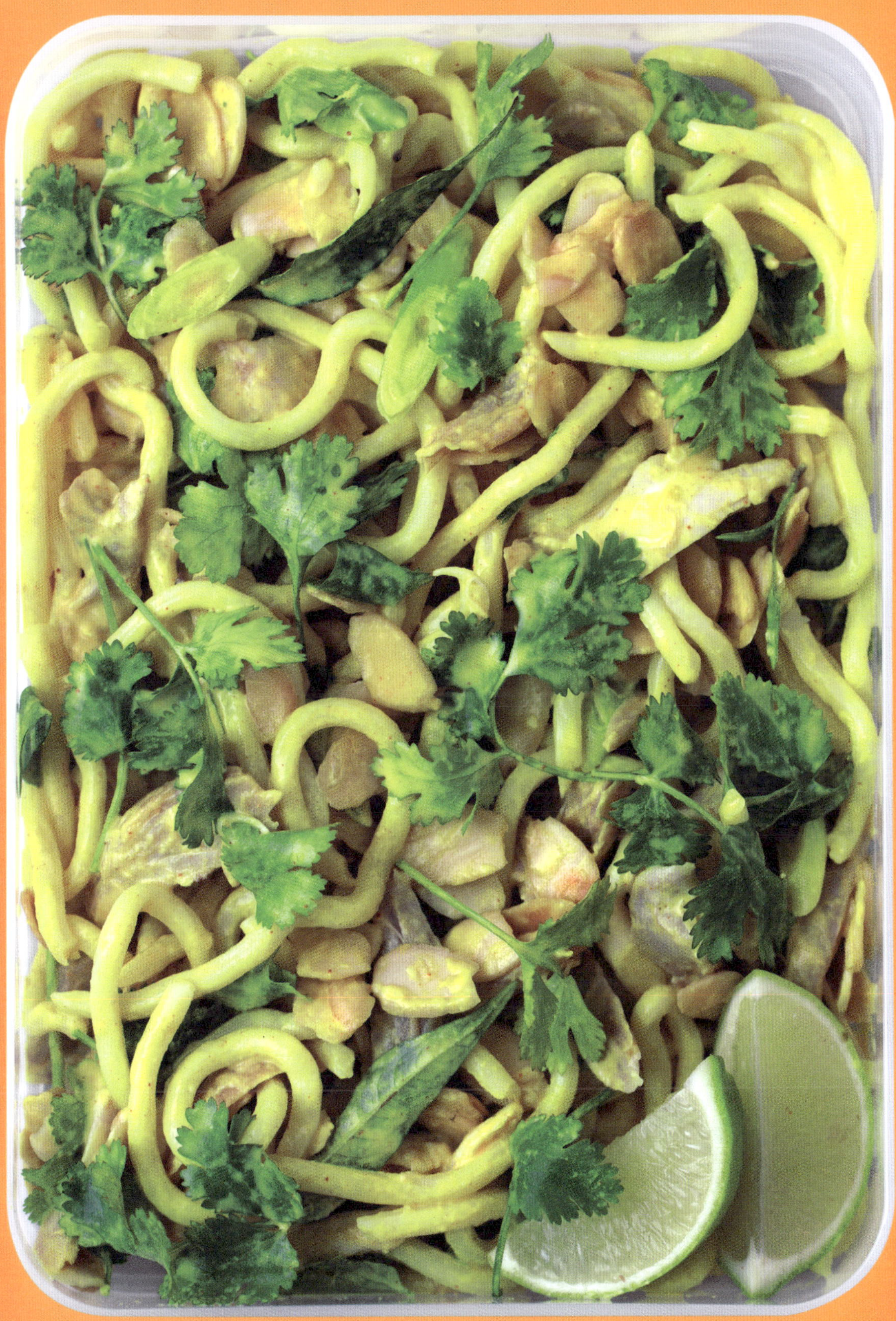

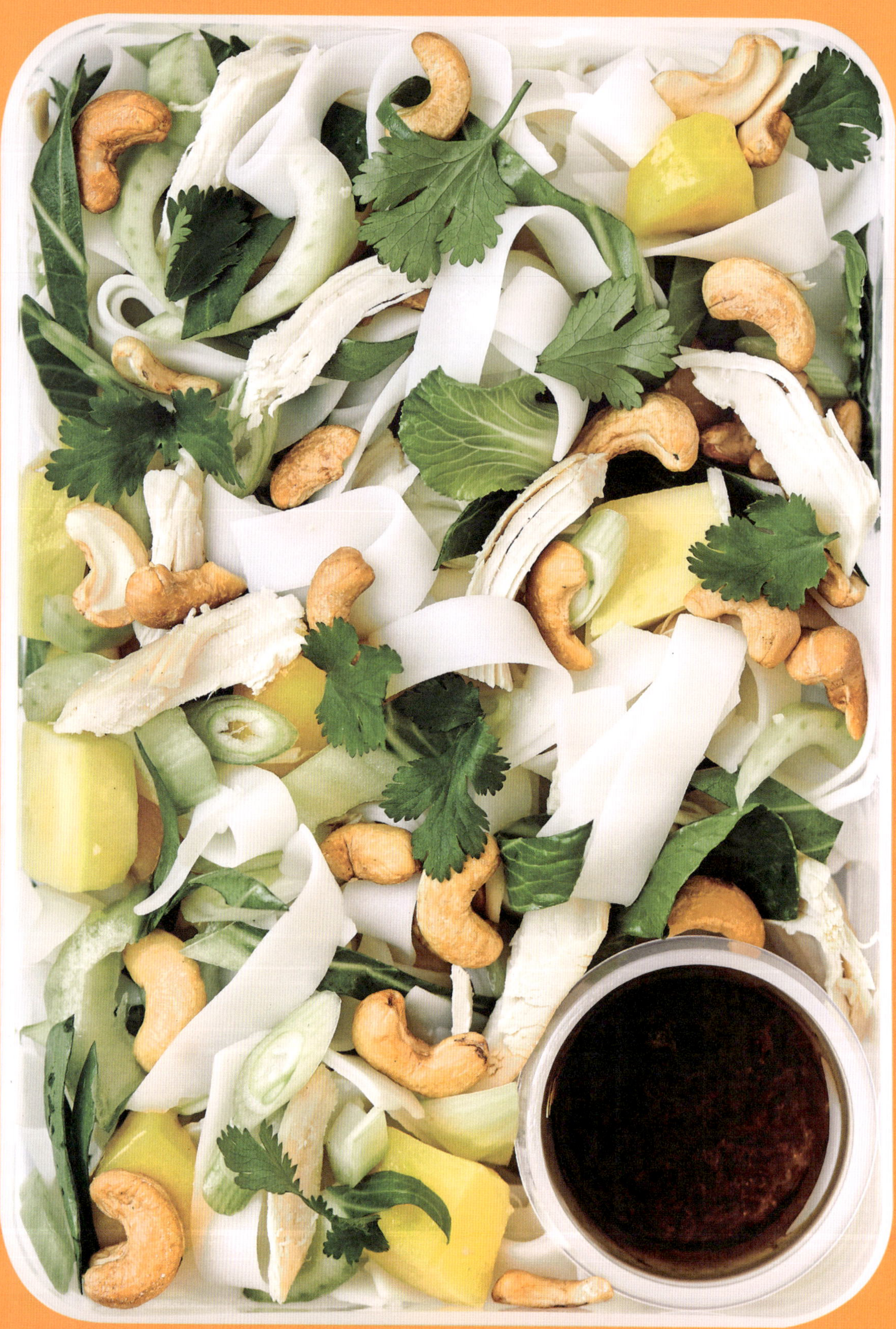

PROTEIN: 43 G NET CARBS: 56 G FAT: 45 G

Chicken, mango & cashew noodle salad

Tender chicken, sweet mango and crunchy cashews are a winning trio. Served with noodles, it's a salad that feels both refreshing and satisfying. You can replace the bok choy with another leafy green, such as baby spinach, if that's already on hand.

- 80 g (2¾ oz) dried wide rice noodles, prepared as per packet instructions
- 100 g (⅔ cup) shredded cooked chicken
- 1 baby bok choy (pak choy), washed well and finely sliced
- ½ mango, diced
- 1 small spring onion (scallion), finely sliced
- small handful of coriander (cilantro) leaves
- 40 g (¼ cup) roasted cashews, chopped

TAMARI-GINGER DRESSING

- 4 teaspoons olive oil
- 1 tablespoon rice vinegar
- 1 tablespoon tamari
- 1 teaspoon toasted sesame oil
- 1 teaspoon minced ginger

1. Place the salad ingredients in a bowl and toss lightly.
2. Combine the dressing ingredients in a small bowl.
3. Pour the dressing over the salad just before serving and toss well to coat.

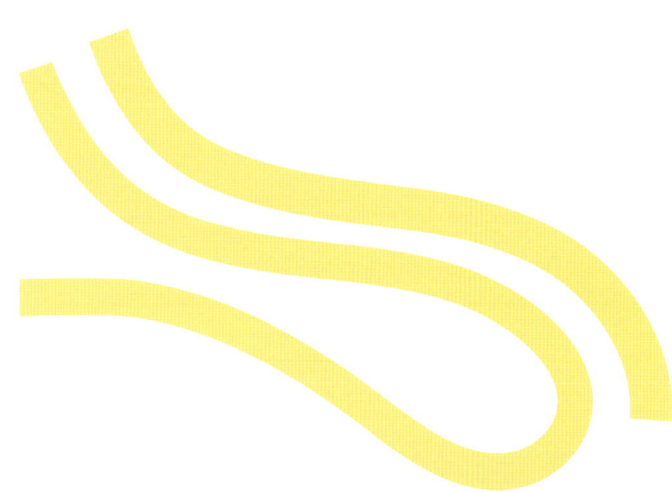

PROTEIN: 27 G NET CARBS: 45 G FAT: 16 G

Sashimi seaweed noodle salad

This salad relies on getting the very freshest sashimi-grade white fish you can find, and is best made the day the salad is to be eaten. Look for seaweed salads at Japanese grocers or sushi stores.

- 100 g (3½ oz) dried wide rice noodles, prepared as per packet instructions
- 80 g (2¾ oz) seaweed salad (store-bought)
- 1–2 radishes, finely sliced
- 1 small green chilli, finely sliced
- 2 tablespoons wasabi peas, crushed
- 50 g (1¾ oz) snow pea (mangetout) sprouts
- 100 g (3½ oz) raw white-fish sashimi, sliced

SOY & PICKLED GINGER DRESSING

- 2 tablespoons soy sauce
- 1 tablespoon rice vinegar
- 1 teaspoon sesame oil
- 1 teaspoon pickled ginger, diced

1. Place the salad ingredients in a bowl, except the sashimi, and toss lightly. Arrange the sashimi slices on top.
2. Combine the dressing ingredients in a small bowl.
3. Drizzle the dressing over the salad just before serving.

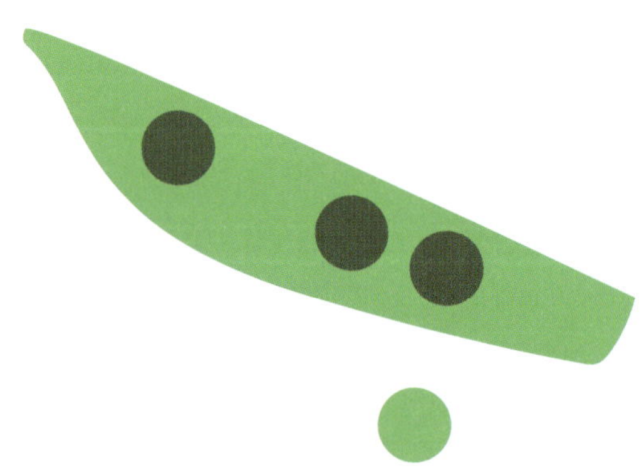

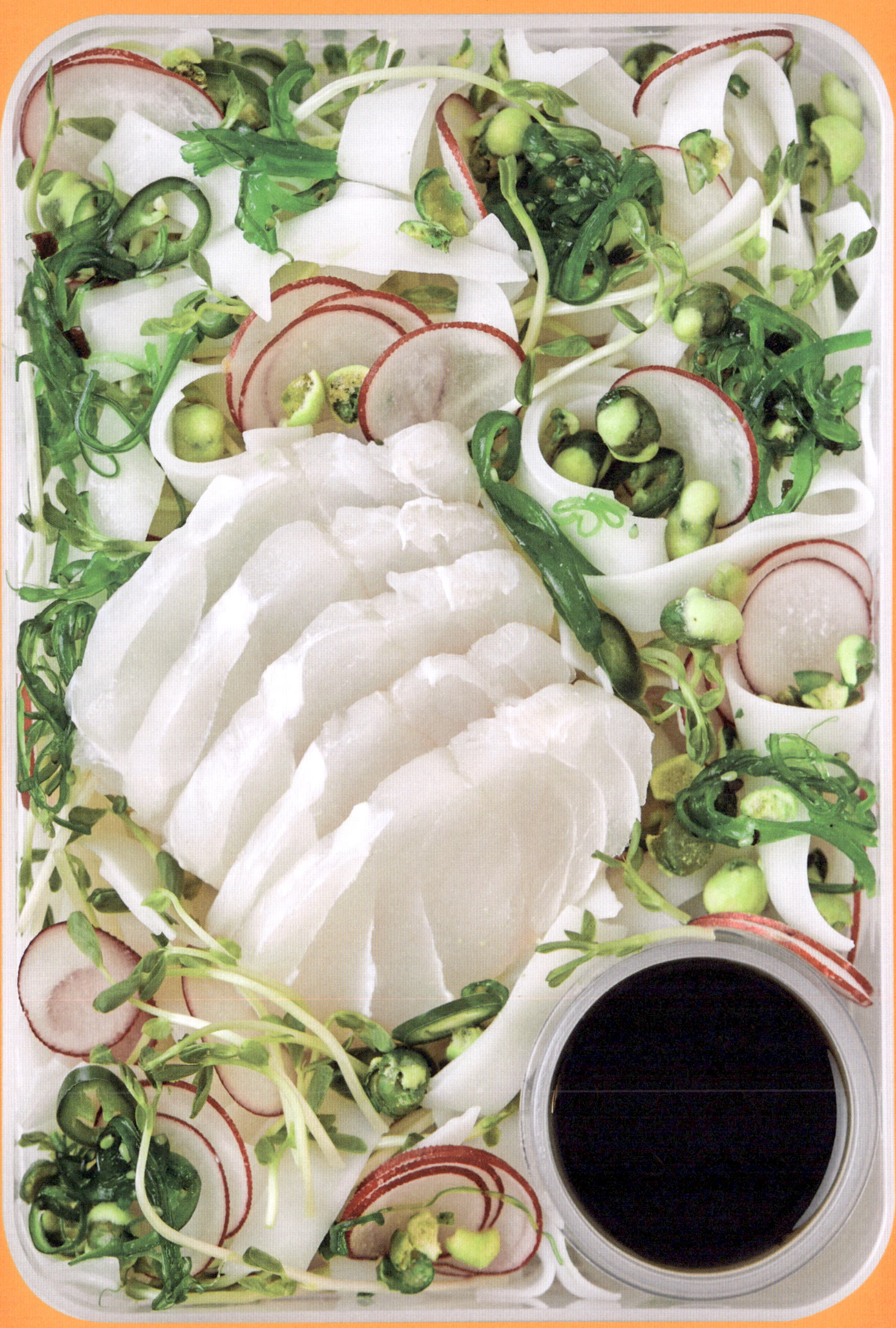

PROTEIN: 33 G NET CARBS: 47 G FAT: 10 G

Green tea noodles with salmon & crunchy greens

Green tea noodles bring subtle flavour and colour, while salmon adds richness. With crisp greens, it's a modern spin on a nourishing noodle salad.

180 g (6½ oz) cooked, rinsed and drained green tea soba noodles

50 g (1¾ oz) green beans, sliced and blanched

85 g (3 oz) raw sashimi-grade salmon, sliced

½ short cucumber, finely sliced

SESAME-MISO DRESSING

1 tablespoon white (shiro) miso paste

1 tablespoon rice vinegar

1 tablespoon mirin

2 teaspoons toasted sesame seeds

1 teaspoon minced ginger

1. Place the salad ingredients in a bowl and toss lightly.
2. Combine the dressing ingredients in a small bowl, then season to taste with salt and pepper.
3. Pour the dressing over the salad just before serving and toss well to coat.

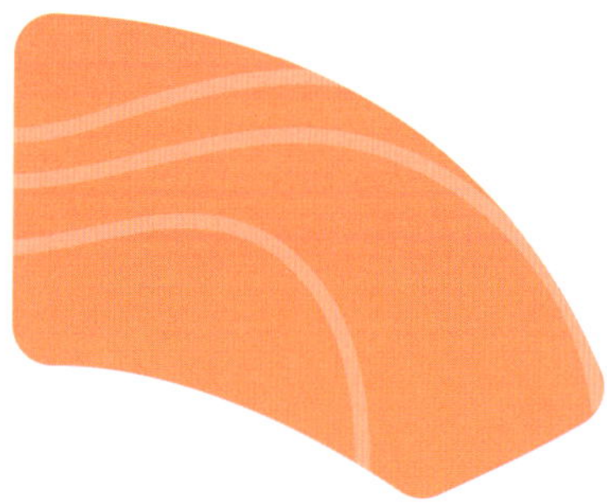

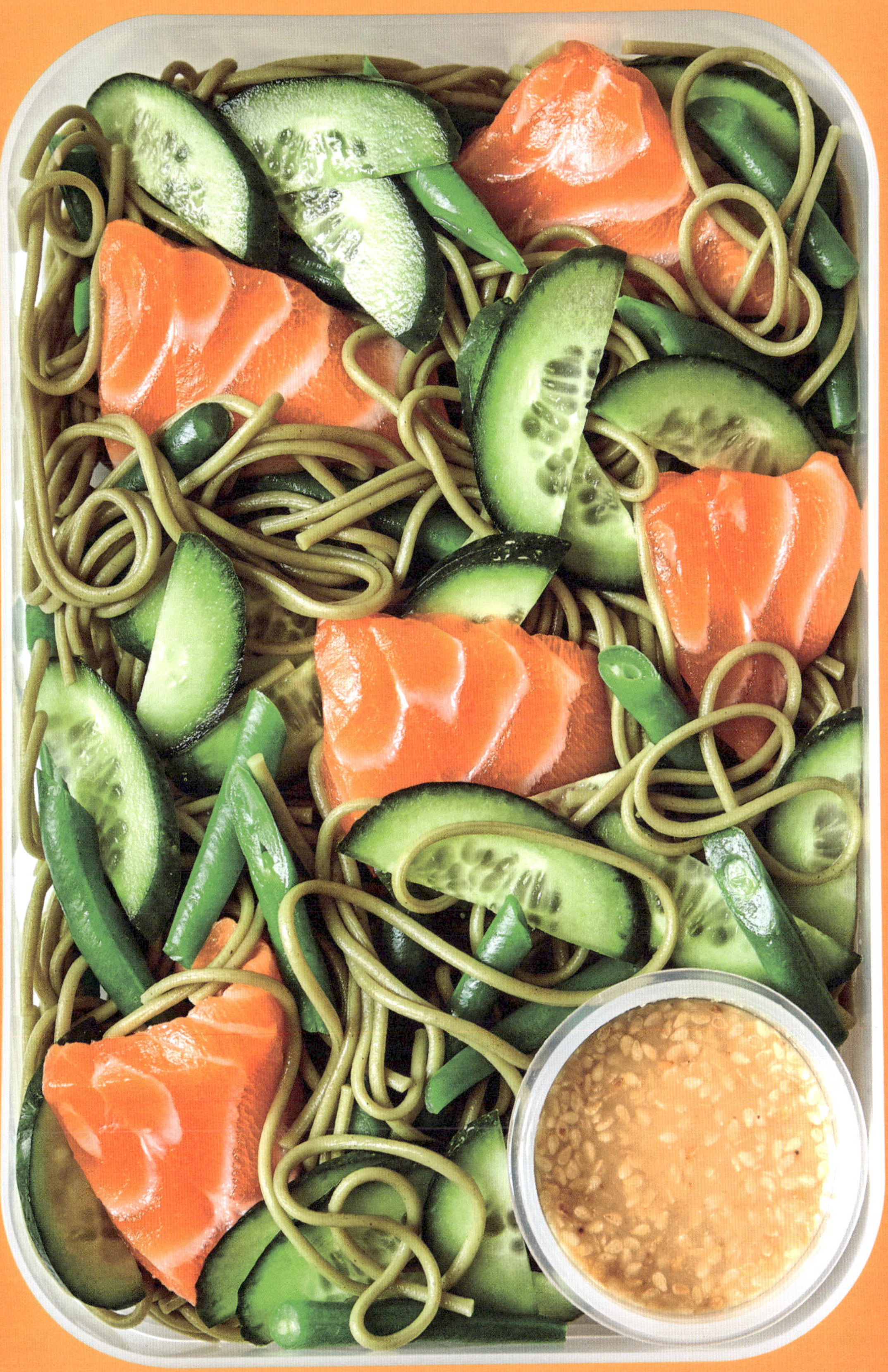

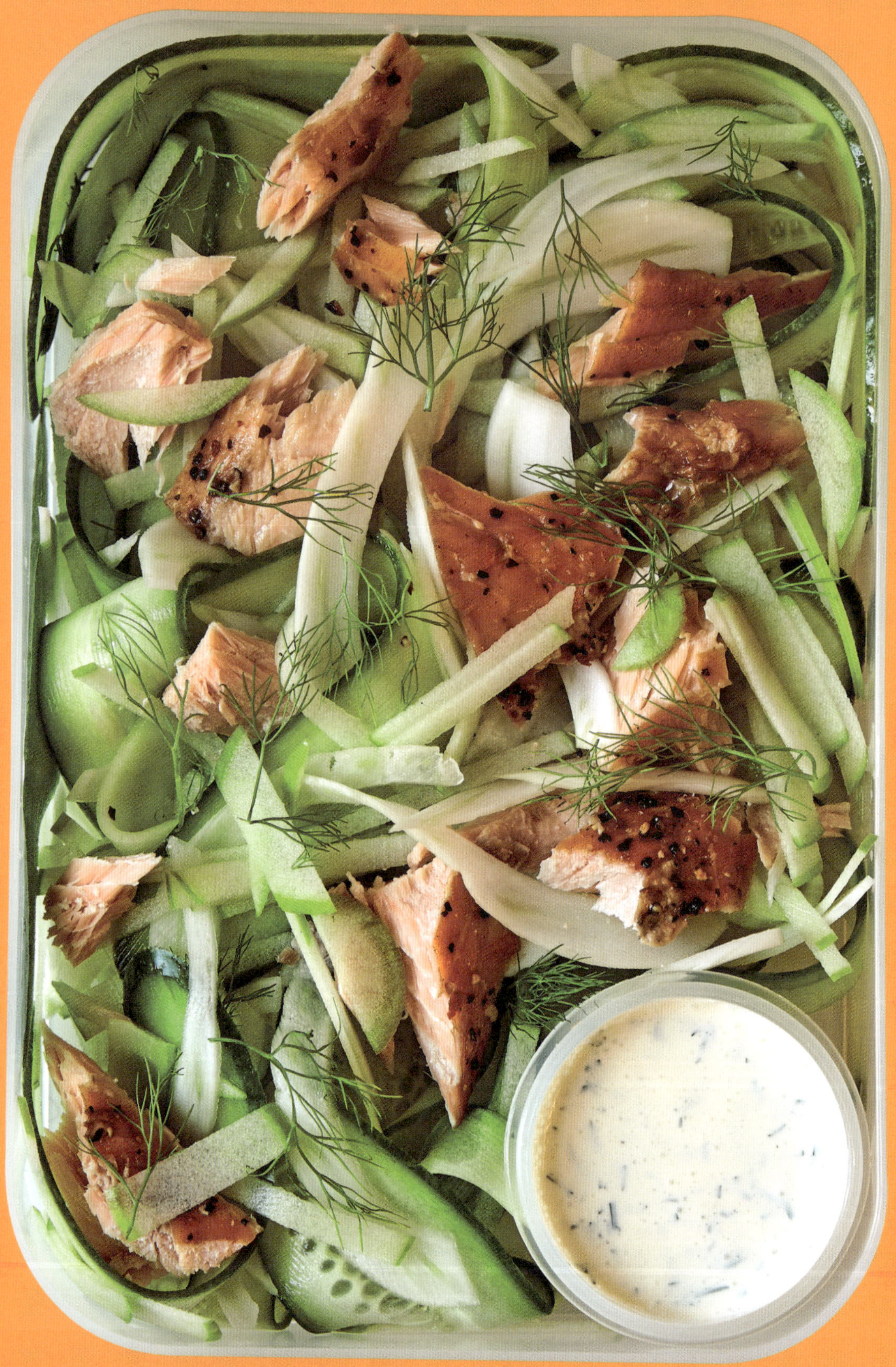

PROTEIN: 26 G NET CARBS: 9 G FAT: 7 G

Cucumber & green apple zoodles with salmon

Cucumber and apple keep things sharp and refreshing, with salmon providing substance. Depending on where you live, hot-smoked salmon is often available in various styles in the cooler section of supermarkets. This recipe calls for pepper-crusted salmon, but you can also use the plain version.

- 120 g (4½ oz) hot-smoked pepper-crusted salmon, flaked
- 1 short cucumber, spiralised into wide ribbons
- 1 small granny smith apple, cored and spiralised
- ½ baby fennel, finely shaved, plus a few fronds

CREAMY LEMON & HERB DRESSING

- 3 tablespoons high-protein Greek-style yoghurt
- 2 teaspoons lemon juice
- 2 teaspoons finely chopped dill leaves
- 2 teaspoons finely chopped mint leaves

1. Place the salad ingredients in a bowl and toss lightly.
2. Combine the dressing ingredients in a small bowl, then season to taste with salt and pepper.
3. Pour the dressing over the salad just before serving and toss well to coat.

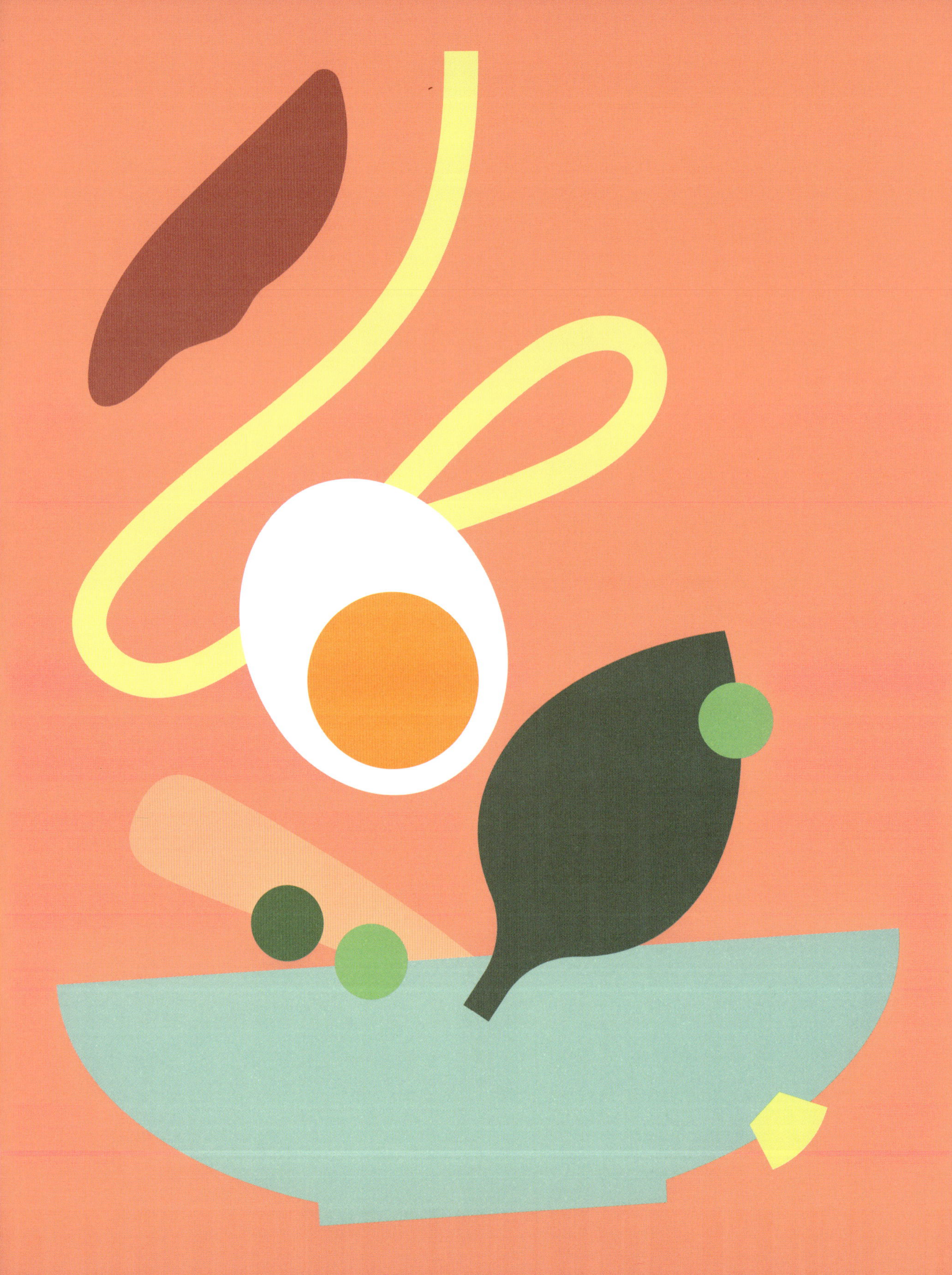

hearty

hits

PROTEIN: 25 G NET CARBS: 85 G FAT: 30 G

Chorizo, chickpea & roasted pepper noodle salad

Chorizo is a Spanish-style cured pork sausage that comes in many forms – including fresh and cured varieties. Fresh chorizo needs to be sliced and fried for a few minutes before use, while cured varieties require no cooking. Either can be used in this recipe.

- 180 g (6½ oz) thin hokkien noodles, prepared as per packet instructions
- 1 roasted red bell pepper (capsicum), finely sliced
- 50 g (1¾ oz) dried or smoked chorizo, finely sliced
- 85 g (3 oz) tinned chickpeas (garbanzo beans), drained and rinsed
- ⅛ small red onion, finely sliced
- 100 g (3½ oz) cherry tomatoes, halved
- 30 g (1 cup) rocket (arugula) leaves

SHERRY VINAIGRETTE

- 1 tablespoon extra virgin olive oil
- 2 teaspoons sherry vinegar
- 1 teaspoon dijon mustard
- 1 teaspoon agave syrup, honey or maple syrup

1. Place the salad ingredients in a bowl and toss lightly.
2. Combine the vinaigrette ingredients in a small bowl, then season to taste with salt and pepper.
3. Pour the vinaigrette over the salad just before serving and toss well to coat.

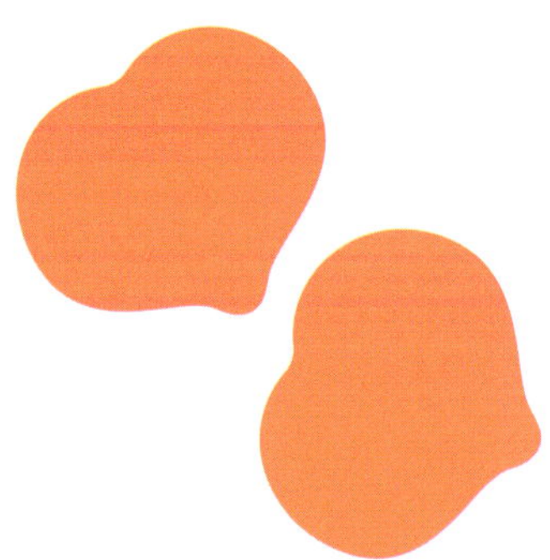

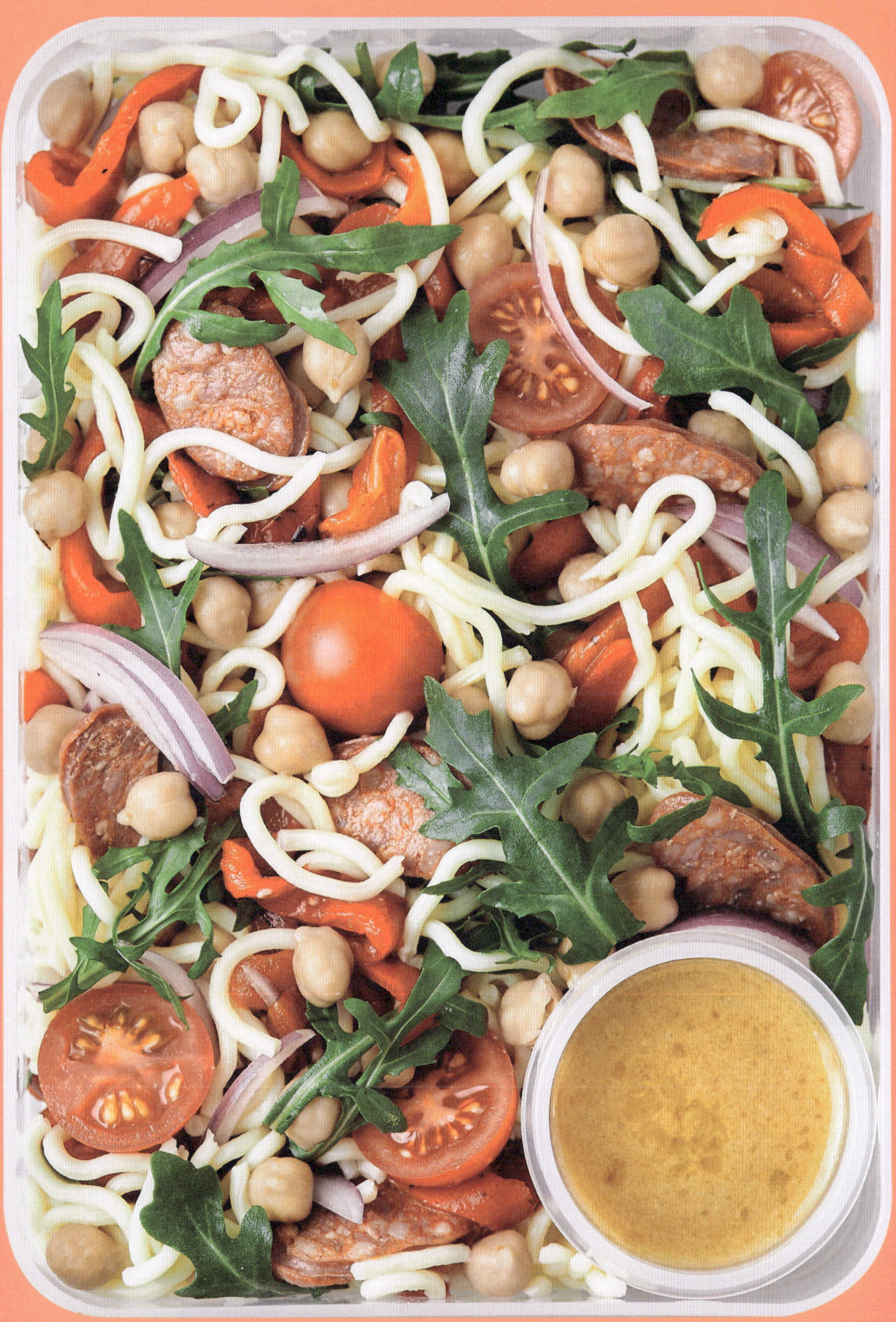

PROTEIN: 36 G NET CARBS: 10 G FAT: 60 G

Roast beef & zucchini salad with smoked almonds

The smoked almonds give this salad a lovely flavour that pairs so well with the roast beef. You can buy smoked almonds from most good supermarkets, but you can easily substitute plain roasted almonds. This recipe is great with roast beef from your deli, but even better made with leftovers from a Sunday roast.

- 1 small zucchini (courgette), cut into ribbons using a vegetable peeler
- 1 teaspoon lemon juice
- 100 g (3½ oz) sliced roast beef, torn into pieces
- 100 g (3½ oz) grape (baby plum) tomatoes, halved
- handful of parsley leaves, chopped
- 30 g (1 oz) smoked almonds, chopped

LEMON & CHILLI DRESSING

- pinch of chilli flakes
- juice of ½ lemon
- 1 teaspoon dijon mustard
- 2 tablespoons extra virgin olive oil

1. Place the zucchini ribbons in a bowl and gently toss in the lemon juice. Add the remaining salad ingredients, except the smoked almonds, and toss lightly. Season to taste with salt and pepper.
2. Combine the dressing ingredients in a small bowl.
3. Pour the dressing over the salad just before serving and toss well to coat. Top with the smoked almonds.

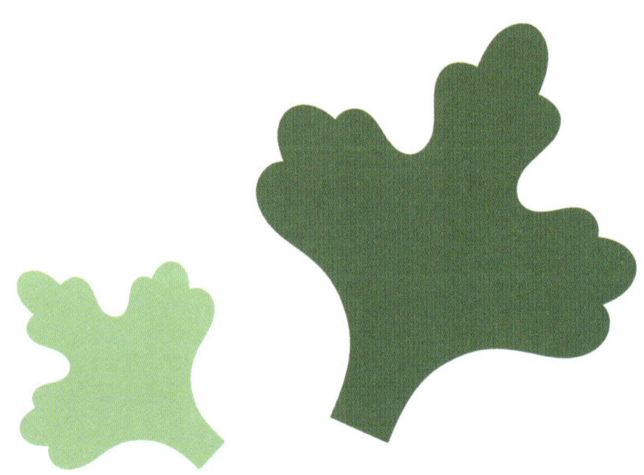

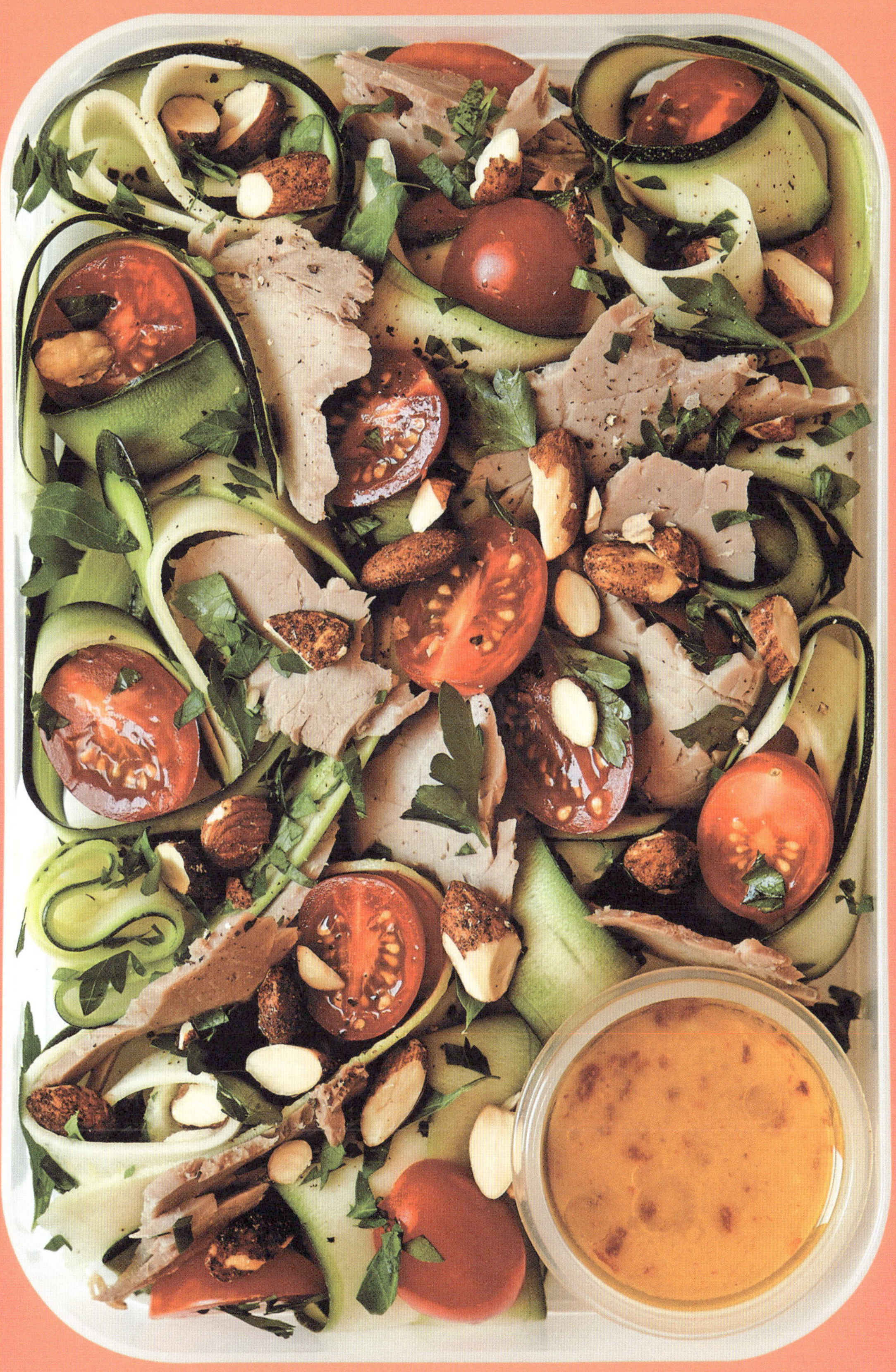

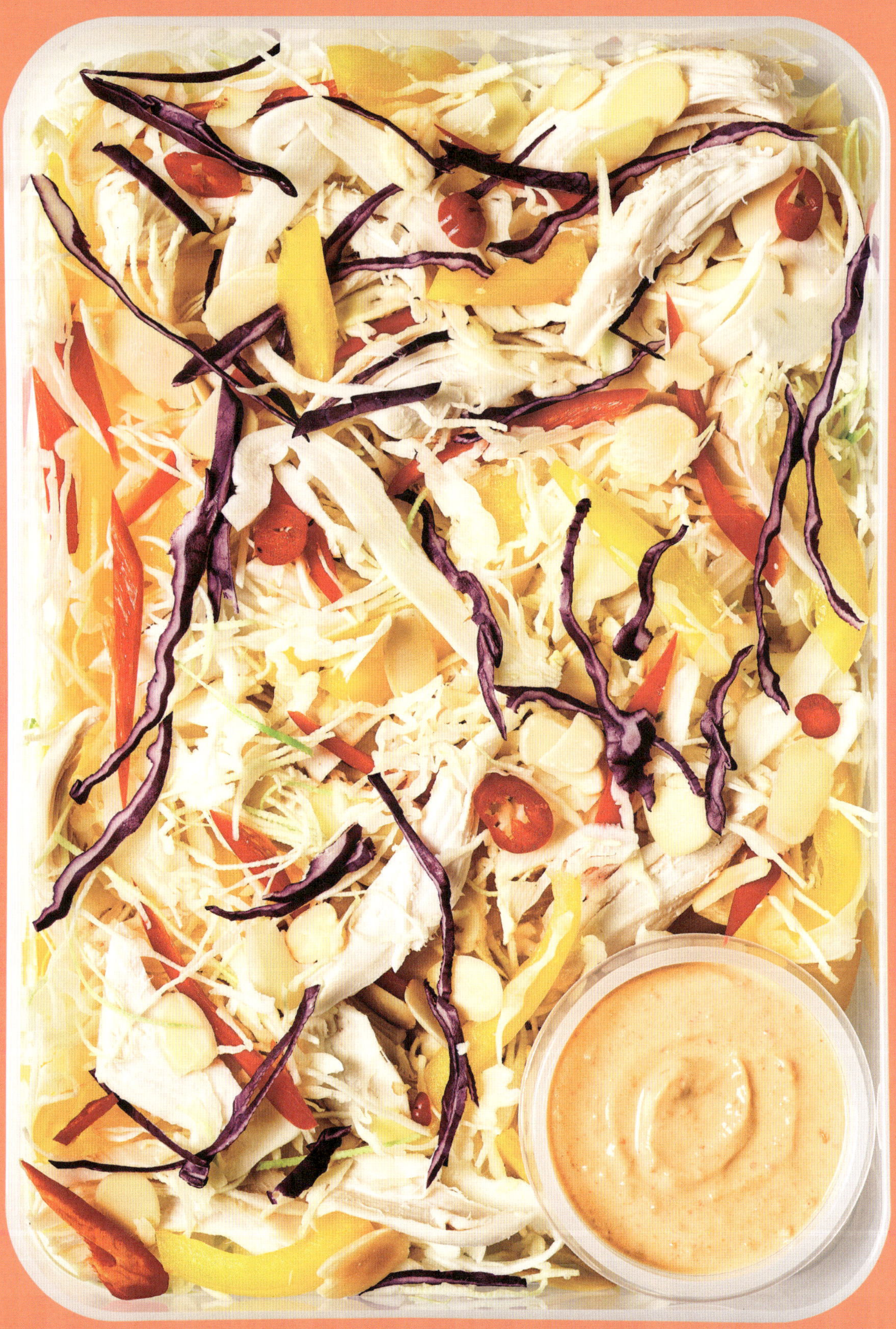

PROTEIN: 36 G NET CARBS: 19 G FAT: 33 G

Spicy roast chicken cabbage salad

Crunchy, smoky, moreish, this salad is the perfect dish for using left-over roast chicken. The dressing has some robust flavours, but is surprisingly balanced – with sweetness from the coconut yoghurt, fattiness from the almond butter, tanginess from the lime and a bit of heat from the sriracha.

110 g (¾ cup) shredded cooked chicken

100 g (⅔ cup) sliced red and yellow bell pepper (capsicum)

75 g (1 cup) finely shredded cabbage

2 tablespoons toasted flaked almonds

1 small red chilli, sliced

SPICY COCONUT DRESSING

2 tablespoons coconut yoghurt

1 tablespoon almond butter

1 tablespoon lime juice

1 teaspoon sriracha chilli sauce

1. Place the salad ingredients in a bowl and toss lightly.
2. In a small bowl, whisk the dressing ingredients until smooth.
3. Pour the dressing over the salad just before serving and toss well to coat.

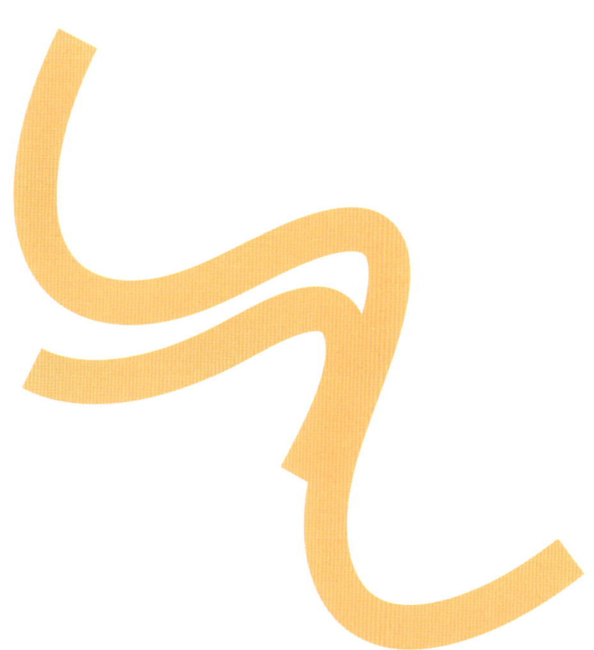

PROTEIN: 26 G NET CARBS: 33 G FAT: 51 G

Chorizo, roasted red pepper & borlotti bean salad

Borlotti beans add creaminess and protein to smoky chorizo and sweet roasted bell pepper while rocket and a zingy dressing keeps it fresh.

170 g (6 oz) tinned borlotti (cranberry) beans, drained and rinsed

90 g (3 oz) smoked chorizo, sliced

2 marinated roasted red bell peppers (capsicums), sliced

60 g (2 cups) rocket (arugula) leaves

PARSLEY & PAPRIKA DRESSING

1½ tablespoons extra virgin olive oil

1½ tablespoons sherry vinegar

1 tablespoon chopped parsley leaves

½ teaspoon smoked paprika

1. Place the salad ingredients in a bowl and toss lightly.
2. Combine the dressing ingredients in a small bowl, then season to taste with salt and pepper.
3. Pour the dressing over the salad just before serving and toss well to coat.

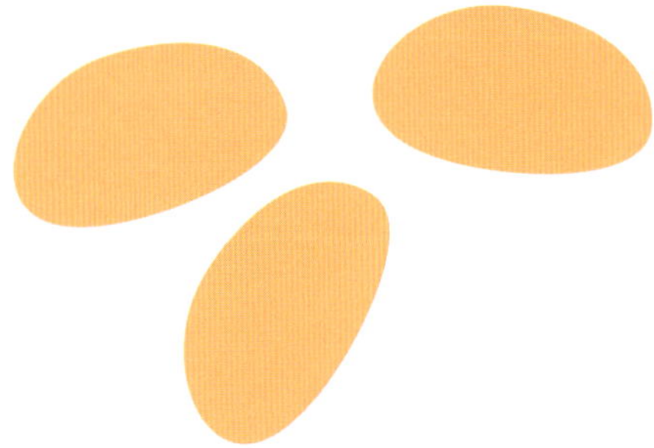

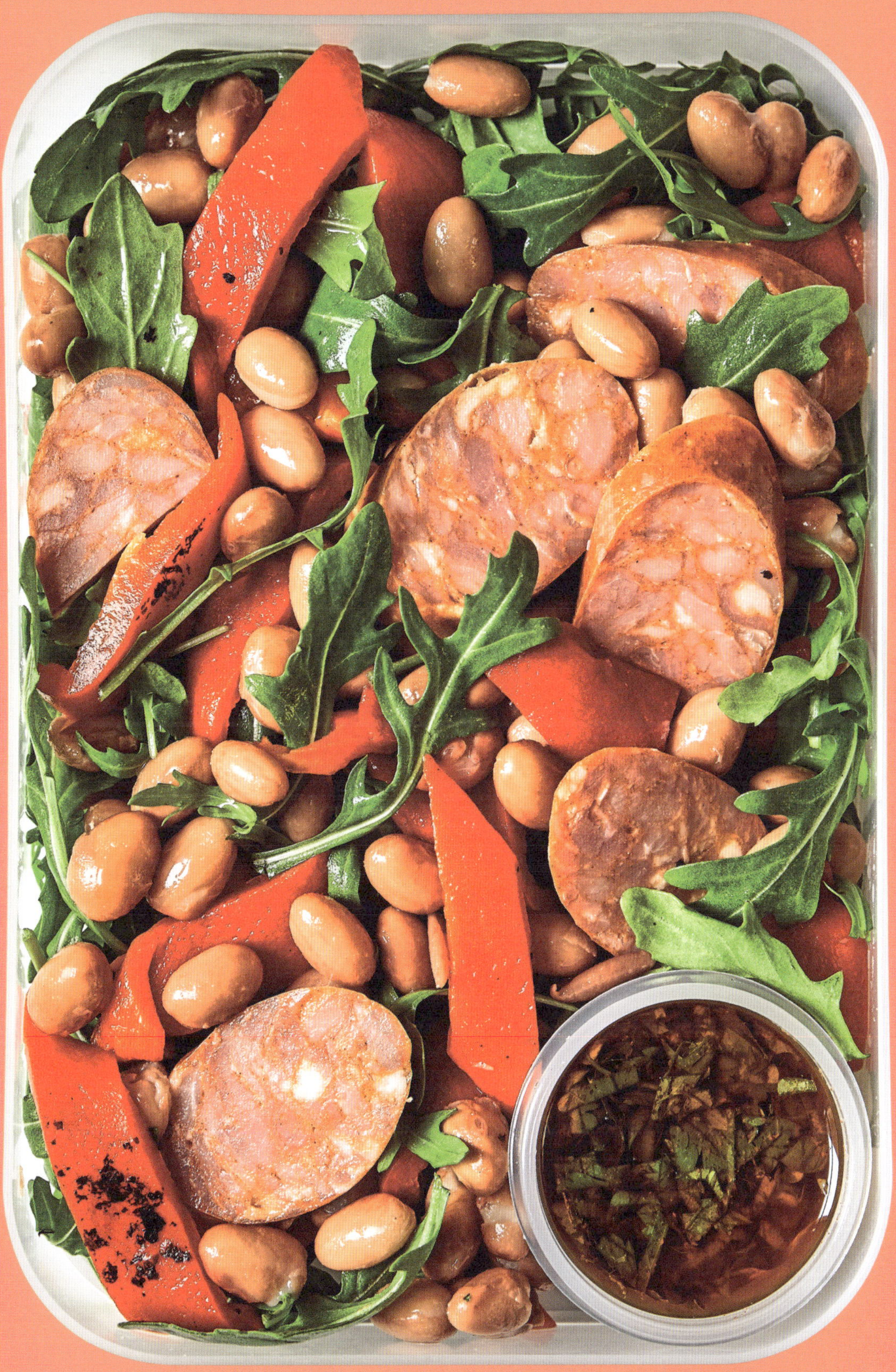

PROTEIN: 35 G NET CARBS: 43 G FAT: 32 G

Hot 'n' spicy prawn & chive noodles

Prawns cook in minutes, bringing lean strength to this noodle bowl. A spicy sauce and a sprinkle of chives tie it together for an easy weeknight fix.

- 180 g (6½ oz) cooked ramen noodles, prepared as per packet instructions
- 120 g (4½ oz) cooked prawns (shrimp), peeled and deveined
- 2 tablespoons chopped chives
- 1 small spring onion (scallion), finely sliced
- 85 g (3 oz) cherry tomatoes, halved
- small handful of coriander (cilantro) leaves
- 1½ teaspoons toasted sesame seeds

SWEET SOY-CHILLI DRESSING

- 2 tablespoons chilli crisp oil
- 2 teaspoons kecap manis (sweet soy sauce)
- 2 teaspoons water
- 1½ teaspoons rice vinegar

1. Place the salad ingredients in a bowl and toss lightly.
2. Combine the dressing ingredients in a small bowl.
3. Pour the dressing over the salad just before serving and toss well to coat.

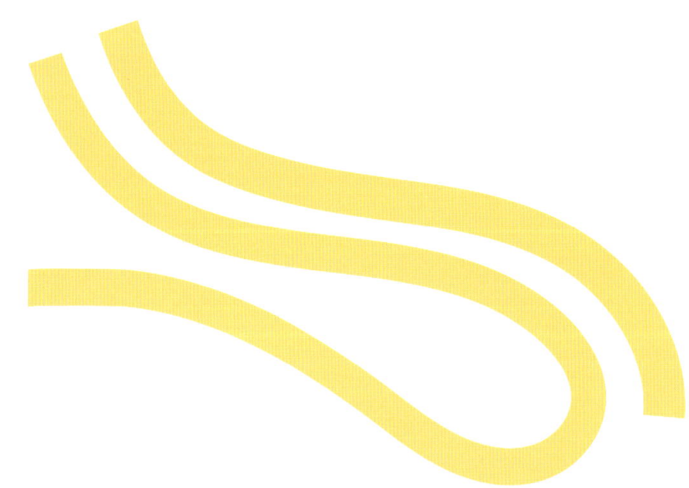

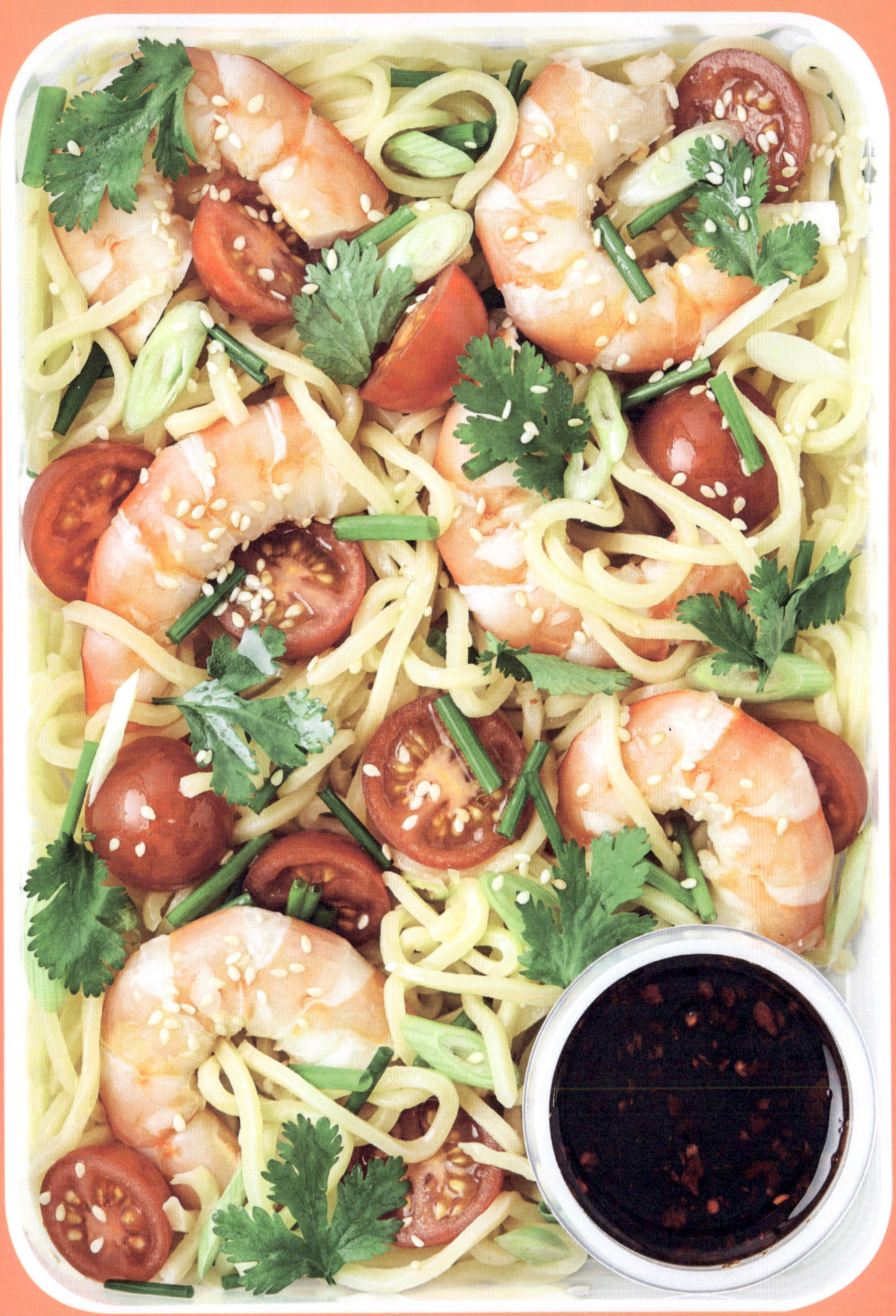

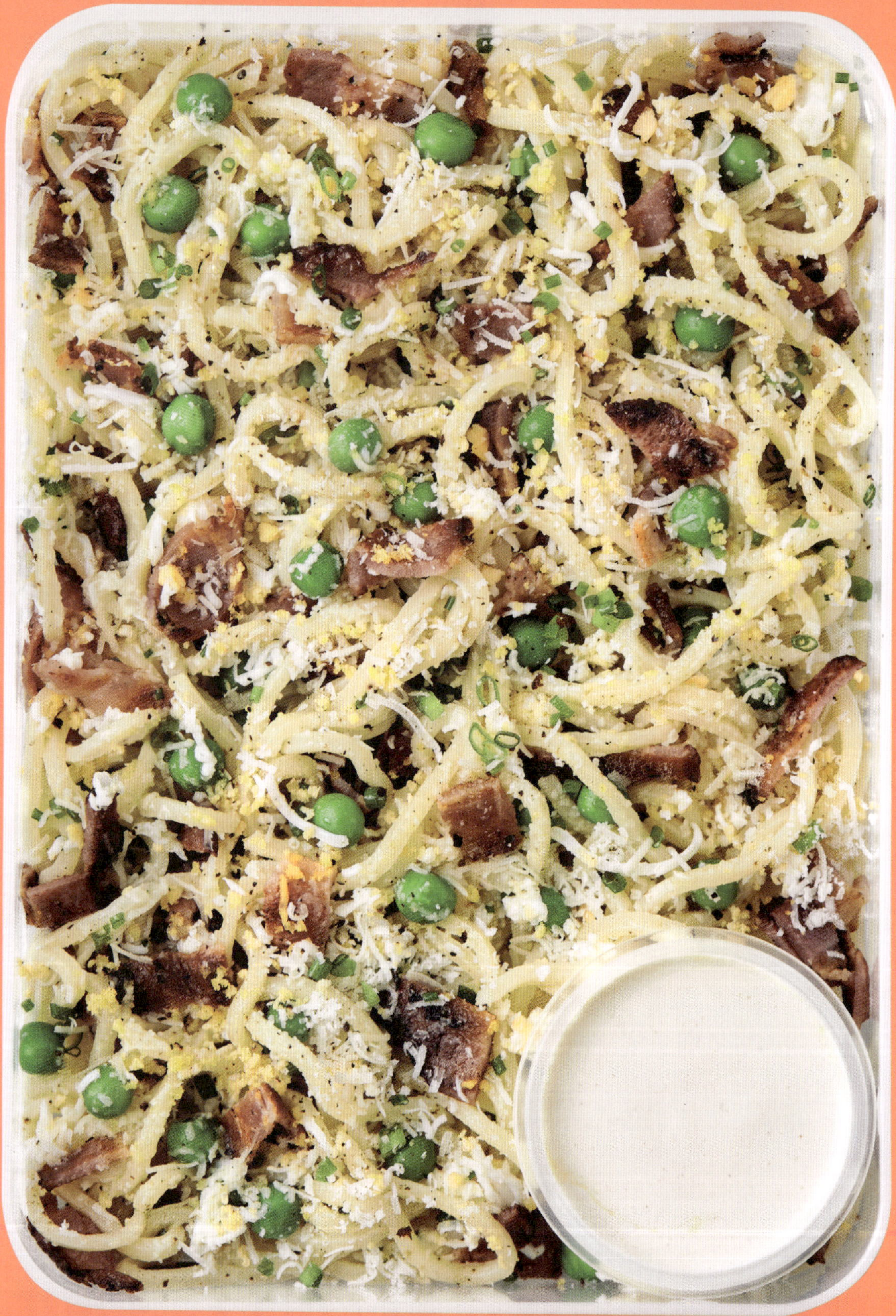

PROTEIN: 39 G NET CARBS: 29 G FAT: 25 G

Carbonara ramen noodle salad

This playful twist uses ramen in place of pasta. Eggs, bacon and parmesan echo the flavours of a classic Italian carbonara, turning instant noodles into a substantial meal.

2 bacon slices, cut into small dice

180 g (6½ oz) cooked ramen noodles, prepared as per packet instructions

1 hard-boiled egg, finely grated

40 g (¼ cup) peas, blanched

25 g (¼ cup) finely grated parmesan

2 tablespoons finely sliced chives

CREAMY DIJON DRESSING

3 tablespoons blended cottage cheese (2% fat)

1½ teaspoons white wine vinegar

½ teaspoon dijon mustard

¼ teaspoon minced garlic

1. Place the bacon in a non-stick frying pan and cook over high heat for 3–4 minutes, until crispy. Allow to cool.
2. Place the bacon, along with the remaining salad ingredients, in a bowl and toss lightly. Season to taste with salt and pepper.
3. Combine the dressing ingredients in a small bowl.
4. Pour the dressing over the salad just before serving and toss well to coat.

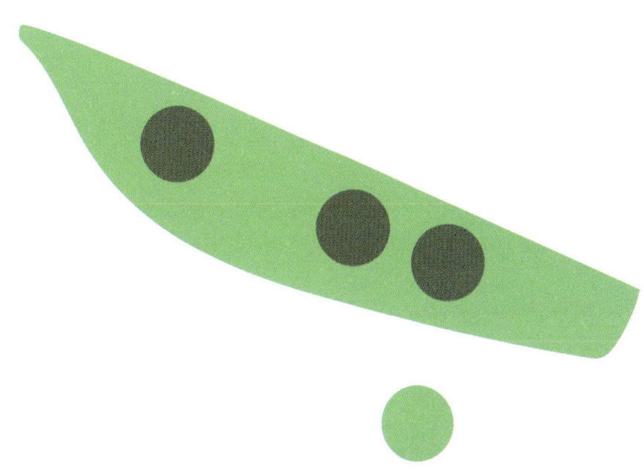

PROTEIN: 32 G NET CARBS: 38 G FAT: 45 G

Chilli tuna & stuffed red pepper pappardelle

Tinned tuna is the fast protein here, stirred through broad pasta ribbons. Sweet roasted bell pepper adds body, while chilli lifts the flavour. If you want to bump up the protein even more, look for pulse pastas that you can substitute for the pappardelle.

- 100 g (3½ oz) fresh pappardelle pasta
- 95 g (3¼ oz) tinned tuna in chilli oil, undrained
- 4 feta-stuffed baby red bell peppers (capsicums), halved
- handful of parsley leaves

RED ONION & CAPER DRESSING

- 2 tablespoons lemon juice
- 1½ tablespoons extra virgin olive oil
- 1½ tablespoons finely chopped red onion
- 1½ teaspoons baby capers

1. Cook the pasta in a saucepan of boiling salted water for 2–3 minutes, until cooked, then drain and cool.
2. Place the pasta, along with the remaining salad ingredients, in a bowl and toss lightly.
3. Combine the dressing ingredients in a small bowl, then season to taste with salt and pepper.
4. Pour the dressing over the salad just before serving and toss well to coat.

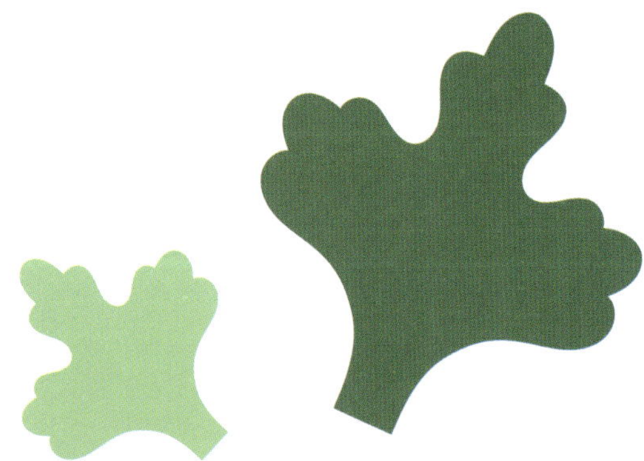

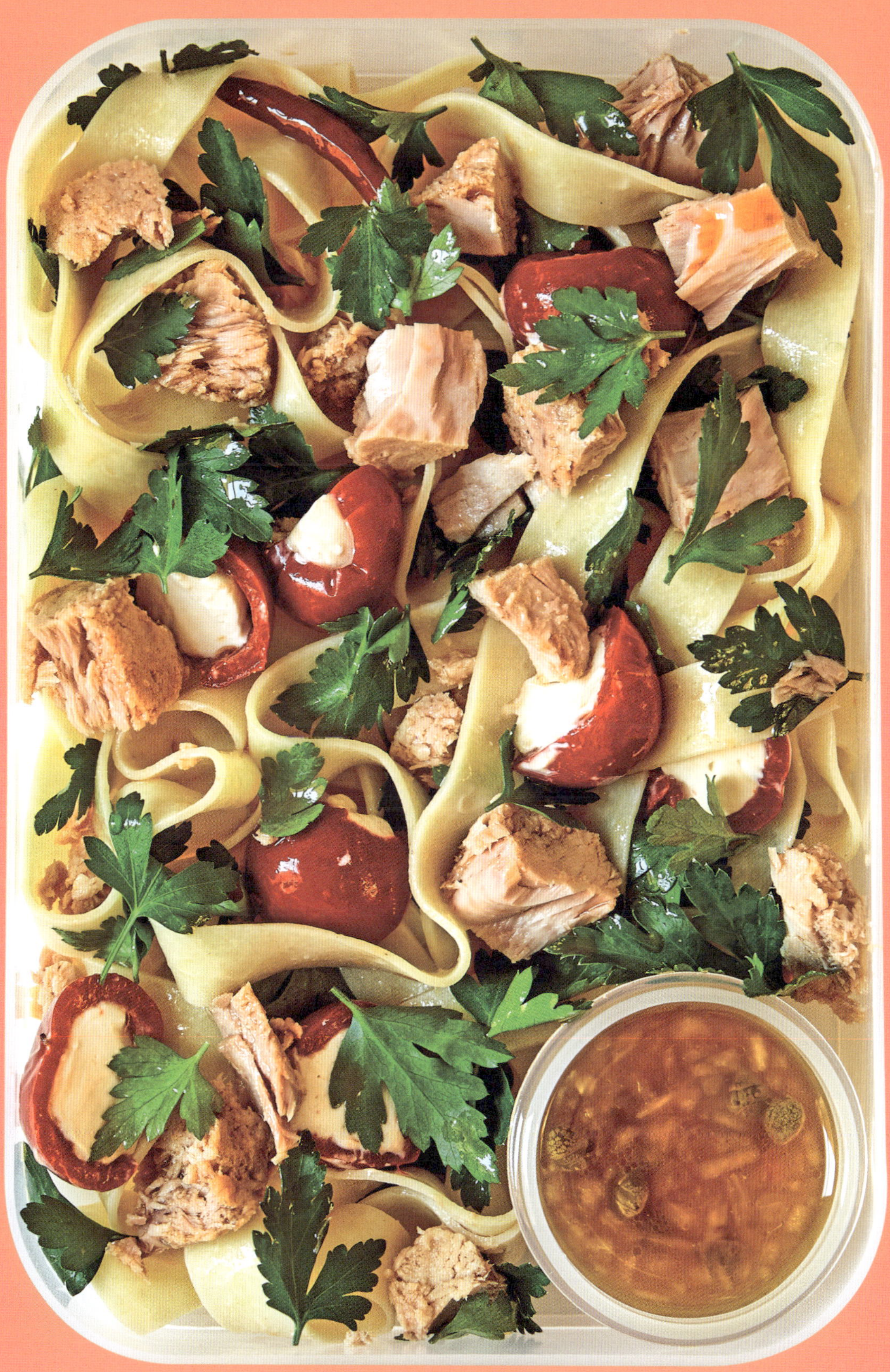

PROTEIN: 57 G NET CARBS: 71 G FAT: 36 G

Satay chicken noodle salad

Chicken and noodles become something special with a peanut satay sauce. It's rich and filling, with lime and herbs cutting through the creaminess.

- 180 g (6½ oz) thin hokkien noodles, prepared as per packet instructions
- 100 g (⅔ cup) shredded cooked chicken
- 1 small spring onion (scallion), finely sliced
- ½ short cucumber, finely sliced
- ¼ red bell pepper (capsicum), finely sliced
- 2 tablespoons peanuts
- small handful of coriander (cilantro) leaves
- pinch of chilli flakes

SATAY DRESSING

- 3 tablespoons peanut butter
- 1½ tablespoons rice vinegar
- juice of ½ lime
- 1 teaspoon kecap manis (sweet soy sauce)
- 1 teaspoon sriracha sauce

1. Place the salad ingredients in a bowl and toss lightly.
2. Combine the dressing ingredients in a small bowl, adding a little water if needed to thin it out.
3. Pour the dressing over the salad just before serving and toss well to coat.

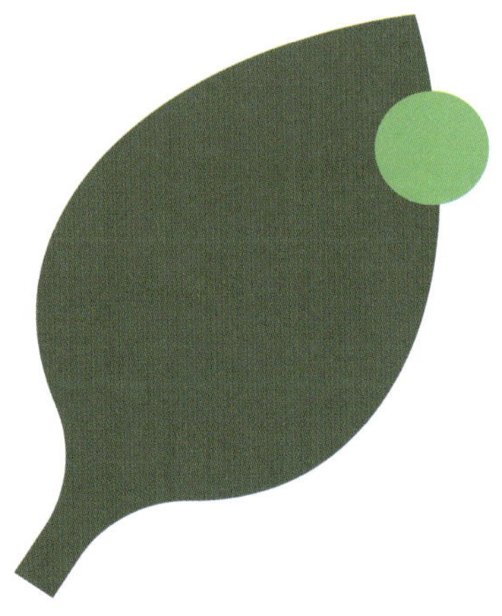

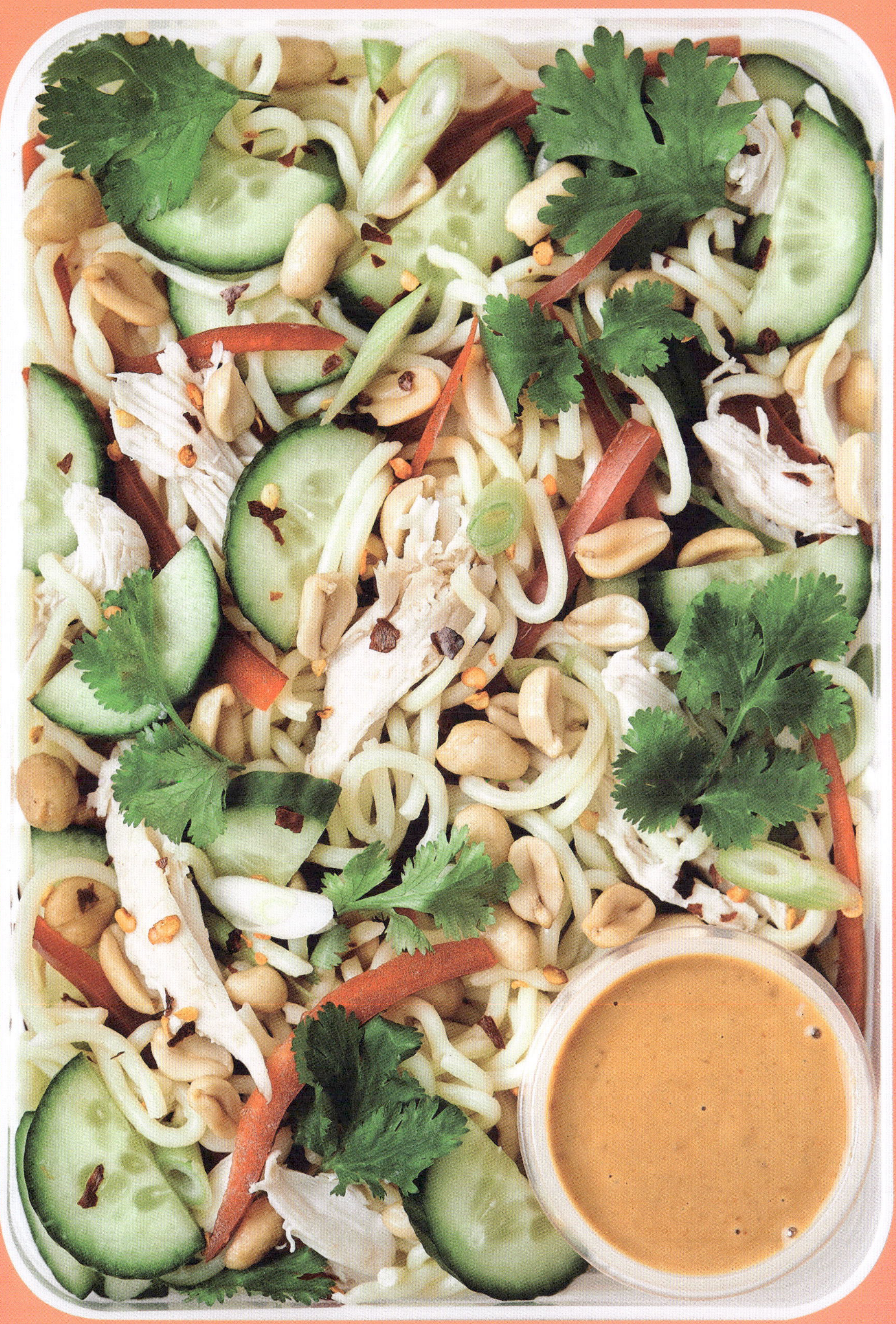

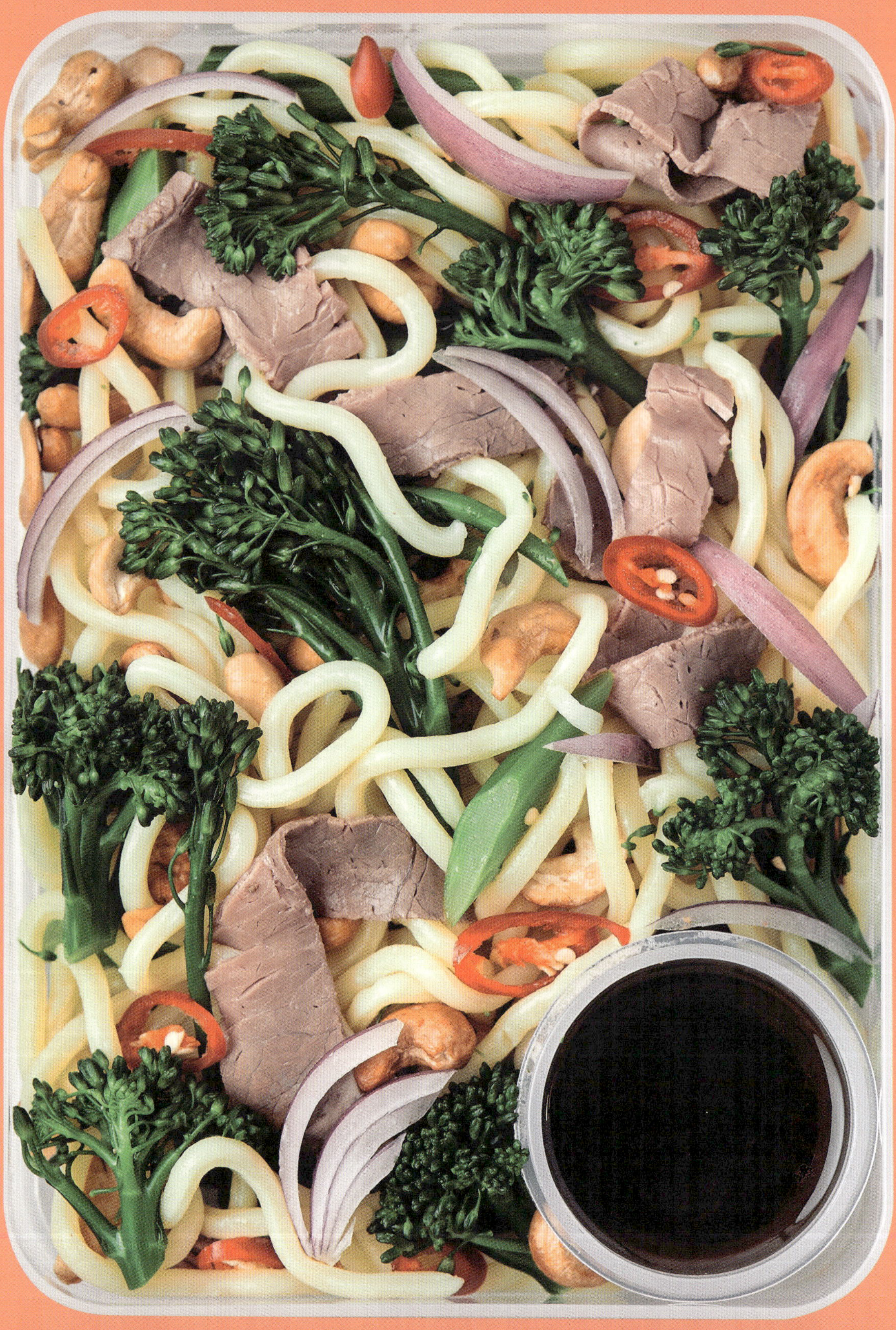

PROTEIN: 46 G NET CARBS: 80 G FAT: 44 G

Beef & broccolini cashew noodle salad

Roast beef strips pair neatly with nutty cashews. Tossed through noodles and greens, it's a balanced dish with both crunch and chew. These days you can buy slices of roast beef from good-quality delicatessens or butchers to toss through this deliciously hearty salad. Simply omit the bird's eye chilli or choose a milder long red chilli if you prefer less spice.

180 g (6½ oz) hokkien noodles, prepared as per packet instructions

100 g (3½ oz) sliced roast beef, cut into strips

3 broccolini stems, cut into 5 cm (2 in) pieces, blanched

⅛ small red onion, finely sliced

1 red bird's eye chilli, sliced

40 g (¼ cup) roasted cashews

SESAME, SOY & GINGER DRESSING

2 teaspoons sesame oil

2 teaspoons soy sauce

2 teaspoons rice vinegar

2 teaspoons honey

¼ teaspoon minced garlic

¼ teaspoon minced ginger

1. Place the salad ingredients in a bowl and toss lightly.
2. Combine the dressing ingredients in a small bowl.
3. Pour the dressing over the salad just before serving and toss well to coat.

PROTEIN: 43 G   NET CARBS: 71 G   FAT: 12 G

Chicken & pineapple noodles with gochujang

Juicy pineapple balances the spice of gochujang, while chicken and noodles keep it hearty. It's a bright, punchy salad with Korean inspiration. Gochujang is a Korean red chilli paste that can be variously spicy, savoury and sweet, depending on the brand. You'll find it in most supermarkets and Asian grocers.

- 180 g (6½ oz) hokkien noodles, prepared as per packet instructions
- 100 g (⅔ cup) shredded cooked chicken
- 50 g (⅓ cup) chopped pineapple
- 1 spring onion (scallion), finely sliced
- 2 teaspoons toasted black sesame seeds
- small handful of mint leaves

GOCHUJANG DRESSING

- 1 tablespoon gochujang paste
- 1 teaspoon kecap manis (sweet soy sauce)
- 1 teaspoon rice vinegar
- 1 teaspoon soy sauce
- 1 teaspoon toasted sesame oil
- ½ teaspoon water

1. Place the salad ingredients in a bowl and toss lightly.
2. Combine the dressing ingredients in a small bowl.
3. Pour the dressing over the salad just before serving and toss well to coat.

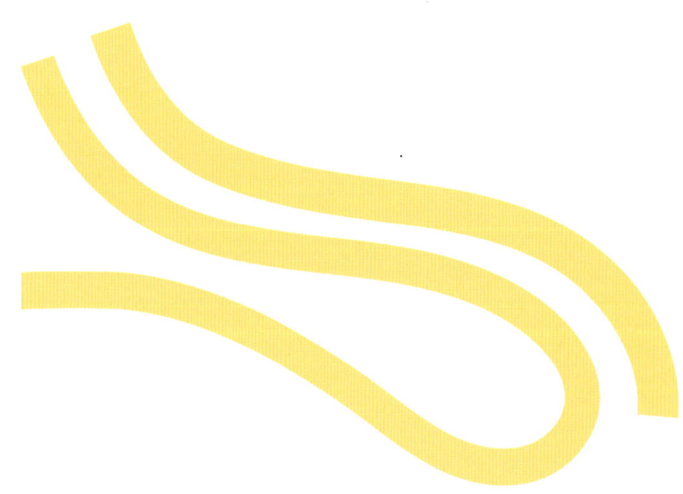

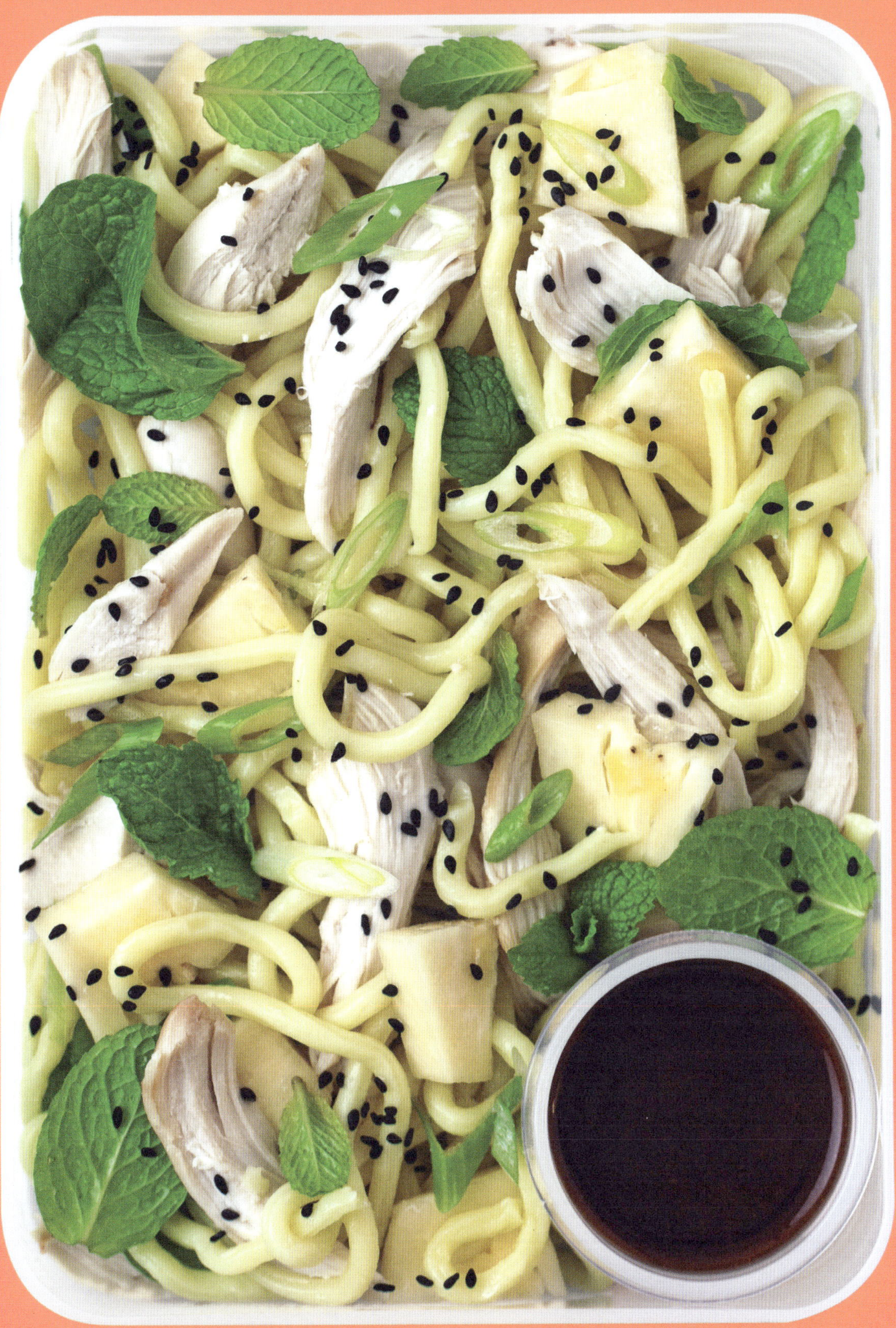

PROTEIN: 44 G NET CARBS: 38 G FAT: 62 G

Chicken ramen with coriander & peanut pesto

Ramen noodles are dressed in a quick coriander–peanut pesto, making them vibrant and nutty. Shredded chicken adds bulk without weighing it down.

- 180 g (6½ oz) cooked ramen noodles, prepared as per packet instructions
- 100 g (⅔ cup) shredded cooked chicken
- ½ short cucumber, diced
- ¼ avocado, diced
- small handful of mint leaves
- 40 g (¼ cup) chilli roasted peanuts
- lime wedge, to serve

CORIANDER & PEANUT PESTO

- 30 g (1 cup) coriander (cilantro) leaves
- 3 tablespoons roasted peanuts
- 3 tablespoons lime juice
- 2½ tablespoons sesame oil
- 1 tablespoon sweet chilli sauce
- 1 small garlic clove, peeled

1. Place the pesto ingredients in a small blender and blend until well combined. Taste and add a little more lime juice if desired.
2. Place the noodles in a bowl, pour the pesto over and toss to combine.
3. Add the remaining ingredients to the noodles, except the lime wedge. Toss to combine.
4. Squeeze the lime over just before serving.

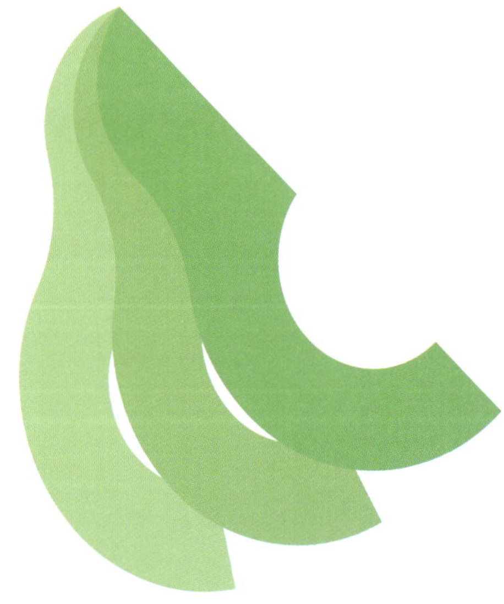

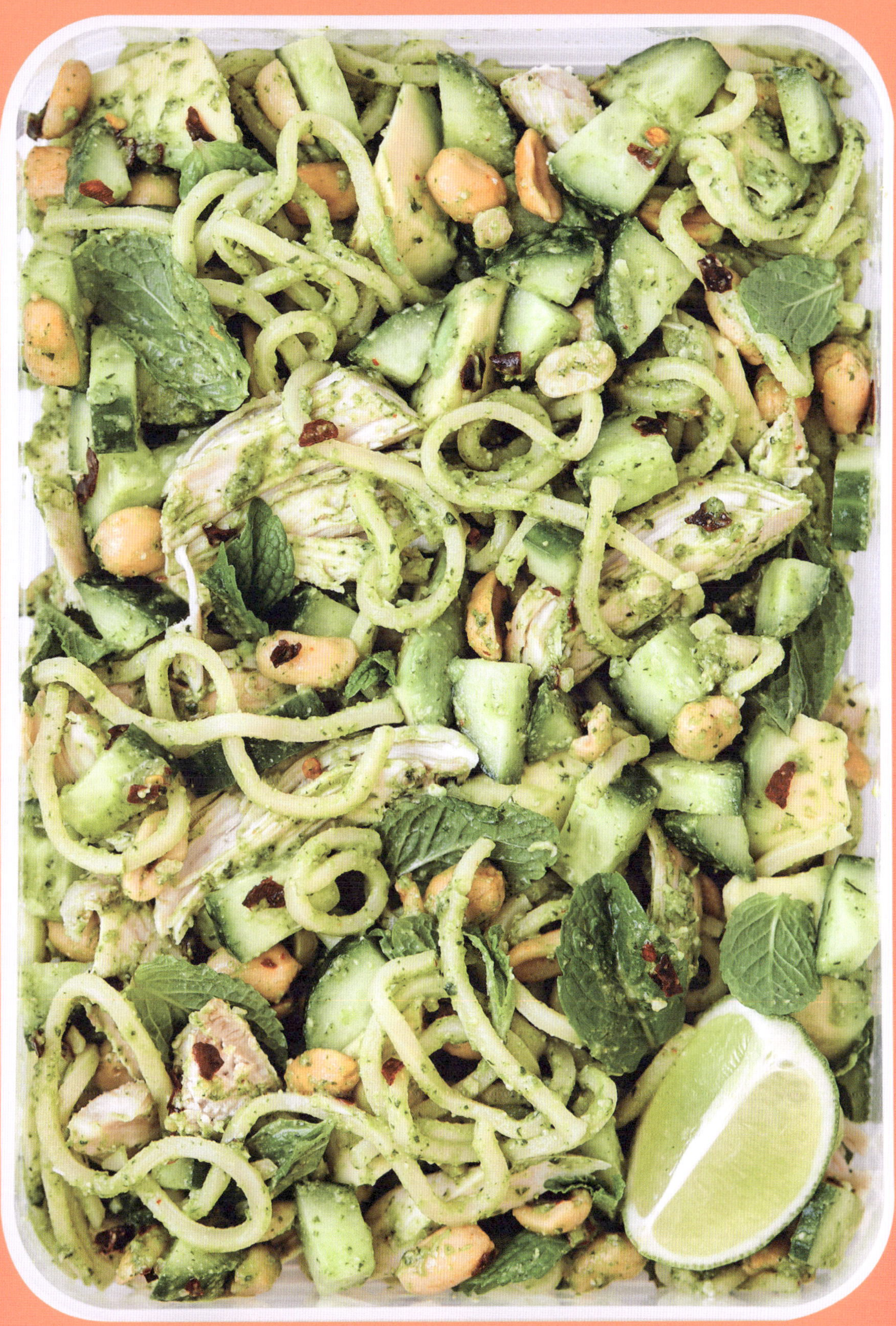

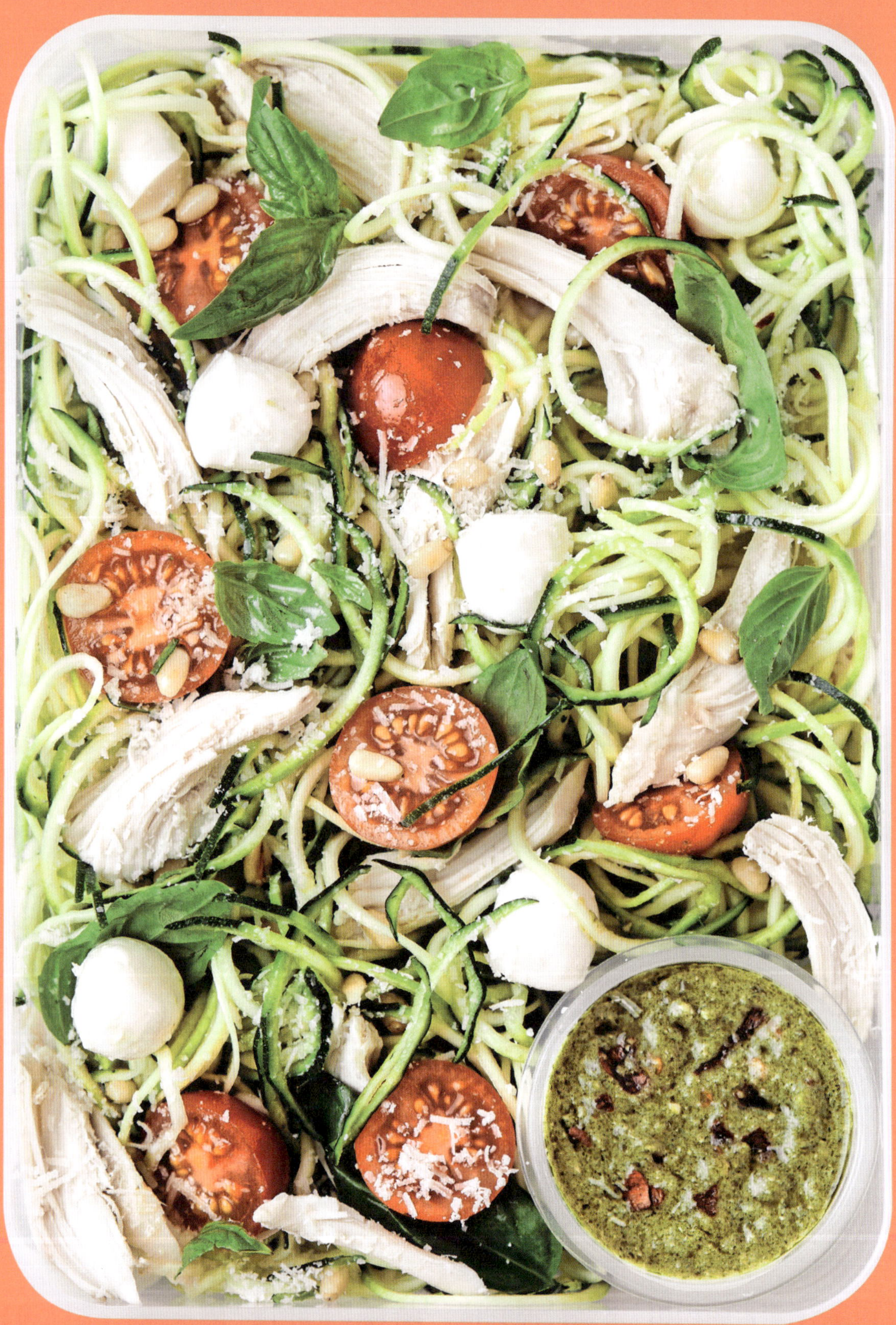

PROTEIN: 48 G   NET CARBS: 12 G   FAT: 42 G

Chicken & basil pesto zoodles

The pesto dressing is central to the flavour of this chicken and zucchini salad, so search out a good-quality option – or make your own and store it until ready to use.

- 1 zucchini (courgette), spiralised
- 100 g (⅔ cup) shredded cooked chicken
- 6 baby bocconcini
- 80 g (2¾ oz) cherry tomatoes, halved
- 2-3 tablespoons finely grated parmesan
- 2 tablespoons toasted pine nuts
- small handful of basil leaves

LEMON PESTO DRESSING

- 3 tablespoons pesto (homemade or store-bought)
- 1 tablespoon lemon juice
- pinch of chilli flakes (optional)

1. Place the salad ingredients in a bowl and toss lightly.
2. Combine the dressing ingredients in a small bowl.
3. Pour the dressing over the salad just before serving and toss well to coat.

PROTEIN: 36 G NET CARBS: 60 G FAT: 25 G

Hokkien noodles with tuna & chilli oil

Tinned tuna and hokkien noodles are pantry standbys that come together fast. The chilli brings heat, while spring onions give freshness. Ponzu is a classic Japanese condiment with a citrus-like taste, giving this salad a deliciously tart–tangy flavour. Seek out good-quality tinned tuna with good texture – it can really lift this recipe.

- 180 g (6½ oz) hokkien noodles, prepared as per packet instructions
- 95 g (3¼ oz) tinned tuna in chilli oil, undrained
- 100 g (3½ oz) cherry tomatoes, halved
- ¼ red bell pepper (capsicum), finely sliced
- 30 g (¾ cup) mixed salad greens
- sliced chilli, to taste

PONZU DRESSING

- 1 tablespoon ponzu sauce
- 2 teaspoons rice vinegar
- 1½ teaspoons sesame oil

1. Place the salad ingredients in a bowl and toss lightly.
2. Combine the dressing ingredients in a small bowl.
3. Pour the dressing over the salad just before serving and toss well to coat.

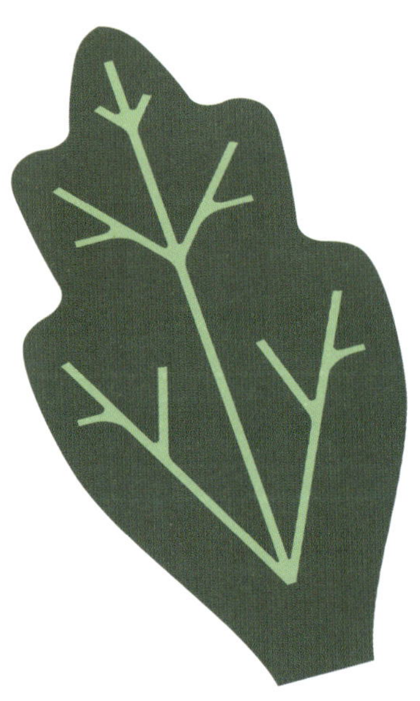

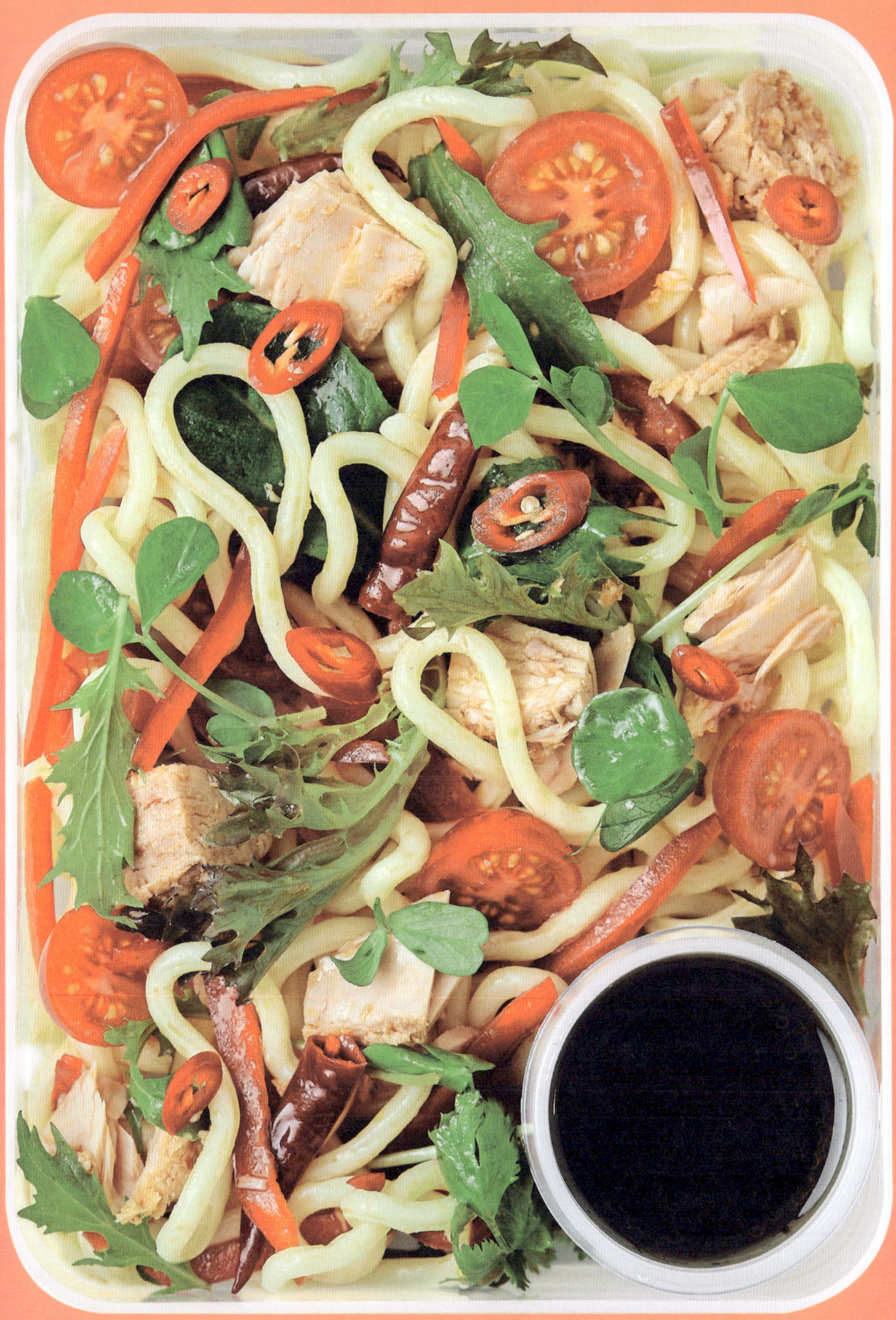

PROTEIN: 37 G NET CARBS: 51 G FAT: 53 G

Duck noodle salad with ginger & hoisin

Duck breast is rich and satisfying, especially when sliced into a noodle salad. Ginger and hoisin dressing provide sweetness and depth.

- 80 g (2¾ oz) dried rice vermicelli noodles, prepared as per packet instructions
- 100 g (3½ oz) shredded cooked Chinese duck
- 3 radicchio leaves, shredded
- 1 plum, sliced into wedges
- 1 small spring onion (scallion), sliced
- 30 g (¼ cup) chopped toasted pecans
- 1 tablespoon dried tart cherries

GINGER-HOISIN DRESSING

- 1 tablespoon hoisin sauce
- 2 teaspoons kecap manis (sweet soy sauce)
- 2 teaspoons rice vinegar
- 1 teaspoon sesame oil
- ½ teaspoon minced ginger

1. Place the salad ingredients in a bowl and toss lightly.
2. Combine the dressing ingredients in a small bowl.
3. Pour the dressing over the salad just before serving and toss well to coat.

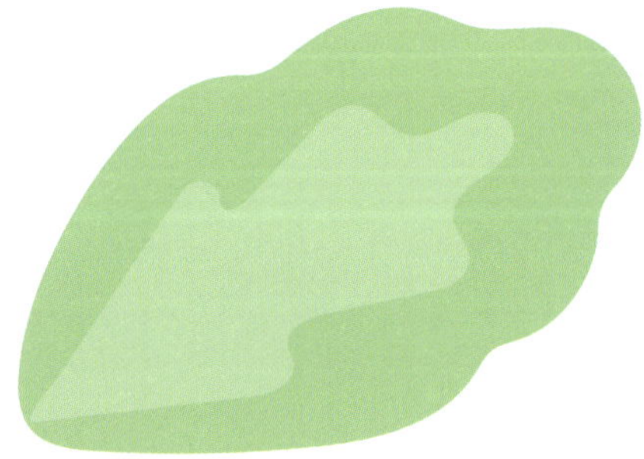

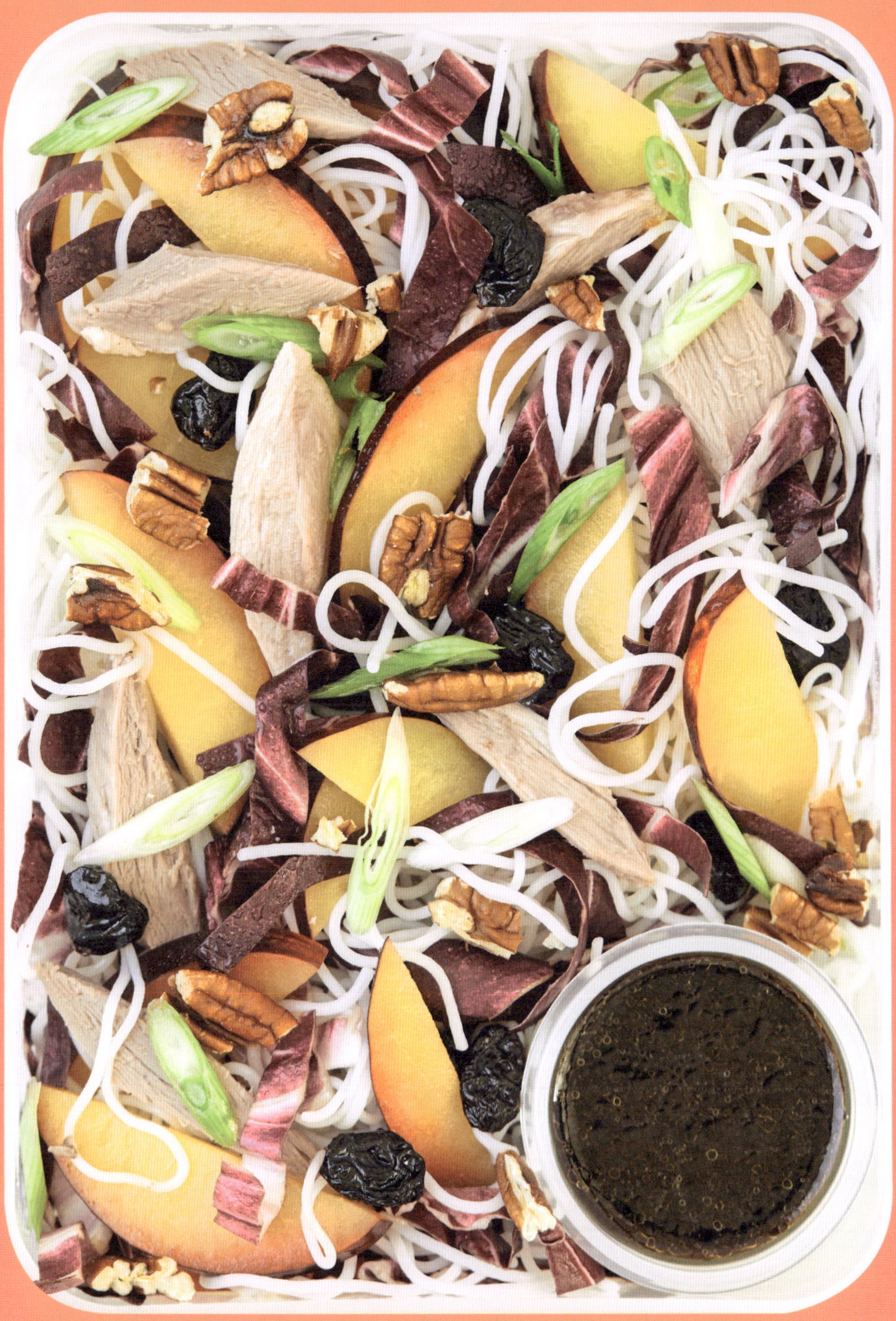

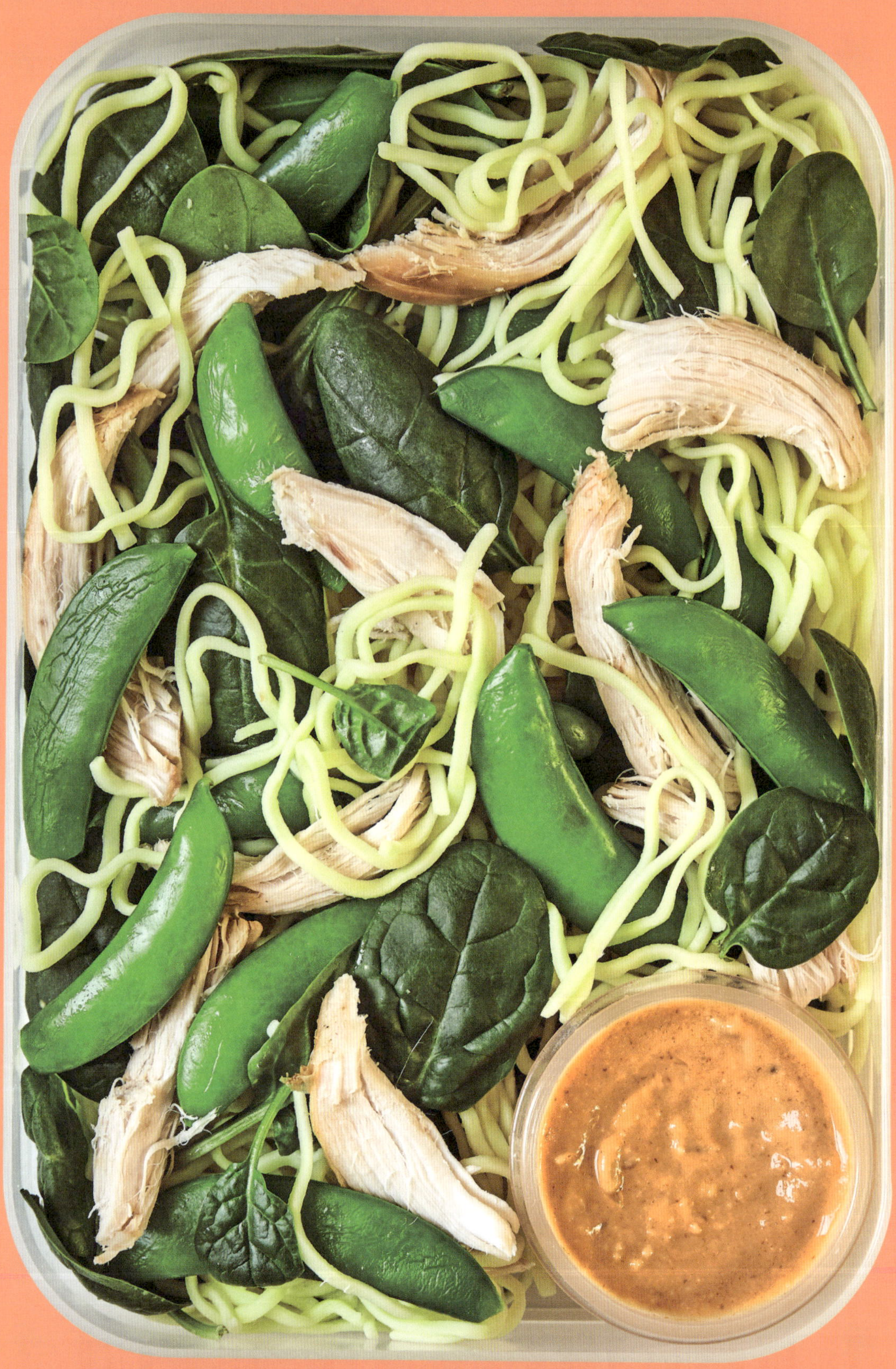

PROTEIN: 50 G NET CARBS: 33 G FAT: 38 G

Spicy ramen noodle & chicken salad

Chicken and ramen noodles make an unfussy base. A chilli-spiked sauce gives it energy, while sugar snap peas and baby spinach keep it fresh. If you prefer to avoid the heat, omit the sriracha sauce and use another sauce instead.

- 200 g (7 oz) cooked ramen noodles, prepared as per packet instructions
- 50 g (1¾ oz) sugar snap peas, blanched
- 100 g (⅔ cup) shredded cooked chicken
- 65 g (1¼ cups) baby spinach leaves

SPICY PEANUT DRESSING

- 3 tablespoons peanut butter
- 1½ tablespoons rice vinegar
- 1 teaspoon toasted sesame oil
- 1 teaspoon sriracha sauce
- juice of ½ lime

1. Place the salad ingredients in a bowl and toss lightly.
2. Combine the dressing ingredients in a small bowl, then season to taste with salt and pepper.
3. Pour the dressing over the salad just before serving and toss well to coat.

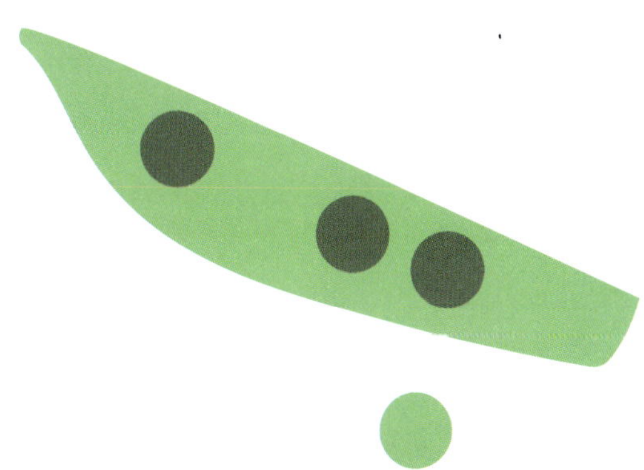

PROTEIN: 40 G NET CARBS: 12 G FAT: 31 G

Tuna niçoise with cucumber noodles

Tuna niçoise is an iconic French salad that combines salad leaves, green beans, egg, olives, potato and tuna. Here we've switched the potatoes for crunchy radishes and slippery cucumber ribbons. For a spicier salad, use tuna steeped in chilli oil.

- 1 short cucumber, sliced into ribbons
- 60 g (2 oz) green beans, blanched
- 1 hard-boiled egg, quartered
- 95 g (3¼ oz) tinned tuna in olive oil, drained
- 2 anchovy fillets in olive oil (optional)
- 2 radishes, sliced
- 85 g (3 oz) cherry tomatoes, halved
- ⅛ small red onion, finely sliced
- 30 g (1 cup) mixed salad leaves
- 30 g (¼ cup) pitted black olives

MUSTARD-GARLIC VINAIGRETTE

- 1 tablespoon extra virgin olive oil
- 2 teaspoons red wine vinegar
- ½ teaspoon dijon mustard
- ¼ teaspoon minced garlic

1. Place the salad ingredients in a bowl and toss lightly.
2. Combine the vinaigrette ingredients in a small bowl, then season to taste with salt and pepper.
3. Pour the vinaigrette over the salad just before serving and toss well to coat.

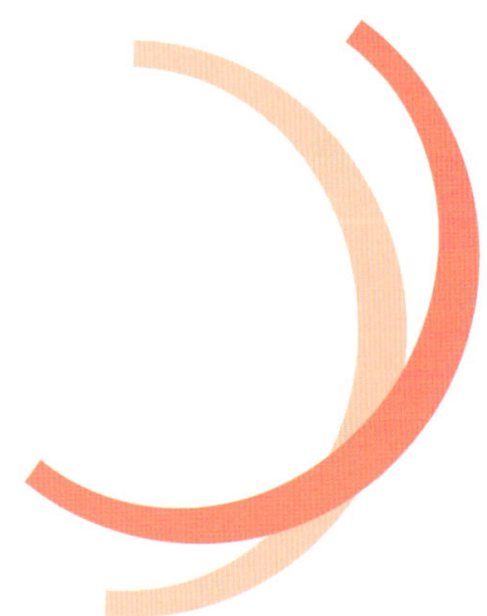

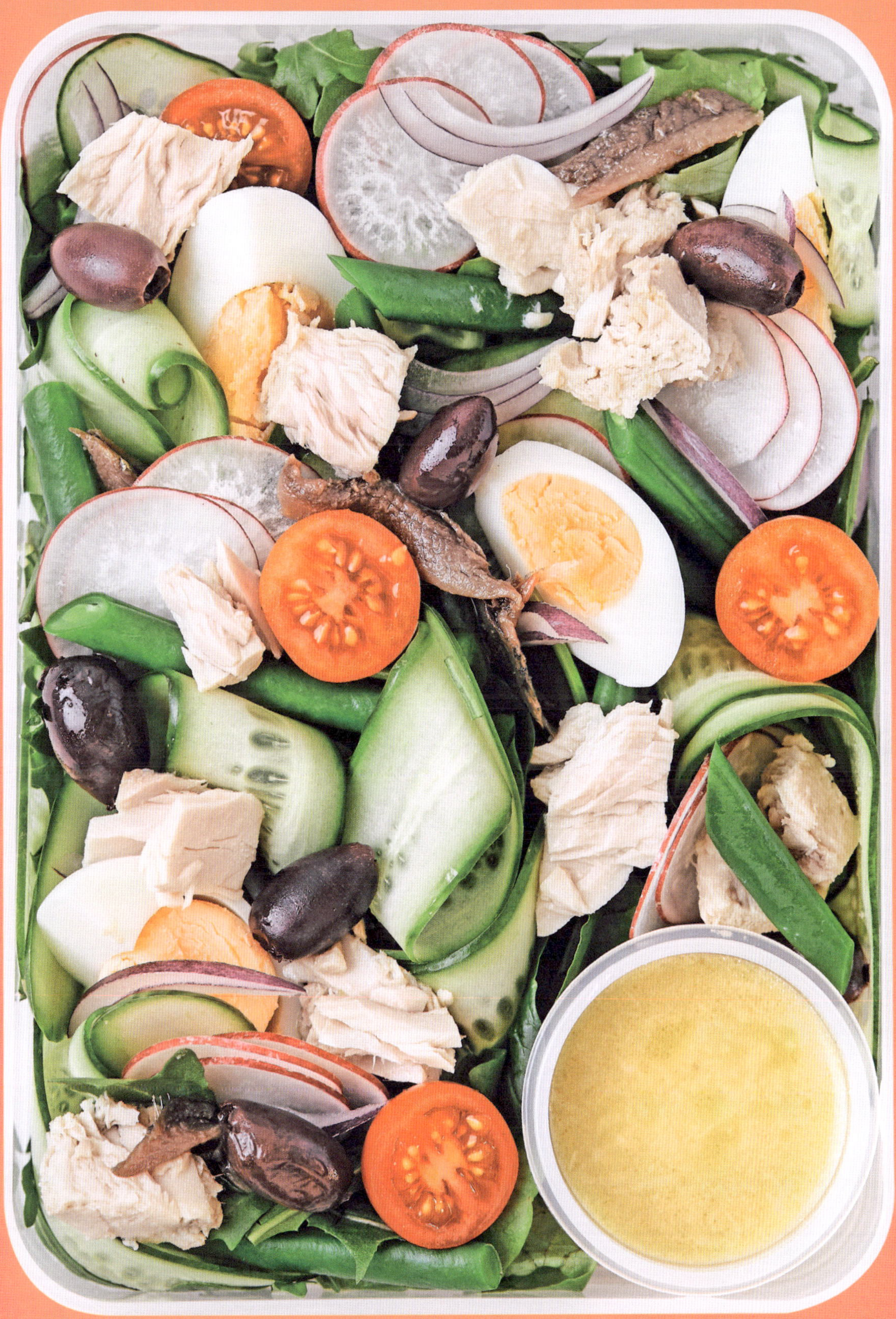

PROTEIN: 41 G NET CARBS: 46 G FAT: 40 G

Kohlrabi noodles with smoked trout, apple & toasted pecans

Smoked trout and pecans bring satisfying richness to crisp kohlrabi noodles. Kohlrabi – a relative of cabbage, cauliflower and broccoli – has a sweet, peppery flavour and can be eaten raw or cooked.

- 150 g (5½ oz) kohlrabi, spiralised
- 100 g (3½ oz) smoked trout, flaked
- 1 small apple, cored and finely sliced
- 25 g (¼ cup) toasted pecans, roughly chopped
- 25 g (1 oz) dried cranberries

HONEY CIDER DRESSING

- 2 teaspoons extra virgin olive oil
- 2 teaspoons apple cider vinegar
- 1 teaspoon dijon mustard
- 1 teaspoon honey

1. Place the salad ingredients in a bowl and toss lightly, then season to taste with salt and pepper.
2. Combine the dressing ingredients in a small bowl.
3. Pour the dressing over the salad just before serving and toss well to coat.

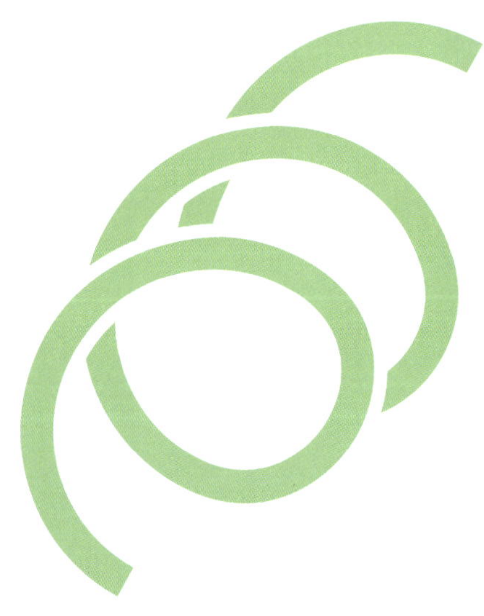

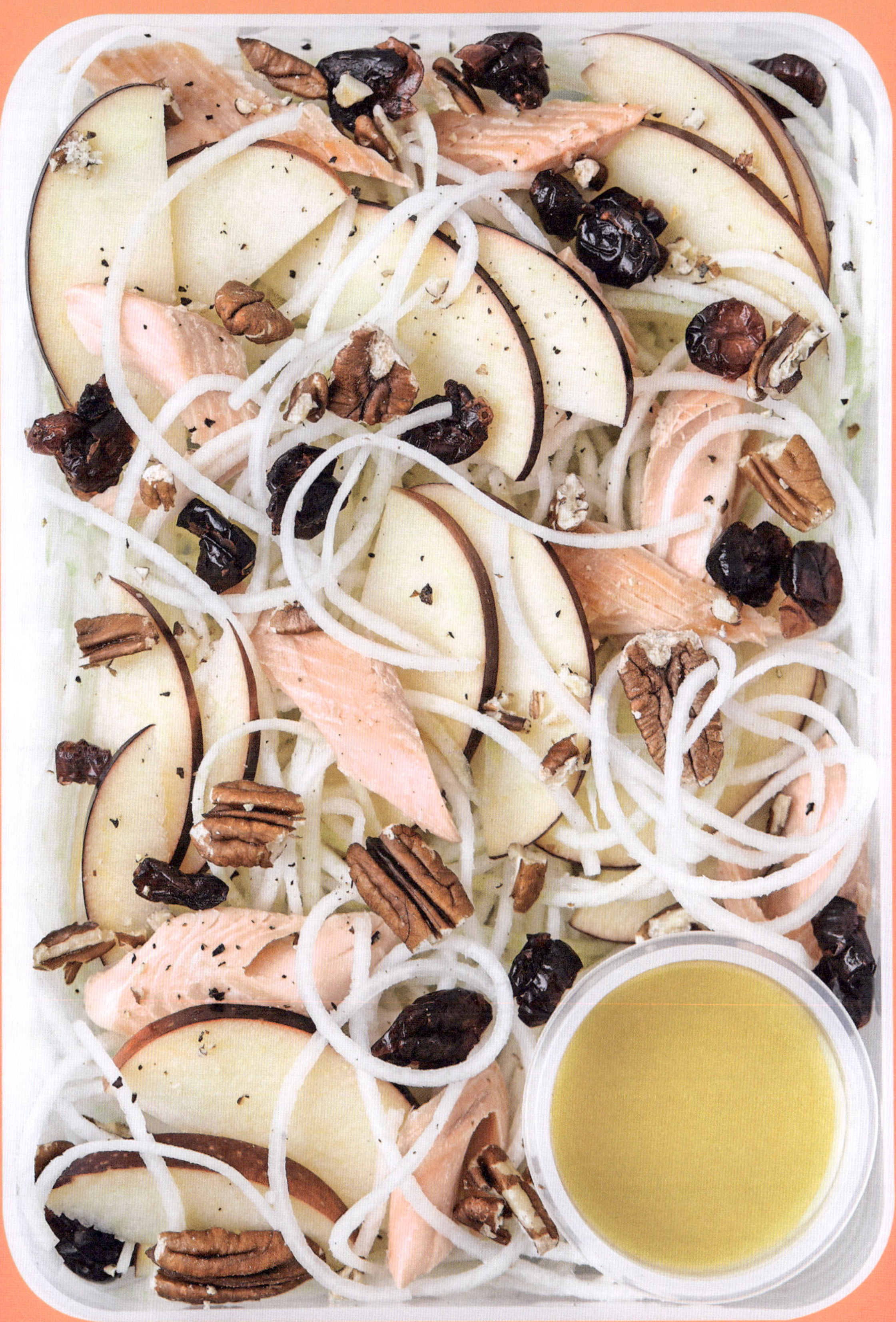

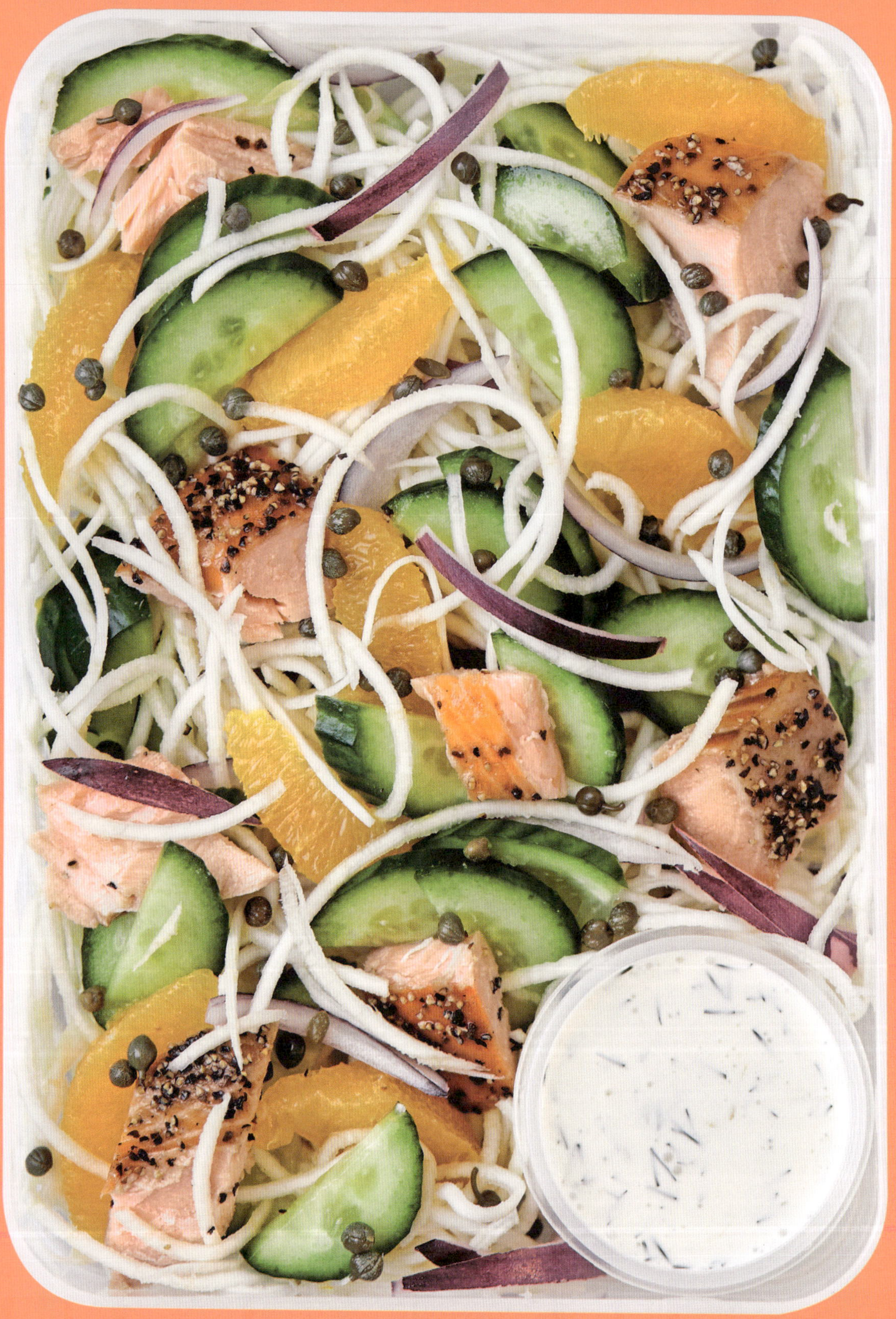

PROTEIN: 28 G NET CARBS: 27 G FAT: 7 G

Salmon & celeriac noodles with creamy dill dressing

Salmon gives this dish weight, while celeriac noodles keep it interesting. Celeriac is a root vegetable that can be eaten raw or cooked. When eaten raw, it has an incredible crunch, with a nutty, celery-like flavour. Here it provides the perfect foil for the hot-smoked salmon. A creamy dill dressing ties everything together with freshness and tang.

- 150 g (5½ oz) celeriac, spiralised
- 110 g (4 oz) hot-smoked pepper-crusted salmon, flaked
- ½ short cucumber, sliced
- ⅛ small red onion, sliced
- 1 small orange, peeled and segmented
- 1 teaspoon baby capers

CREAMY DILL DRESSING

- 3 tablespoons high-protein Greek-style yoghurt
- zest and juice of ½ lemon
- 2 teaspoons chopped dill

1. Place the salad ingredients in a bowl and toss lightly.
2. Combine the dressing ingredients in a small bowl, then season to taste with salt and pepper.
3. Pour the dressing over the salad just before serving and toss well to coat.

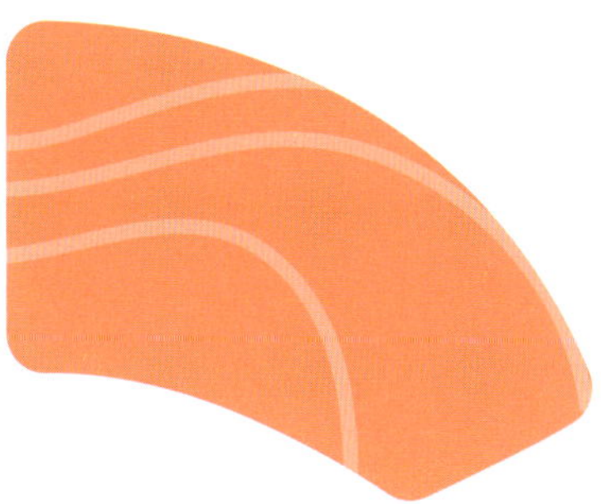

Index

D

E/F

G

H

I

J/K

L

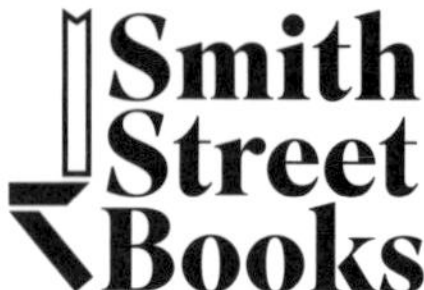

Published in 2026 by Smith Street Books
Naarm (Melbourne) | Australia
smithstreetbooks.com

Distributed outside of ANZ, North & Latin America by
Thames & Hudson Ltd., 6–24 Britannia Street, London, WC1X 9JD
thamesandhudson.com

EU Authorised Representative: Interart S.A.R.L.
19 rue Charles Auray, 93500 Pantin, Paris, France
productsafety@thameshudson.co.uk; www.interart.fr

ISBN: 978-1-9235-0310-6

Smith Street Books respectfully acknowledges the Wurundjeri People of the Kulin Nation, who are the Traditional Owners of the land on which we work, and we pay our respects to their Elders past and present.

Publisher: Paul McNally
Project manager: Elena Callcott
Recipes: Deborah Kaloper
Introduction text: Elena Callcott and Ana Jacobsen
Editor: Ana Jacobsen
Design concept: Double Slice Studio (Amelia Leuzzi and Bonnie Eichelberger)
Design layout: Nikola Roberts
Photographers: Chris Middleton, Daniel Herrmann-Zoll, Jacinta Moore
Proofreader: Pamela Dunne
Food stylist: Deborah Kaloper
Production manager: Aisling Coughlan
Indexer: Max McMaster
Prepress: Megan Ellis

Recipes in this book have previously appeared in *The 5-Minute Salad lunchbox* (2019), *The 5-Minute, 5-Ingredient Lunchbox* (2021), *The 5-Minute Noodle Salad Lunchbox* (2024) and *The 5-Minute Keto Salad Lunchbox* (2025), published by Smith Street Books.

Printed & bound in China by C&C Offset Printing Co., Ltd.

Book 447
10 9 8 7 6 5 4 3 2 1

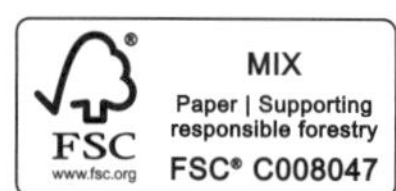